BRIEF COGNITIVE-BEHAVIORAL THERAPY
FOR SUICIDE PREVENTION

Also Available

Treating Suicidal Behavior:
An Effective, Time-Limited Approach

M. David Rudd, Thomas E. Joiner,
and M. Hasan Rajab

BRIEF COGNITIVE-BEHAVIORAL THERAPY
FOR SUICIDE PREVENTION

Craig J. Bryan
M. David Rudd

THE GUILFORD PRESS
New York   London

The authors have checked with sources believed to be reliable in their efforts to provide information
that is complete and generally in accord with the standards of practice that are accepted at the time of
publication. However, in view of the possibility of human error or changes in behavioral, mental health,
or medical sciences, neither the authors, nor the editors and publisher, nor any other party who has been
involved in the preparation or publication of this work warrants that the information contained herein
is in every respect accurate or complete, and they are not responsible for any errors or omissions or the
results obtained from the use of such information. Readers are encouraged to confirm the information
contained in this book with other sources.

Library of Congress Cataloging-in-Publication Data

Names: Bryan, Craig J., author. | Rudd, M. David, author.
Title: Brief cognitive-behavioral therapy for suicide prevention / Craig J. Bryan, M. David Rudd.
Description: New York : The Guilford Press, [2018] | Includes bibliographical references and index.
Identifiers: LCCN 2018002529| ISBN 9781462536665 (pbk.) | ISBN 9781462536672 (hardcover)
Subjects: LCSH: Suicide—Prevention. | Suicidal behavior—Treatment. | Cognitive therapy. |
    Behavior therapy.
Classification: LCC RC569 .B78 2018 | DDC 616.85/8445—dc23
LC record available at *https://lccn.loc.gov/2018002529*

About the Authors

Craig J. Bryan, PsyD, ABPP, is Executive Director of the National Center for Veterans Studies and Associate Professor in the Department of Psychology and the Department of Psychiatry at the University of Utah. He is an associate editor of the journal *Suicide and Life-Threatening Behavior* and previously served on the board of directors of the American Association of Suicidology. Dr. Bryan has received honors including the Charles S. Gersoni Military Psychology Award from Division 19 (Society for Military Psychology) and the Peter J. N. Linnerooth National Service Award from Division 18 (Psychologists in Public Service) of the American Psychological Association, as well as the Edwin S. Shneidman Award from the American Association of Suicidology. He is a University of Utah Presidential Scholar and Beacon of Excellence recipient. From 2005 until 2009, he served on active duty in the U.S. Air Force as a clinical psychologist, including a deployment to Iraq in 2009. Dr. Bryan's primary research interests include suicide prevention and posttraumatic stress disorder. He has published over 150 scientific articles and several books, most of which focus on suicide prevention, trauma, and military mental health.

M. David Rudd, PhD, ABPP, is President of the University of Memphis, where he is also Distinguished University Professor of Psychology. He is also Co-Founder and Scientific Director of the National Center for Veterans Studies at the University of Utah. Dr. Rudd is a Fellow of the American Psychological Association, the International Academy of Suicide Research, and the Academy of Cognitive Therapy, and has been elected a Distinguished Practitioner and Scholar of the National Academies of Practice in Psychology. He previously served as chair of the Texas State Board of Examiners of Psychologists, president of the Texas Psychological Association, president of the American Association of Suicidology, and a member of the American Psychological Association's Council of Representatives. Dr. Rudd's research focuses on the treatment of suicidal patients. He has published over 200 scientific articles and numerous books on the clinical care of suicidal individuals, and is considered an international leader in suicide prevention.

Contents

PART III

PHASE ONE:
EMOTION REGULATION AND CRISIS MANAGEMENT

PART IV

PHASE TWO:
UNDERMINING THE SUICIDAL BELIEF SYSTEM

PART V

PHASE THREE: RELAPSE PREVENTION

Purchasers of this book can download and print the reproducible forms,
handouts, and clinician tools at *www.guilford.com/bryan2-materials*
for personal use or use with individual clients (see copyright page for details).

PART I

BACKGROUND AND CONCEPTUAL FOUNDATION

CHAPTER 1

Why Brief Cognitive-Behavioral Therapy to Prevent Suicide?

In 2014, more than 41,000 individuals died by suicide in the United States (Centers for Disease Control and Prevention, 2016). From 1970 to 2000, the U.S. general population suicide rate declined approximately 20% from an estimated 13.2 per 100,000 to 10.4 per 100,000. Around the turn of the century, however, this downward trend reversed and the suicide rate steadily increased to 13.4 per 100,000 in 2014. Though suicide rates have increased across most demographic subgroups, the most pronounced increase has occurred among middle-aged (i.e., 45–64 years) white men. Similar trends have been observed globally, although differences by age groups have been noted (Chang, Stuckler, Yip, & Gunnell, 2013). In Europe, for instance, suicides increased most dramatically among young men ages 15 to 24 years. For each death by suicide, there are an estimated 10 to 30 suicide attempts (Centers for Disease Control and Prevention, 2016). In light of these trends, there has been increased interest in identifying and developing interventions and prevention strategies that reduce death by suicide and suicidal behavior more generally.

Within the United States, research focused on the understanding and treatment of suicidal individuals began in earnest during the 1950s, driven in large part by Edwin Schneidman and Norman Farberow, both clinical psychologists, and Robert Litman, a psychiatrist, at the Los Angeles Suicide Prevention Center. Although the number of suicide researchers has since grown rapidly, it was not until the 1990s that clinical researchers, both within the United States and around the world, started to apply rigorous scientific methods to develop and critically evaluate the efficacy of treatments for reducing suicide ideation and preventing suicide attempts. Despite these efforts, the suicide rate of the U.S. general population started to rise in 1999 and in 2014 reached its highest point in nearly 30 years (Centers for Disease Control and Prevention, 2016).

Traditional approaches to treating suicidal patients have largely been influenced by a *risk factor model* of suicide, which seeks to understand suicidal thoughts and behaviors by identifying and describing their correlates. For example, several well-established correlates of suicidal thoughts and behaviors include male gender, white or Caucasian race, age above 45 years, and psychiatric diagnoses (Franklin et al., 2017). Within the general category of psychiatric diagnoses, mood disorders and substance abuse disorders have traditionally been implicated (Kessler, Borges, & Walters, 1999; May & Klonsky, 2016; Nock et al., 2008). The risk factor model does not necessarily propose any specific underlying process or cause for suicidal behavior, but rather assumes that it is the accumulation of multiple risk factors that contributes to suicidal thoughts and behaviors. Treatment informed by this model aims to reduce these risk factors under the assumption that doing so will reduce the incidence and/or severity of suicidal thoughts and behaviors. Countering this assumption are the results of a recent meta-analysis of 50 years of research studies in which the risk factor model was found to have relatively little impact on suicide prevention or the development of effective treatments (Franklin et al., 2017). The utility of the risk factor model of suicide has increasingly been called into question.

The *psychiatric syndromal model,* in which suicidal thoughts and behaviors are conceptualized as symptoms of psychiatric illness, is a specific subcategory of the more general risk factor model. From this perspective, suicidal thoughts and behaviors are described and organized according to observable characteristics and surface features of the behaviors (e.g., method, lethality, and intent), similar to the syndromal classification schemes commonly used in the mental health and medical professions (e.g., the World Health Organization's *International Classification of Diseases,* the American Psychiatric Association's *Diagnostic and Statistical Manual*). In the medical field, a syndrome is reclassified as a disease once the characteristics and surface features of the syndrome are linked to their underlying processes and causes. As applied to suicide, the psychiatric syndromal model implicates the central role of psychiatric illness when treating suicidal patients: that is, treat the psychiatric illness and suicide risk will resolve. By extension, if a suicidal patient is diagnosed with depression, then the clinician should treat the depression to prevent suicide attempts; if a suicidal patient has posttraumatic stress disorder, however, then the clinician should treat the trauma. Although the psychiatric syndromal model has predominated in our clinical understanding of suicide for decades and is the perspective from which most clinicians approach the treatment of suicidal patients, accumulating evidence has failed to support the effectiveness of this conceptual framework (e.g., Tarrier, Taylor, & Gooding, 2008). This may be due in part to the fact that most psychiatric disorders are correlated with suicidal *thoughts* but not suicidal *behaviors* (Kessler et al., 1999; May & Klonsky, 2016; Nock et al., 2008). This suggests that treatments that prioritize psychiatric disorders may not be sufficiently specific to the mechanisms that give rise to suicidal behavior. As a result, they reduce psychiatric symptoms but not the risk for suicide attempts.

A third general framework for understanding suicidal behaviors is the *functional model.* According to this model, suicidal thoughts and behaviors are conceptualized as the outcome of underlying psychopathological processes that specifically precipitate and maintain suicidal thoughts and behaviors over time (Hayes, Wilson, Gifford, Follette, & Strosahl, 1996). From this perspective, suicidal thoughts and behaviors are not the result of any particular psychological process per se (e.g., psychiatric illness); rather, they are the result of how the psychological process is experienced by the individual within the context of his or her personal history, immediate environment, and behavioral responses. Clinically, the functional model suggests that the primary target of treatment with suicidal individuals is not the psychiatric illness itself, but rather it is the context that surrounds the emergence and maintenance of suicide risk over time.

To highlight the differences between these models, consider two separate women diagnosed with major depression secondary to marital problems. Both individuals have comparable levels of depression severity, but one of these women (Patient A) makes a suicide attempt following an argument with her partner, whereas the second woman (Patient B) experiences suicide ideation following a similar argument but does not make a suicide attempt. According to the risk factor and the psychiatric syndromal models, the suicidal symptoms experienced by both women are explained in part by underlying depression. There is no clear explanation for why only one of these two women made a suicide attempt, but both models would generally presume that, since Patient A made a suicide attempt but Patient B did not, Patient A must have a greater number of risk factors than Patient B. The risk factor model would suggest that the differential risk factor profiles for both women would need to be identified in order to develop a treatment plan for each. These treatment plans would generally seek to reduce or eliminate each woman's risk factors. The psychiatric syndromal model would take a similar, albeit more focused approach: the indicated treatment approach for both women should focus on reducing depression. Because Patient A made a suicide attempt, the psychiatric syndromal model would presume she has a more severe clinical profile overall as compared to Patient B. Patient A might therefore be more likely than Patient B to receive treatment in an inpatient setting because she is more likely to be seen as requiring a higher level of care.

In contrast to these two approaches, the functional model would assume that the suicidal symptoms experienced by both women are explained only in part by their depression; a more complete explanation is provided by considering their depression within the context of each woman's history and the circumstances surrounding the emergence of their suicidal episodes. To understand why Patient A made a suicide attempt but Patient B did not, we would therefore seek to identify differences in how the two women responded to the argument with their spouses across several domains: cognition (e.g., Why does she think the argument happened? What does she believe the argument says about her relationship and/ or her as a person?), emotion (e.g., Which emotions did she experience?), behavior (e.g., What actions did she take after the argument? How did she attempt to manage her emotions?), and somatic (e.g., What bodily sensations did she experience during and after the argument?). In short, Patient A made a suicide attempt not because she was depressed, but rather because she experienced the argument in a way that was shaped by previous life experiences and a general deficiency in effective self-regulation and coping. Outpatient treatment for Patient A is therefore likely to be different from treatment for Patient B, and would focus on these deficits in self-regulation and coping instead of focusing exclusively on depression.

The superiority of treatment approaches based on the functional model relative to treatment approaches based on a risk factor or psychiatric syndromal model are now well established empirically. In a meta-analysis of 24 studies investigating treatment effectiveness for suicide ideation and suicide attempts, for instance, treatments that directly targeted suicidal thoughts and behaviors as the primary outcome (i.e., a functional approach) contributed to statistically significant and larger improvements in suicide risk relative to treatments that primarily targeted psychiatric diagnosis (Tarrier et al., 2008). In light of such studies, the general consensus among suicide researchers is that the treatment of suicidal individuals should focus directly on suicide risk itself as opposed to psychiatric diagnosis. Unfortunately, despite the scientific evidence that supports this perspective, the majority of mental health professionals continue to be influenced heavily by the psychiatric syndromal model of treatment, a situation that is due in large part to insufficient education and training for clinicians in newer and better models of care (Schmitz et al., 2012).

THE EVOLUTION OF COGNITIVE-BEHAVIORAL THERAPY TO PREVENT SUICIDE ATTEMPTS

Although clinical suicide researchers as a whole hail from a remarkably diverse range of disciplines (e.g., psychology, social work, psychiatry, sociology) and clinical traditions (e.g., biomedical, psychodynamic, cognitive-behavioral, interpersonal), the most significant advances in the development of effective treatments for suicidal patients have arguably come from the cognitive-behavioral tradition. This is not to say that important knowledge has not been gained from clinical researchers trained in different theoretical perspectives and traditions, but rather that cognitive-behavioral models may "fit" more readily with the functional approach to conceptualizing suicide. Indeed, the functional model's emphasis on understanding the contextual antecedents and consequences of suicidal thoughts and behaviors (e.g., thoughts, emotions, and behavioral responses) parallels the core conceptual principles of cognitive-behavioral theory.

When considering treatment efficacy for suicidal behaviors in general, it should first be noted that no treatments have been shown to prevent suicide *death*. This is due in large part to the very high cost that would need to be incurred to conduct and implement such a study; death by suicide occurs with such infrequency that it would require a very large sample of participants to examine death as an outcome. To put this in perspective, across two studies of brief cognitive-behavioral therapy (Brown, Ten Have, et al., 2005; Rudd et al., 2015), only 3 out of a total of 272 participants died by suicide during the study period. In other words, only 1% of patients died by suicide. This low base rate is quite notable when one considers that approximately 90% of the participants in these two studies had made at least one suicide attempt during their lives (in most cases, the suicide attempt was within the past month), which means these participants were very high risk. Researchers would therefore need to enroll a very large number of high-risk individuals (over 1,500) into a study to show that a treatment could reduce the risk for death by suicide by half. Tragically, the cost of conducting such a large-scale study, which would necessitate the collaborative participation of multiple research sites, is much higher than what many funding agencies would consider practical.

Because death by suicide is not (yet) a feasible outcome for the purposes of research, treatment efficacy studies typically use proxies for suicide death that occur with greater frequency, such as suicide attempts and suicide ideation. Studies that evaluate the effects of treatment on suicide attempts as the primary outcome are generally considered to be more rigorous and informative than studies that consider treatment effects on suicide ideation, whereas studies that evaluate the effects of treatment on psychiatric diagnoses and other suicide risk factors are generally considered to be the least informative. This is because suicide attempts are a much closer approximation to suicide death than suicide ideation or psychiatric diagnosis (one must make a suicide attempt in order to die by suicide) and because suicide attempts are a stronger risk factor for later death by suicide than suicide ideation and psychiatric diagnosis. For example, in the classic meta-analysis of 249 studies investigating suicide as an outcome of psychiatric illness, Harris and Barraclough (1997) found that individuals with a history of suicide attempt had a standardized mortality ratio of approximately 40, which means that individuals who have attempted suicide are 40 times more likely to die by suicide than individuals with no such history. By comparison, the standardized mortality ratios for psychiatric disorders commonly associated with suicide were much lower: 20 for major depressive disorder, 19 for substance use disorder, 15 for bipolar disorder, and 8.5 for schizophrenia. Suicide attempt is therefore considered to be the best available proxy for suicide death.

Another important consideration with respect to treatment efficacy is the nature of the control or comparison treatment condition, without which it is not possible to determine if a treatment is effective. Because it is unethical to *not* treat acutely suicidal individuals, studies of suicidal patients *must* include an active treatment as the control condition. The most common control condition in treatment studies to prevent suicide attempts is *treatment as usual*, also known as *usual care*. Treatment as usual entails standard mental health treatment delivery as it is typically provided by mental health professionals. In most studies, treatment as usual generally entails some combination of individual psychotherapy and psychotropic medications, and may also include group therapy, substance abuse counseling, and case management. In essence, clinicians providing treatment as usual are simply asked to do whatever it is they would normally do with a suicidal patient; they are not asked to change anything about how they conduct treatment. Treatments are only considered to be "effective" for preventing or reducing risk for suicide attempts if they reduce the risk for suicide attempts relative to another active treatment approach that is widely used by mental health clinicians. In other words, an effective treatment is one that has "beaten" another form of treatment in a head-to-head comparison. To date, cognitive-behavioral therapies have garnered the most consistent evidence of efficacy, indicating they have outperformed other forms of therapy in numerous studies.

Brief cognitive-behavioral therapy (BCBT) to prevent suicide is best understood as the "next step forward" in the development and refinement of the cognitive-ehavioral model that been successfully used by clinical researchers over the course of several decades. To date, approximately 30 clinical trials testing the efficacy of cognitive-behavioral therapies to reduce suicide risk have been conducted with varying outcomes (Tarrier et al., 2008). One of the first treatments to demonstrate efficacy for reducing the risk of suicide attempts was dialectical behavior therapy (DBT; Linehan, 1993). Based on the biosocial model of suicide, DBT is a multimodal, structured cognitive-behavioral therapy that entails psychoeducational skills training groups, individual psychotherapy, between-session phone consultation for patients, and regularly occurring clinician supervision. The efficacy of DBT and modi-fied versions of DBT have been replicated in several clinical trials, making it "the most thoroughly studied and efficacious psychotherapy for suicidal behavior" (National Action Alliance Clinical Care & Intervention Task Force, 2012, p. 17). DBT entails training in emo-tion regulation, distress tolerance, problem solving, and cognitive reappraisal skills, accom-plished with a range of cognitive-behavioral interventions such as cognitive restructuring, exposure, and behavioral rehearsal (Lynch, Chapman, Rosenthal, Kuo, & Linehan, 2006).

Results of the first randomized clinical trial of DBT (Linehan, Armstrong, Suarez, All-mon, & Heard, 1991) indicated that patients receiving DBT were 32% less likely to engage in self-directed violence[1] during the 12-month follow-up period than patients receiving treatment as usual (64% in DBT vs. 96% in treatment as usual). Among those patients in DBT who did engage in self-directed violence, the total number of self-directed violence episodes was significantly fewer than for patients in treatment as usual (1.5 episodes in DBT vs. 9.0 episodes in treatment as usual during the 12-month follow-up), and the medi-cal lethality of their behavior was significantly less severe. In terms of treatment utilization, patients in DBT were significantly more likely to start individual therapy than patients in treatment as usual (100% in DBT vs. 73% in treatment as usual) and were significantly more likely to remain in therapy for an entire year (83% in DBT vs. 42% in treatment as usual). Patients in DBT also had significantly fewer psychiatric hospitalization days during the 12-month follow-up than patients in treatment as usual. In terms of depression, hope-lessness, and suicide ideation severity, however, patients in DBT and treatment as usual improved to a comparable degree.

Results of a more recent clinical trial of DBT (Linehan, Comtois, Murray, et al., 2006) were similar to this first study, although in this newer study the control condition was pro-vided by peer-nominated experts from the Seattle Psychoanalytic Society (referred to as *community treatment by experts*) and suicide attempts were assessed separately from non-suicidal self-injury. Patients in DBT were 50% less likely to make a suicide attempt dur-ing the 2-year follow-up period than patients in expert treatment (23% in DBT vs. 46% in expert treatment). Of those who did make suicide attempts, the medical lethality of the attempts was significantly less severe in DBT than in expert treatment. Patients in DBT were significantly more likely to stay in therapy than patients in expert treatment (81% in DBT vs. 43% in expert treatment) and were significantly less likely to be admitted to an inpatient psychiatric hospital. In terms of suicide ideation, depression, and reasons for liv-ing, patients in DBT and expert treatment improved to a similar degree. The results of this later study therefore paralleled the pattern of findings from the first DBT trial.

Although DBT has demonstrated considerable promise as a treatment for preventing suicide attempts, wider implementation of DBT has been hindered by the fact that the treatment is very resource intensive, time-consuming, and difficult to learn. Briefer and less

---

[1] *Self-directed violence* refers to any form of intentional self-injurious behavior without regard to its intent (i.e., suicidal vs. nonsuicidal). It is therefore a general term that includes both suicide attempts and nonsuicidal self-injury. In Linehan and colleagues' (1991) study, the primary outcome was "parasuicide act," a term that has since been replaced by *self-directed violence* and therefore is no longer in widespread use among suicide researchers. Because a parasuicide act could be either nonsuicidal self-injury or a suicide attempt, the primary outcome from this early DBT study is not specific to suicide attempts.

complex cognitive-behavioral treatment models that could be delivered more practically and flexibly were therefore desired. Rudd, Joiner, and Rajab (2001) were among the first clinical researchers to articulate a brief, time-limited cognitive-behavioral therapy for suicidal patients. Based on the *fluid vulnerability theory* of suicide and the concept of the *suicidal mode* (described in detail in Chapter 2), this structured outpatient individual therapy entailed skills training in cognitive reappraisal, problem solving, and emotion regulation. A central component of Rudd and colleagues' treatment approach was the *crisis response plan*, an intervention that provides explicit guidelines outlining the steps that a patient should take during times of crisis to more adaptively cope with and respond to crises (the crisis response plan is described in detail in Chapter 10). Versions of the crisis response plan have since been retained in subsequent refinements of cognitive-behavioral therapies to prevent suicide attempts (e.g., Wenzel, Brown, & Beck, 2009). In addition, the crisis response plan has subsequently been refined and adapted for use as a stand-alone crisis intervention for use across multiple settings including emergency departments, inpatient psychiatric units, outpatient clinics, primary care clinics, and crisis hotlines (Bryan, Mintz, et al., 2017; Stanley & Brown, 2012). The crisis response plan's focus on effective skills use in response to behavioral emergencies has become a central feature of subsequent treatment refinements for preventing suicide attempts.

Empirical evidence supporting the efficacy of a brief, time-limited cognitive-behavioral therapy for preventing suicide attempts was first published by Brown, Ten Have, and colleagues (2005), who used a 10-session outpatient individual cognitive therapy that was similarly based on the concept of the suicidal mode and focused on skills training in cognitive reappraisal, problem solving, and emotion regulation. Similar to the approach described by Rudd and colleagues (2001), the crisis response plan played a central role in this cognitive therapy protocol, although it was subsequently renamed the *safety planning intervention* (Stanley & Brown, 2012). Several new interventions were developed for this treatment, the most notable of which are the survival kit (described in Chapter 15) and the relapse prevention task (described in Chapter 20). In a randomized clinical trial comparing cognitive therapy for suicide prevention to usual care, Brown and colleagues reported results that were very similar to those obtained from the earlier DBT trials. In terms of suicide attempts, patients receiving cognitive therapy were 50% less likely to make a suicide attempt during the 18-month follow-up period than patients receiving usual care (24% in cognitive therapy vs. 42% in usual care), but there were minimal differences between patients in cognitive therapy and usual care in terms of depression, hopelessness, and suicide ideation. Also similar to DBT, patients in cognitive therapy were significantly more likely to remain in treatment (88% in cognitive therapy vs. 60% of usual care during the first 6 months) but were no more likely to be hospitalized during the 18-month follow-up (13% in cognitive therapy vs. 8% in usual care). Many of the refinements and improvements to the cognitive-behavioral model made by Brown and colleagues have been retained in BCBT.

The findings of Brown, Ten Have, and colleagues (2005) marked an important advance in the development of brief cognitive-behavioral therapy, and demonstrated that time-limited treatments had the potential to be just as effective as longer and more complex cognitive-behavioral therapies. Although one might assume that time-limited treatments would be especially ill suited for high-risk patients who tend to have challenging clinical issues such as complex comorbidities and a tendency to refuse or negate help from others (Rudd, Joiner, & Rajab, 1995), meta-analytic results suggest that longer-duration cognitive-behavioral therapies are no more (or less) effective than briefer cognitive-behavioral therapies (Tarrier et al., 2008). Even within DBT, the total number of sessions attended by patients is not associated with clinical outcomes (Linehan et al., 1991; Linehan, Comtois, Murray, et al., 2006). If the duration of treatment has little to do with cognitive-behavioral therapy's ability to prevent suicide attempts, then what aspects of treatment contribute to its efficacy?

Common Elements of Effective Therapies

In light of mounting evidence that some forms of cognitive-behavioral therapy were better than other forms of treatment for reducing the risk for suicide attempts, researchers became interested in identifying the elements or "ingredients" that accounted for these differences. What was it that made some therapies more effective than others? Answering this question would be critical for developing more focused and potent treatments. In recent years, clinical researchers have converged on several common factors that differentiate effective therapies from less effective treatments (Rudd, 2009, 2012). These findings laid the foundation for the specific changes made during the development of the BCBT protocol described in this treatment manual. As will become apparent throughout this manual, BCBT was based on all of these core ingredients.

Simple, Clinically Useful Theoretical Models

All of the most effective treatments are based on simple and practical models that are easily translated to clinical work. For example, DBT is based on a biosocial model of suicide (Linehan, 1993), whereas cognitive therapy for suicide prevention is based on the concept of the suicidal mode (Wenzel et al., 2009). A common feature of these theoretical models is their emphasis on recognizing how the connections among thoughts, emotional processing, and associated behavioral responses contribute to suicidal thoughts and behaviors. By extension, in order to change the suicidal process, the clinician and patient must directly target and alter the connections among these domains. The effectiveness of a treatment is enhanced when it is based on a useful model because the clinician can more easily explain to the patient why he or she desires suicide and why the specific interventions will help. In short, effective therapies provide a conceptual model to help the patient understand "what is wrong" and "what to do about it." Consistent with this principle, BCBT is based on the fluid vulnerability theory of suicide and the concept of the suicidal mode, both of which will be discussed in detail in Chapter 2.

Treatment Protocols and Clinician Fidelity

All of the most effective treatments are protocol driven, which means they specify in advance how to optimally prioritize problems or issues and how to sequence specific interventions most rapidly and effectively. In effective treatments, suicide risk is the highest-priority clinical issue and each intervention is selected to directly target this priority. Treatments that only indirectly target suicide risk (e.g., by targeting the psychiatric diagnosis instead) are not as effective (Tarrier et al., 2008). To ensure the treatment protocol is implemented as intended, effective treatments often employ a manual for clinicians to follow. The notion of a manualized treatment carries a good deal of negative connotation for many clinicians, often because the term "manualized" is taken to mean "fixed" or "rigid," when in reality clinicians have considerable flexibility in determining how to best administer the protocol for each individual patient. Clinicians also receive intensive training and supervision to minimize the tendency to "drift" from the prescribed protocol. The degree to which a clinician follows the protocol is referred to as *clinician fidelity*. Treatments in which clinicians have high fidelity (i.e., they "follow the directions") yield better results than treatments in which clinicians show low fidelity. This is because fidelity reflects reliability: when following the protocol, the clinician delivers the treatment in a consistent manner both for a given patient as well as across multiple patients. Similar to other effective treatments, BCBT is manualized and clinician fidelity is emphasized. This treatment manual therefore outlines the interventions and procedures that have been found to be effective for preventing suicide attempts. Because clinician fidelity is so crucial to effective care, BCBT fidelity checklists are available in Appendix B.1. These fidelity checklists can be used by clinicians to assess their adherence to the BCBT protocol. They are also used by approved BCBT consultants to provide individualized feedback to clinicians learning the treatment.

Patient Adherence

In addition to clearly articulating what is expected of clinicians, effective treatments also articulate what is expected of patients. Of particular importance is the patient's level of engagement in the treatment process. Effective treatments therefore provide a clear plan for what the clinician should do if the patient does not complete assignments, does not participate during therapy sessions, drops out of treatment unexpectedly, or engages in other therapy-interfering behaviors (cf. Linehan, 1993). The emphasis on patient adherence is reflected by findings showing that effective treatments retain patients much better than comparison treatments (Brown, Ten Have, et al., 2005; Linehan et al., 1991; Linehan, Comtois, Murray, et al., 2006). In BCBT, patient adherence is emphasized throughout the treatment, and is crystallized in the commitment to treatment statement (described in Chapter 11), a new intervention added to the BCBT protocol in order to directly target patient adherence.

Skills-Training Focus

Although cognitive-behavioral therapies are, broadly speaking, a form of "talk therapy," the content of effective treatments is not limited to merely talking about problems and solutions. Effective treatments translate these discussions into behavior change through the demonstration of behavioral skills that target identified skill deficits that contribute to and sustain suicidal crises. In addition to telling patients what to do, clinicians therefore also *show* patients what to do and allow ample time in session to practice these skills and receive feedback to problem-solve or troubleshoot difficulties. Patients then practice these new skills in between sessions and report their progress back to their clinicians. The clinician in turn reinforces skill acquisition and mastery and helps the patient to generalize skills across multiple situations. In BCBT, the clinician teaches a new skill or concept in each session, shows the patient how to do the skill, practices the skill with the patient in session, and then sets up a plan for the patient to practice the skill in between sessions.

Patient Responsibility and Autonomy

In traditional approaches to treating suicidal patients, primary responsibility for treatment progress is often assumed to be held by the clinician, whereas in effective treatments the primary responsibility for treatment progress is *shared* between the patient and clinician. Effective treatments therefore emphasize the patient's autonomy and invite the patient to fully participate in treatment planning and crisis management. Clinicians, by comparison, are primarily responsible for administering the protocol reliably (i.e., clinician fidelity) and addressing patient nonadherence when it arises. In BCBT, patient responsibility for treatment progress is exemplified by the crisis response plan (described in Chapter 10), which is aimed at teaching patients how to effectively manage crises on their own. Patient autonomy is also highlighted in interventions like means safety counseling (described in Chapter 13), which invites patients to create and then implement a plan to maximize their safety.

Clear Guidance for Crisis Resolution

Effective treatments teach patients how to identify emerging crises and provide them with clear steps to follow in order to resolve them. Consistent with the principle of personal responsibility and autonomy, these plans prioritize strategies that patients can use themselves. Should these personal steps fail or prove to be inadequate, effective treatments also make sure that patients know how to access professional and/or emergency services as a backup. Critically, effective treatments always dedicate sufficient time to practicing crisis management skills. As previously noted, the crisis response plan serves as the foundation for teaching patients how to identify and effectively manage crises in BCBT. Likewise, all of the interventions and procedures used in BCBT are designed to augment the patient's crises management skill set.

Individual Therapy Format

According to the results of Tarrier and colleagues' (2008) meta-analysis of 28 trials of cognitive-behavioral therapies, treatments that are provided in an individual format alone or in an individual format combined with group sessions (e.g., DBT) are associated with significant reductions in suicide attempts and suicide ideation, but treatments that are provided in a group format only are not associated with better outcomes. Although the exact reasons for this are not yet fully understood, a leading hypothesis is that group therapies that employ a more traditional interpersonal process format do not focus sufficiently on skills training. In light of these findings, BCBT was developed as an individual therapy.

Summary

Overall, several trends have emerged in treatments that effectively prevent suicide attempts. First, effective cognitive-behavioral therapies have several notable similarities that appear to be essential for preventing suicide: a useful theoretical model; manualization and clinician fidelity; emphasis on patient adherence; skills training; respect for patient autonomy; crisis management skills; and a format that includes individual therapy. Second, cognitive-behavioral therapies consistently reduce patients' risk for making a suicide attempt by up to 50% for up to 18 months posttreatment. Third, when a patient in an effective CBT *does* make a suicide attempt, the attempt tends to be less medically severe, which means the patient is more likely to survive. Fourth, risk for suicide attempts is reduced in effective cognitive-behavioral therapies despite the fact that these treatments are not necessarily better than other treatments at reducing psychiatric symptoms or suicide ideation. This lends support to the perspective that a psychiatric syndromal model for understanding suicide risk is inadequate, and suggests that psychiatric symptoms and even suicide ideation may be less useful as indicators of clinical outcome, treatment progress, and overall risk for suicide. Fifth, patients are more likely to stay in effective cognitive-behavioral therapies. When considered in light of evidence that treatment duration and total number of sessions attended do not correlate with outcome, this finding may suggest that some cognitive-behavioral therapies do a better job of undermining patients' hopelessness about treatment and their capacity to change. Finally, effective cognitive-behavioral therapies prevent suicide attempts even though patients are less likely to be hospitalized, suggesting that outpatient therapy is safe and effective as compared to more intensive treatment modalities.

EFFECTIVENESS OF
BRIEF COGNITIVE-BEHAVIORAL THERAPY

As noted above, the BCBT protocol described in this treatment manual is the next incremental step in the advancement of treatments to prevent suicide attempts. During the past 25 years, the cognitive-behavioral approach to preventing suicide attempts has steadily improved from 32% reduced risk (Linehan et al., 1991) to 50% reduced risk (Brown, Ten Have, et al., 2005; Linehan, Comtois, Brown, Heard, & Wagner, 2006). Because it has retained many of the elements found to be effective in these cognitive-behavioral treatments, BCBT has many similarities to DBT and cognitive therapy for suicide prevention. BCBT also contains some refinements and new components intended to improve the overall effectiveness of the treatment based on recent advances in suicide research; these refinements and additions are described in subsequent chapters along with the rationale behind them.

A randomized clinical trial testing the efficacy of this BCBT protocol was recently completed and published (Rudd et al., 2015). Participants in this trial included 152 active-duty military personnel (85% male) with suicide ideation during the past week and/or a suicide attempt within the past month. Participants were referred to the study upon discharge from inpatient hospitalization for suicide risk; half were randomized to receive BCBT and half were randomized to receive treatment as usual. Treatment as usual was determined by the participant's primary mental health clinician (i.e., a licensed psychologist or psychiatrist) and included individual and group psychotherapy, psychiatric medication, substance abuse treatment, and/or support groups. In addition to treatment as usual, participants randomized to BCBT were scheduled to receive 12 outpatient individual BCBT sessions scheduled on a weekly or biweekly basis, with the first session lasting 90 minutes and subsequent sessions lasting 60 minutes. BCBT was administered by two clinical social workers with different levels of professional experience: one who had just recently completed her master's degree and one who had been a licensed practitioner for over 20 years.

With respect to outcomes, results of this study were also consistent with previous clinical trials. As can be seen in Figure 1.1, differences between treatments in suicide attempt rates emerged within 6 months and persisted for up to 2 years after the start of treatment. Over the course of the 2-year study, participants in BCBT were 60% less likely to make a suicide attempt as compared to participants in treatment as usual (14% in BCBT vs. 40% in treatment as usual). In terms of psychiatric symptom severity, participants in BCBT tended to report slightly less severe symptoms over time as compared to those in treatment as usual, but these differences were not statistically significant (see Figure 1.2). This pattern of results therefore aligns with previous studies of DBT and cognitive therapy for suicide prevention. In contrast to previous studies, however, the BCBT trial followed participants for up to 2 years—the longest follow-up conducted to date. The BCBT trial also marked the first study to enroll a predominantly male sample, thereby confirming the model's efficacy for men.

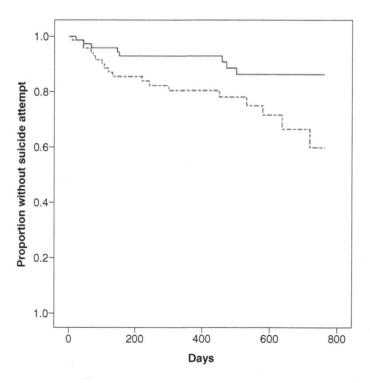

FIGURE 1.1. Survival curves for time to first suicide attempt among participants receiving BCBT (solid line) and participants receiving treatment as usual (dashed line).

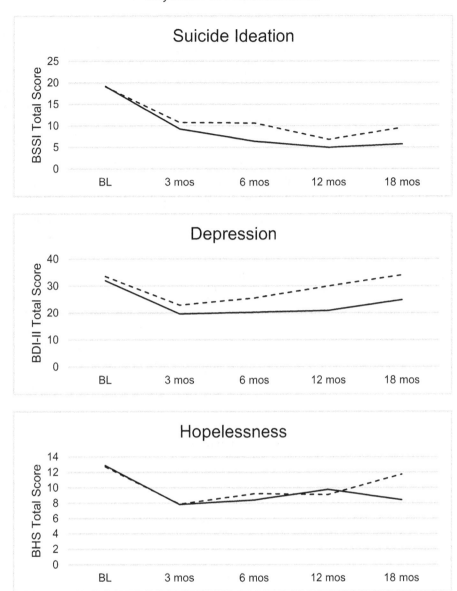

FIGURE 1.2. Differences in severity of suicide ideation, depression, and hopelessness among partici-
pants receiving BCBT (solid line) and participants receiving treatment as usual (dashed line). BSSI, Beck
Scale for Suicide Ideation; BDI-II, Beck Depression Inventory—2nd Edition; BHS, Beck Hopelessness
Scale.

Because this study was conducted in a military setting, the effect of treatment on career
outcomes was also examined. Results showed that participants in BCBT were less likely
to be medically retired from the military than participants in treatment as usual (27% in
BCBT vs. 42% in treatment as usual), suggesting that BCBT may have a positive impact on
social–occupational functioning in addition to its clinical benefits. Overall, participants in
BCBT attended a mean of 12 BCBT sessions and participants in treatment as usual attended
a mean of 12 individual therapy sessions during the first 3 months of the study, suggesting
participants in both treatments received a comparable "dose" of individual therapy. There

were no differences between the two groups in terms of overall treatment utilization (i.e., group therapy, self-help therapy, substance abuse treatment, medication) during the entire study, although participants in BCBT had significantly fewer days of inpatient psychiatric hospitalization (3 days in BCBT vs. 8 days in treatment as usual), similar to previous findings from DBT. Secondary analyses have since been conducted to examine the potential role of dose effects in BCBT (Bryan & Rudd, 2015). Among participants who received fewer than 12 individual therapy sessions, suicide attempt rates during follow-up were 0% in BCBT as compared to 26.3% in treatment as usual. Among those who received 12 or more individual therapy sessions, the suicide attempt rates during follow-up were 19.7% in BCBT as compared to 43.8% in treatment as usual. Of note, suicide attempts were dramatically reduced in BCBT even among those participants who received a much smaller number of individual therapy sessions overall (see Table 1.1), which suggests that even a few sessions of BCBT are better than a large number of sessions of treatment as usual.

Several additional data analyses have since been conducted to determine if BCBT may be more or less effective for different patient subgroups. The results of these analyses are summarized in Table 1.2. As can be seen, BCBT is associated with reduced risk for suicide attempts regardless of gender, history of suicide attempt, and psychiatric diagnosis, which supports the treatment's efficacy across a diverse range of patient characteristics.

In summary, the results of Rudd and colleagues (2015) partially replicated those of Brown, Ten Have, and colleagues (2005) and confirmed the effectiveness of BCBT as a

TABLE 1.1. Estimated Suicide Attempt Probabilities in BCBT and Treatment as Usual by Total Number of Individual Therapy Sessions Attended during Follow-Up

No. of individual therapy sessions	BCBT	Treatment as usual
0–12	0.0%	25.5%
13–24	11.5%	38.5%
25–48	20.9%	21.0%
49+	18.6%	51.0%

TABLE 1.2. Estimated Suicide Attempt Probabilities in BCBT and Treatment as Usual According to Various Patient Characteristics

Subgroup	BCBT	Treatment as usual
Gender		
Women	9%	58%
Men	14%	34%
Diagnosis		
Posttraumatic stress	14%	34%
Substance use	21%	47%
Borderline personality	0%	51%
Prior suicide attempts		
No	0%	54%
Yes	15%	32%

viable alternative to longer and more time-intensive treatments like DBT. Perhaps more importantly, the 60% reduction in risk for suicide attempts among individuals receiving BCBT was the largest magnitude reduction in suicide attempt risk to date, which hints at the possibility of further incremental improvement in the effectiveness of cognitive-behavioral therapies over time. Although efforts to further refine BCBT continue, the protocol described in this book currently represents the latest and most effective treatment for preventing suicide attempts developed to date.

OVERVIEW OF
THE BRIEF COGNITIVE-BEHAVIORAL THERAPY MANUAL

This manual describes all of the procedures and interventions that comprise the BCBT protocol tested by Rudd and colleagues (2015).

The first part of this manual provides a discussion of the theoretical and conceptual principles that underlie BCBT and its implementation. The fluid vulnerability theory of suicide and its embedded notion of the suicidal mode are first described in detail. Core principles and strategies for establishing an effective therapeutic alliance with high-risk patients are next reviewed, followed by procedures for approaching the informed consent process. The following chapter describes strategies and tips for assessing a patient's risk for suicide and subsequently documenting a suicide risk assessment. Next comes a description of various methods for monitoring progress during BCBT, including recommended methods for addressing suicide attempts and psychiatric hospitalizations that occur during the course of treatment. Part I concludes with an overview of BCBT, including a discussion of two issues that are commonly raised by clinicians as concerns when working with suicidal patients: substance use and psychotropic medication use.

The second part of this manual focuses on the first session of BCBT, the most structured session of the entire treatment. The chapters in this section describe the specific sequence of procedures comprising the first session: describing BCBT, conducting a narrative assessment of the suicidal crisis, explaining the treatment log, completing the case conceptualization in collaboration with the patient, and creating a crisis response plan.

Part III describes the procedures and interventions that comprise the first phase of BCBT, which generally spans Sessions 2 to 5. This phase begins with the development of a treatment plan and the use of the commitment to treatment statement, the latter of which directly targets patient adherence. Strategies for addressing the patient's safety and risk for repeat suicide attempts are next described via means safety counseling. Subsequent chapters describe a variety of procedures and interventions used during the first phase of BCBT: stimulus control and sleep hygiene, relaxation, mindfulness, reasons for living, and the survival kit. This aligns with BCBT's overarching approach, which prioritizes emotion regulation and crisis management skills training in order to rapidly reduce symptomatic distress and short-term risk of suicide attempts. In contrast to other manualized therapies that prescribe a particular sequence of procedures, BCBT allows for the flexible selection of procedures and interventions that optimally fit with the patient's needs and treatment goals. In this way, the clinician can customize the delivery of specific procedures to the unique needs of their patient while maintaining fidelity to the model. Despite this flexibility, we have found that some sequences often work better than others. As a result, we ordered the chapters in this section to reflect the sequence of procedures that seems to work best for both patients and clinicians.

The fourth part of this manual describes the procedures and interventions that comprise the second phase of BCBT, which generally spans Sessions 6 to 10. In this phase of the treatment, the focus shifts to the patient's suicidal belief system, which is comprised of automatic thoughts, assumptions, and core beliefs that contribute to and sustain suicidal thoughts and behaviors. As is discussed in Chapter 2, the suicidal belief system is hypothesized to be a chief mechanisms of vulnerability that underlies the patient's risk for future suicidal behavior. The procedures described in this section are based on the worksheets developed by Resick, Monson, and Chard (2017) for cognitive processing therapy for posttraumatic stress disorder (PTSD) and are designed to teach the patient how to identify the relationships among life circumstances, beliefs, and negative emotions, and how to adopt more helpful thoughts: ABC worksheets, challenging questions, and patterns of problematic thinking. Also described here are activity planning and coping cards, two behavioral strategies that complement and support cognitive change. As with the first phase, we ordered the chapters in the sequence that seems to work best for patients and clinicians, although clinicians have the flexibility to use an alternative sequencing pattern.

The fifth part of this manual describes the sole procedure that constitutes the third and final phase of BCBT: the relapse prevention task, which entails a guided imagery exercise that typically spans Sessions 11 and 12. In this final procedure, the patient demonstrates his or her ability to implement the skills learned during BCBT to successfully resolve emotional crises and reduce the likelihood that suicidal behavior will be used as a coping strategy in the future. Also covered in this part is determining when a patient should be considered ready to end BCBT, with suggestions for wrapping up the treatment.

The manual concludes with two appendices that provide specific tools and resources for successfully implementing BCBT. Appendix A includes copies of all patient forms and handouts required for BCBT, and Appendix B includes copies of clinician tools such as fidelity checklists, suicide risk assessment documentation templates, and relaxation and mindfulness scripts. (The materials in Appendices A and B are also available for downloading; see the box at the end of the table of contents.)

To facilitate ease of learning by clinicians, the concepts and procedures described in this manual are supplemented by sample scripts that can be used as a guide for clinicians learning BCBT. These scripts are not necessarily intended to be followed exactly; rather, they provide examples of language and structure that a clinician might use when implementing BCBT. In addition, several case studies are introduced and followed throughout the manual to provide examples of how BCBT can be implemented with patients reflecting a range of risk levels and clinical complexity. These case studies are based on actual patients who completed the BCBT protocol, although details have been changed to preserve privacy and confidentiality. Finally, this manual includes "tips and advice" sections throughout to highlight important lessons learned during the course of our clinical research, collaborations with other suicide researchers, supervision of clinicians learning to use BCBT, and our own personal experience treating suicidal patients with BCBT.

CHAPTER 2

Conceptualizing Suicide
The Suicidal Mode

As noted in Chapter 1, a common element of treatments that work is having a simple and practical theoretical model upon which the treatment is based. In most cases, the models that underlie effective treatments conceptualize suicide as the outcome of the interactions among life events, internal psychological states (i.e., cognition and emotion), and behaviors, such that suicide can be understood as being the result of the interplay among individual-level and environmental-level factors. BCBT is based on the conceptual model known as the *suicidal mode,* which is embedded within the *fluid vulnerability theory* of suicide (Rudd, 2006). Several core assumptions of the fluid vulnerability theory are listed in Figure 2.1, of which the chief assumption is that suicide risk is characterized by both stable and dynamic properties, which are often referred to as baseline risk and acute risk.

Baseline risk entails the individual's "set point" or general propensity for becoming suicidal or making a suicide attempt. To that end, baseline risk refers to the individual's predispositions to suicide, which include historical and trait-like factors that remain relatively constant over time or tend to resist change over time. For example, risk factors such as gender, trauma exposure, and past suicidal behavioral are unchangeable historical risk factors whereas emotional lability, cognitive reactivity, and problem-solving style are trait-like factors that, although modifiable, tend to resist change. In addition to risk factors associated with increased vulnerability for suicide, baseline risk predispositions can also include the absence of protective factors associated with decreased vulnerability for suicide, such as social support, trait optimism, or cognitive flexibility. The fluid vulnerability theory proposes that baseline risk varies from individual to individual based on one's unique constellation of risk and protective factors. Baseline risk would therefore be higher for those with

1. Suicide risk comprises stable and dynamic properties referred to as *baseline risk* and *acute risk*. Baseline risk entails the chronic or more persistent aspect of risk whereas acute risk entails the state-based or more transient aspect of risk.

2. Suicidal episodes are time-limited.

3. Baseline risk varies from individual to individual based on one's unique constellation of historical and development predispositions. These predispositions determine an individual's threshold for activation in response to triggering events.

4. Acute suicidal episodes occur among sufficiently vulnerable individuals when they experience a sufficiently stressful trigger.

   a. Individuals with high baseline risk have low thresholds for activation and therefore experience frequent and long-lasting suicidal episodes even when experiencing mild stress.

   b. Individuals with low baseline risk have high thresholds for activation and therefore rarely experience suicidal episodes even when experiencing extreme stress.

5. Multiple suicide attempts and nonsuicidal self-injury are the clearest markers of elevated baseline risk and vulnerability to persisting risk.

6. Acute suicide risk resolves when the aggravating factors that maintain the suicidal mode are deactivated or reduced.

7. After resolution of an acute suicidal episode an individual returns to his or her baseline risk level.

FIGURE 2.1. Core assumptions of the fluid vulnerability theory.

many predisposing risk factors combined with few protective factors, whereas baseline risk would be lower for those with few predisposing risk factors combined with many protective factors. When faced with stressful life events, individuals with higher baseline risk are more likely to become suicidal and to make a suicide attempt than individuals with lower baseline risk. The baseline dimension of risk therefore corresponds to the stable aspect of suicide risk that tends to persist over time.

Acute risk, in contrast, entails short-term fluctuations in suicide risk that occur in response to external events such as life stressors or triggering experiences. Acute risk includes relatively transient, state-dependent thoughts (e.g., "This is unfair"; "I messed up again"; "I can't take this anymore"), emotions (e.g., depression, anger, guilt), and physiological experiences (e.g., agitation, sleep disturbance, bodily pain) that are associated with the stress response. Acute risk is also associated with the consequent behaviors that the individual takes in reaction to this stress response (e.g., substance use, social withdrawal). These behaviors are often aimed at reducing or escaping from emotional distress, although they may not be the most effective strategies for achieving this goal. In contrast to baseline risk factors, acute risk factors tend to be dynamic in nature and are generally modifiable. According to the fluid vulnerability theory, resolving an active suicidal crisis is achieved most efficiently by targeting the acute risk factors that are most directly related to the suicidal crisis over time. The acute dimension of risk therefore corresponds to the dynamic aspect of risk that fluctuates from moment to moment.

THE SUICIDAL MODE

Over the past several decades, hundreds, if not thousands, of risk and protective factors have been identified for suicide. In the absence of a simple conceptual model, the existence of so many risk and protective factors can make the task of understanding suicide seem overwhelming. In BCBT, risk and protective factors are therefore structurally organized using the concept of the *suicidal mode* (see Figure 2.2). A visual depiction of the suicidal mode is also available in Appendix A.1. Many clinicians find it helpful to print a copy of Appendix A.1 for easy reference when working with suicidal patients. The visual depiction of the suicidal mode can help clinicians to conceptualize cases in "real time" and to better organize clinical information as it is acquired.

The suicidal mode provides a cognitive-behavioral framework for describing the characteristics and features of suicidal episodes (which may or may not include an actual suicide attempt), and serves as the underlying theoretical foundation for BCBT. Structurally, the suicidal mode is comprised of four interactive and mutually influential domains: cognitive, behavioral, emotional, and physical. These four domains are conceptualized across two levels corresponding to the stable (i.e., *baseline*) and dynamic (i.e., *acute*) dimensions of risk described by the fluid vulnerability theory of suicide. This reflects the fact that there are stable and dynamic aspects of cognitive risk factors, stable and dynamic aspects of behavioral risk factors, and so on. For example, a prior mood disorder diagnosis serves as a baseline risk factor because it is historical in nature and reflects a vulnerability to mood disturbance. Because mood fluctuates over time (e.g., individuals have good days and bad days), depression also functions as an acute risk factor. In Figure 2.2, "psychiatric disorder" is therefore listed in the emotional domain of baseline risk and "depression" is listed in the emotional domain of acute risk.

The baseline dimension of the suicidal mode is therefore comprised of relatively stable risk factors that persist over time. Within the cognitive domain, baseline risk factors include internalized and implicit self-perceptions including shame, self-hatred, and perceived defectiveness; deficits in cognitive flexibility that impair executive functioning and the ability to quickly generate potential solutions to problems; problem-solving deficits such as the tendency to discount past experiences and to prefer short-term rewards even at the cost of bigger long-term rewards; and a pessimistic style in which the likelihood of positive outcomes is underestimated. Within the behavioral domain, baseline risk factors include skills deficits in the areas of distress tolerance, emotion regulation, and interpersonal communication, each of which increases the likelihood of maladaptive coping in response to stressful situations and triggering events. Within the emotional domain, baseline risk factors include a history of psychiatric disorders, especially recurrent or chronic conditions like psychotic and mood disorders, and emotional lability that may be related to hypothalamic–pituitary–adrenal (HPA) axis dysfunction. Within the physical domain, baseline risk factors include demographic and/or historical characteristics like gender, race, sexual orientation, and history of trauma exposure; genetic and biological vulnerabilities associated with the *SKA2* gene and putamen gray matter; and medical conditions like chronic pain.

The suicidal mode also comprises state-based or dynamic factors that fluctuate over time in response to situational factors and triggers. These acute factors can similarly be

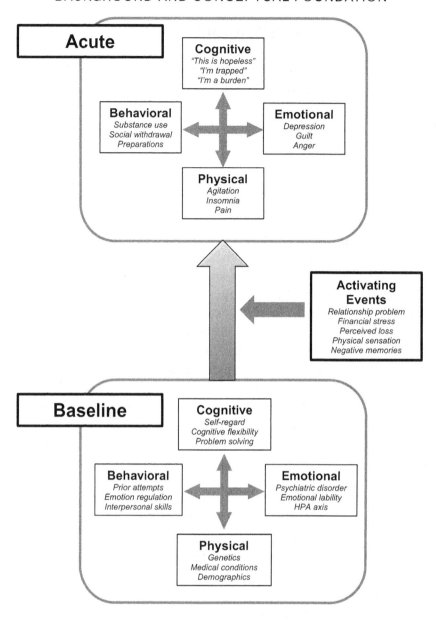

FIGURE 2.2. The suicidal mode.

organized across cognitive, behavioral, emotional, and physical domains. Within the cognitive domain, acute risk factors include automatic thoughts and assumptions that occur in response to stressful situations, such as hopelessness, feeling trapped, perceived burdensomeness, and self-deprecation. Within the behavioral domain, acute risk factors include the specific coping strategies that an individual employs to avoid or reduce emotional distress, such as substance use, social withdrawal, and taking steps to prepare for a suicide attempt (e.g., counting pills, tying a noose, driving to the location of the intended attempt). Within the emotional domain, acute risk factors include dysphoric and uncomfortable affective experiences that are common to the suicidal state, such as depression, guilt, and anger.

Within the physical domain, acute risk factors include somatic experiences commonly associated with emotional distress such as agitation, insomnia, pain, and muscle tension.

These various domains are interactive in nature, such that activation of one domain is often associated with activation of another domain. Risk factors are therefore intertwined with one another, such that they are constantly pushing and pulling on each other as part of a complex network of activity. This pushing and pulling behavior is represented in Figure 2.2 by the four-way arrows that fall in between the four domains and accounts for the "downward spiral" or "snowball effect" that many suicidal individuals describe; it is the sequence of thoughts, emotions, physical sensations, and behavioral responses leading up to a suicidal crisis. Although the mutual interaction of multiple domains within the suicidal mode can lead to a cascade effect that ends with the emergence of suicidal behavior, this cascade effect can also be used for the purposes of recovery: *deactivation* of a risk domain can lead to the deactivation of other risk domains. This latter point highlights the primary rationale for the design and structure of BCBT: improvement in one area will typically lead to improvements in other areas. By targeting multiple domains of risk, BCBT can reduce long-term vulnerability to the reemergence of suicidal behaviors.

Activating Events and Sensitization to Suicide Risk

According to the fluid vulnerability theory, predispositions will only lead to an acute suicidal crisis if the individual's predispositions are activated or "turned on" by a contextual stimulus, sometimes referred to as "triggers." Activating events can include environmental stressors like relationship problems, financial stress, or perceived losses, or they can include internal experiences like physical sensations (e.g., pain) or psychological experiences (e.g., traumatic memories, negative emotions). The relationships among baseline risk factors, activating events, and acute risk factors are depicted in Figure 2.2 by two arrows. The first arrow flows from baseline risk to acute risk, which represents the vulnerability to experiencing suicidal thoughts and behaviors that arise from the individual's unique constellation of stable risk factors. Practically speaking, this means that the structural features of a suicidal crisis will often be related to the individual's stable risk factors. Among individuals with chronic medical conditions, for instance, an acute suicidal crisis is much more likely to reflect medical or health-related concerns than an acute suicidal crisis experienced by individuals without chronic medical conditions. Acute risk factors for such individuals may be marked by somatic symptoms like pain or physical discomfort, self-perceptions characterized by perceived defectiveness or "being broken," and the use of medications (e.g., narcotics) as a coping strategy. In the same way, individuals with histories of trauma are more likely to experience acute risk factors that reflect stable trauma-related risk factors: self-conscious and self-derogatory statements (e.g., "It's all my fault"), sleeplessness secondary to trauma-related nightmares, emotions marked by guilt and shame, and rejection of social support due to difficulties with trust.

The second arrow in Figure 2.2 flows from the activating events to the arrow connecting baseline risk factors to acute risk factors. This reflects the perspective that an individual's baseline risk factors would only be expected to lead to an acute suicidal episode within the context of sufficient activating events. In other words, the likelihood of a suicidal crisis emerging among individuals with many baseline risk factors depends on the quantity and/ or intensity of the activating event. Said another way, suicidal episodes occur only when the stress associated with an activating event exceeds the individual's threshold of tolerance. Individuals with many baseline risk factors have lower thresholds of tolerance, so they experience suicidal episodes with relatively little provocation. Such individuals tend to experience frequent suicidal episodes that last for extended periods of time, even in response to seemingly mild or benign stressors. In contrast, individuals with few baseline risk factors have higher thresholds of tolerance, so they tend to be quite resilient to suicidal episodes, even when they experience very extreme activating events. If an activating event is sufficiently stressful or chronic, however, individuals with very low baseline risk can nonetheless experience an active suicidal crisis. To understand why some individuals become suicidal and others do not, one must therefore consider how the unique features and characteristics of an activating event are experienced within the context of the individual's unique cluster of baseline risk factors.

The Suicidal Belief System and the Nature of Persisting Risk

From the perspective of the fluid vulnerability theory, behavioral and cognitive risk factors warrant particular attention in treatment because enacting change across these two domains can directly and reliably adjust baseline risk for suicide, which in turn reduces the individual's risk for future suicide attempts. By extension, patients who do not make sufficient changes within these two domains will maintain an elevated level of baseline risk, even after the conclusion of treatment. Change in baseline behavioral and cognitive risk factors is therefore believed to be a primary mechanism of change in BCBT. Support for this assertion comes from studies showing that reduced risk for suicide attempts following cognitive therapy is associated with improvements in problem solving and reductions in careless or impulsive decision making (Ghahramanlou-Holloway, Bhar, Brown, Olsen, & Beck, 2012). Research also indicates that internalized and implicit negative self-perceptions including shame, self-hatred, and perceived defectiveness predict future suicide attempts better than acute risk factors including depression and suicide ideation (Bryan, Rudd, Wertenberger, Etienne, et al., 2014; Nock et al., 2010), and differentiate individuals who have attempted suicide from those who have engaged in nonsuicidal self-injury (Bryan, Rudd, Wertenberger, Etienne, et al., 2014). These latter findings in particular implicate suicide-specific cognitive risk factors such as perceived burdensomeness (e.g., "People would be better off without me"), self-hatred (e.g., "I deserve to be punished"; ""I am unworthy of love), and perceived incompetence (e.g., "I can't handle this"; "I fail at everything."). Because these suicide-specific schemas increase the likelihood of suicidal mode activation and sustain the suicidal mode over time, they are collectively referred to in BCBT as the *suicidal belief system*.

To illustrate the importance of predisposing cognitive and behavioral risk factors for long-term risk reduction, consider the example of a young woman named Mary who lacks basic stress management skills and has a number of negative self-schemas consistent with the suicidal belief system (e.g., "I'm a failure": "I'm completely unworthy of love"; "I don't deserve to be forgiven for my mistakes"; "I'm worthless"). Following a major conflict with her romantic partner, Mary intentionally takes an overdose of sleep medication requiring medical treatment, after which she is briefly hospitalized. During her inpatient stay, Mary and her partner resolve the conflict and her emotional distress returns to baseline. Because Mary no longer feels suicidal, she is discharged from the hospital. Although she is now "stabilized," Mary nonetheless still possesses her behavioral (i.e., poor stress management skills) and cognitive (i.e., suicidal beliefs) predispositions. Thus, even though her active suicidal mode has been deactivated, Mary's long-term risk for suicide persists "beneath the surface" as a lingering vulnerability that will go largely unobserved until she experiences a new activating event, which will likely result in a new suicidal crisis. If, however, Mary acquired some basic stress management skills (e.g., relaxation, mindfulness) and learned to replace her critical self-perceptions with a more positive cognitive style marked by optimism (e.g., "Things will be OK"), perceived competence (e.g., "I can handle this"; "I'm going to be OK"), and pride (e.g., "I'm worthy of respect"), she would be much less likely to become suicidal again in the future in response to activating events (Bryan, Andreski, McNaughton-Cassill, & Osman, 2014; Bryan, Ray-Sannerud, Morrow, & Etienne, 2013b, 2013c; Hirsch & Conner, 2006). If these changes were to occur, Mary's baseline risk for suicide would be reduced, which would lead to a long-term reduction in her risk for making another suicide attempt.

BCBT was specifically designed to reduce baseline risk for suicide attempts that can persist over the long term, even when an individual is not in acute distress. BCBT accomplishes this goal by focusing on the acquisition of new skills and coping strategies that enable the patient to respond more effectively to life stressors (i.e., behavioral predispositions) and replacing the suicidal belief system with more positive and adaptive schemas that promote resiliency and decrease vulnerability to suicidal crises (i.e., cognitive predispositions).

CLINICAL IMPLICATIONS

The suicidal mode serves as the central organizing principle for the BCBT protocol; all interventions flow directly from it. The suicidal mode not only provides a simple and straightforward way for the patient to understand why he or she wants to die by suicide and/ or made a suicide attempt, it also provides the patient with a rationale for each procedure and intervention used during treatment. To this end, when introducing and teaching a new intervention to the patient, the clinician should be sure to tie the concept or skill directly to the suicidal mode. Patients who clearly understand why they are being asked to use a skill and how it is supposed to work are much more likely to use the skill effectively.

The fluid vulnerability theory also has important implications for understanding the emergence and resolution of suicide risk over time. As noted previously, individuals with many baseline risk factors are more easily activated when they experience activating events than individuals with fewer baseline risk factors. Furthermore, it takes longer for individuals with many baseline risk factors to resolve their suicidal crises as compared to individuals with fewer baseline risk factors. These dynamics are illustrated in Figure 2.3, which plots out the fluctuations in suicide risk for a low-baseline-risk individual (Person A, solid line) and a high-baseline-risk individual (Person B, dotted line). Note that both individuals

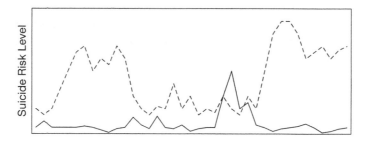

FIGURE 2.3. Emergence and resolution of suicide risk over time for an individual with low baseline risk for suicide (Person A, depicted by solid line) and an individual with high baseline risk for suicide (Person B, depicted by dashed line).

remain at their respective baseline risk levels until they experience an activating event, which leads to an acute suicidal episode. The relative magnitudes of the suicidal episodes are equal for both Person A and Person B, but Person B is at greater risk overall during this crisis because he was higher risk to begin with. As the crises resolve, both individuals eventually return to their baseline levels of risk, but Person A resolves faster than Person B because she has fewer baseline risk factors and is therefore "better equipped" to handle the crisis. This figure highlights a critical implication of the fluid vulnerability theory: even when Person B is at his baseline risk level, he nonetheless possesses higher risk overall than Person A. Furthermore, Person A's risk severity during an acute suicidal crisis is not much higher than Person B's risk severity at baseline. Thus, Person B's "relative best" is not much lower risk than Person A's "relative worst." This highlights a critical implication of the fluid vulnerability theory: when formulating a patient's overall suicide risk level (e.g., during a suicide risk assessment interview), clinicians should consider both the baseline *and* acute dimensions of risk, as opposed to considering only the acute dimension. This is because acute risk is superimposed on top of baseline risk; high-baseline individuals continue to be high risk even when they are at their relative best.

The importance of baseline risk is supported by considerable research finding stronger associations of suicide ideation and attempts with stable risk factors as compared to their associations with acute risk factors. For instance, previous suicide attempts and nonsuicidal self-injury are among the strongest predictors of current and future suicide attempts, and consistently outperform other acute risk factors like depression and hopelessness (Bryan, Bryan, Ray-Sannerud, Etienne, & Morrow, 2014; Joiner et al., 2005; Klonsky, May, & Glenn, 2013). Considerable evidence indicates that individuals who have made two or more suicide attempts, in particular, are among the highest-risk patients. Multiple suicide attempts are therefore considered to be the clearest marker of elevated baseline risk (Bryan & Rudd, 2006) because a history of multiple suicide attempts generally serves as a proxy indicator of other relevant baseline risk factors including history of psychopathology, impaired problem solving, and emotion regulation skills deficits (Forman, Berk, Henriques, Brown, & Beck, 2004; Rudd, Joiner, & Rajab, 1996). Newer research suggests that nonsuicidal self-injury should also be considered a marker of elevated baseline risk (Bryan, Bryan, May, & Klonsky, 2015; Bryan, Rudd, Wertenberger, Young-McCaughon, & Peterson, 2014; Guan, Fox, & Prinstein, 2012; Wilkinson, Kelvin, Roberts, Dubicka, & Goodyer, 2011). Given the strong role that baseline risk plays in the emergence of suicidal thoughts and behaviors, clinicians should be careful not to underestimate a patient's risk level by minimizing or overlooking the importance of stable risk factors.

Another core assumption of the fluid vulnerability theory is that individuals return to their baseline risk levels following the resolution of acute suicidal episodes. Although this may seem like an obvious conclusion, this has important clinical implications when working with high-baseline patients. Referring back to Figure 2–3, note that although both Person A and Person B return to their respective baseline risk levels following their acute suicidal episodes, Person B's overall level of risk remains elevated. As mentioned before, Person B's baseline risk level is not much lower than Person A's peak risk level, indicating that Person B's *relative best* is therefore not much different from Person A's *relative worst*. As applied to treatment planning, this suggests that clinicians (and patients) who overlook the role of baseline risk could establish expectations or treatment goals that are unrealistic or unattainable. For example, some high-baseline patients (especially those who have made multiple suicide attempts) experience low-intensity suicide ideation with high frequency (e.g., "I think about suicide hundreds of times a day but the suicidal thoughts just kind of jump in and then out of my mind real quick"), even when they are not in crisis. For such patients, setting "no suicidal thoughts" as a treatment goal could be a recipe for failure because this criterion may be unrealistic for some patients, even when they are doing reasonably well. By comparison, a treatment goal such as "reduced risk for suicide attempt" is much more realistic and achievable regardless of the patients' baseline risk level.

Implicit in the above points is that suicide risk is an intrinsically dynamic construct. Even within the context of treatment, suicide risk will fluctuate in intensity, sometimes very quickly or unexpectedly. Although this might seem obvious, it nonetheless bears explicit mention: although suicide risk by and large decreases during treatment, transient increases in risk can also occur. These fluctuations are especially likely to occur among patients who have made multiple suicide attempts (Bryan & Rudd, 2017). Clinicians should therefore anticipate that *most* patients will experience an upsetting setback at some point in treatment, *many* will fail to learn new skills or try new ideas as quickly as desired, *some* will experience a new suicidal episode, and a *few* will make a suicide attempt. In very rare cases, patients who make a suicide attempt while in treatment will die by suicide. In light of this unsettling and anxiety-provoking reality of clinical work with suicidal patients, BCBT was designed to flexibly respond to the needs of patients no matter where they are in the suicidal process: before, during, or after a crisis.

INTEGRATING OTHER CONCEPTUAL MODELS OF SUICIDE WITH THE FLUID VULNERABILITY THEORY

Although BCBT's development was based largely on the fluid vulnerability theory and the notion of the suicidal mode, other conceptual models of suicide that have been described in the clinical literature are also relevant to BCBT. Two models in particular—the interpersonal psychological theory of suicide (Joiner, 2005) and the integrated motivational–volitional model (O'Connor, 2011)—have been especially influential for clinical researchers during the past decade. Each of these models, similar to the fluid vulnerability theory, are couched within the ideation-to-action framework (Klonsky & May, 2015) in that they clearly distinguish suicidal ideation and its risk factors from suicidal behaviors and their (distinct) risk factors. As noted by May and Klonsky (2016), many well-documented risk factors of suicide are actually correlates of suicidal ideation but do not distinguish between those who think about suicide and those who actually try to kill themselves. The ideation-to-action framework represents an important recent advance in the field of suicide prevention in general and the clinical treatment of suicidal patients in particular, as it provides an explanation for a remarkably consistent pattern across clinical trials: treatments that significantly reduce the incidence of suicidal behaviors, including BCBT, are not necessarily superior with respect to reducing suicidal ideation and other psychiatric symptoms (Brown, Ten Have, et al., 2005; Gysin-Maillart, Schwab, Soravia, Megert, & Michel, 2016; Linehan et al., 1991, 2006; Rudd et al., 2015). Effective treatments therefore impact suicidal behaviors and suicidal thoughts in unique ways.

Although the interpersonal psychological theory and the integrated motivational–volitional model offer alternative perspectives for understanding suicidal behavior, these approaches have considerable overlap with the fluid vulnerability theory. Critically, these alternative conceptual approaches do not necessarily present competing ideas, but rather they emphasize different pathways by which individuals transition from suicidal thought to action. Thus, each model has unique implications for the care of suicidal individuals that are critical for the implementation of BCBT. Each model is therefore described briefly, as is its implications for BCBT.

The Interpersonal Psychological Theory

Joiner's (2005) interpersonal psychological theory of suicide is arguably the most familiar of the contemporary theories of suicide. According to this model, suicidal behavior requires two necessary conditions—the desire to kill oneself and the capability to do so—neither of which are sufficient by themselves. The interpersonal psychological theory therefore provides a simple and straightforward model for differentiating those who think about suicide from those who act upon these thoughts. The desire for suicide (i.e., suicidal ideation) entails the combination of two key thought processes: perceived burdensomeness and thwarted belongingness. *Perceived burdensomeness* entails the perception that one is a liability to others and/or that others would benefit from one's absence or death (e.g., "Others would be better off without me"), whereas *thwarted belongingness* entails the perception that one is isolated and alone, and/or does not fit in with others (e.g., "No one cares about me"). When an individual experiences elevated levels of both perceived burdensomeness and thwarted belongingness and perceives this psychological state as never-ending (e.g., "This will never change"), active suicidal ideation is likely to emerge. Suicidal desire therefore entails a combination of perceived burdensomeness, thwarted belongingness, and hopelessness, all of which are specific features of the suicidal mode's cognitive domain.

From the perspective of the interpersonal psychological theory, however, the presence of suicidal ideation is not enough for an individual to make a suicide attempt; the suicidal individual must also possess the *capability* for suicide. Suicidal capability contains several components that begins with fearlessness about death, which facilitates the emergence of suicidal intent among those with suicidal ideation. If the suicidal individual with elevated intent also possesses elevated pain tolerance, the likelihood of transitioning to suicidal behavior increases (Van Orden, Witte, Gordon, Bender, & Joiner, 2008). These two latent constructs that underlie suicidal capability—fearlessness about death and pain tolerance—cut across multiple domains of the suicidal mode: cognitive appraisal processes specific to threat and discomfort, whether physical or psychological; emotional processes including affect regulation; and the behavioral responses pursued in response to these cognitive, affective, and physiological experiences (specifically, approach or avoidance).

Suicidal capability was initially thought to be acquired over the course of an individual's lifespan as a result of exposure to painful and provocative experiences such as violence, aggression, and trauma (Joiner, 2005; Selby et al., 2010; Van Orden et al., 2008). Recent prospective studies have not provided much support for this assumption, however, and suggest instead that suicidal capability may have trait-like properties that remain stable over time, even following exposure to violent and potentially traumatic experiences (e.g., Bryan, Sinclair, & Heron, 2016). These newer findings suggest that suicidal capability aligns with the fluid vulnerability theory's notion of baseline risk. As a construct, suicidal capability encompasses several key predisposing vulnerabilities for suicide articulated by the fluid vulnerability theory, notably emotion regulation (i.e., fearlessness, pain tolerance) and cognitive appraisal (i.e., perceived burdensomeness, thwarted belongingness). The interpersonal psychological theory is therefore a conceptual model that is compatible with the fluid vulnerability theory and the embedded concept of the suicidal mode.

From a clinical perspective, the interpersonal psychological theory supports the need to target suicidal desire and/or suicidal capability. The first of these two tasks has received a considerable amount of attention by clinicians and researchers and can be accomplished via cognitive interventions aimed at undermining perceived burdensomeness and thwarted belongingness (e.g., Joiner, Van Orden, Witte, & Rudd, 2009). The second task, reducing suicidal capability, has received very little clinical or empirical attention by comparison, although in recent years a shift toward increased recognition of the value of limiting access to potentially lethal means for suicide, especially firearms, has occurred (Britton, Bryan, & Valenstein, 2016; Bryan, Stone, & Rudd, 2011). Consistent with these implications, BCBT includes cognitive strategies aimed at undermining suicidal beliefs including perceived burdensomeness and thwarted belongingness and directly targets access to lethal means via means restriction counseling and crisis response planning.

The Integrated Motivational–Volitional Model

A significant limitation of many existing theoretical models is their relatively narrow focus on a small number of domains of risk, and in some cases, only a single domain of risk (O'Connor, 2011). For example, Baumeister (1990) has emphasized the importance of escape from the self as the primary motive for suicidal behavior, whereas Wenzel and Beck (2008) have emphasized hopelessness and other cognitive schemas. To address these limitations, the integrated motivational–volitional model of suicidal behavior (O'Connor, 2011) was developed to synthesize several models of suicidal behavior, and it has many similarities to the fluid vulnerability theory and the concept of the suicidal mode.

Consistent with the ideation-to-action framework, the integrated motivational–volitional model seeks to provide a model for understanding how individuals become suicidal and, in some cases, transition to suicidal behavior. This model is organized into three phases: premotivational, motivational, and volitional. The *premotivational* phase includes background factors (e.g., demographics, personality traits, previous trauma), environmental contingencies (e.g., social support, access to resources), and life events (e.g., relationship problems, financial strain) that exist prior to the emergence of suicidal thoughts or behaviors. These premotivational factors interact with each other and determine whether or not suicidal thoughts and intent will emerge. Similar to the fluid vulnerability theory's baseline dimension of risk, the integrated motivational–volitional model argues that individuals have unique thresholds for activation that are determined in large part by their background factors, especially previous experiences with suicidal thoughts and behaviors. Individuals who have been suicidal in the past are therefore sensitized to additional suicidal crises in the future. Likewise, individuals who have attempted suicide previously are sensitized to make additional suicide attempts.

The second phase of the model, the *motivational* phase, entails the formation of suicidal ideation and intent. The central hypothesized pathway to suicidal thinking and subsequent behavior surrounds defeat, humiliation, and entrapment. Specifically, individuals with many background vulnerabilities are sensitized to signals of defeat (e.g., "I'm a failure") and humiliation (e.g., "I feel embarrassed"). For example, individuals with high levels are perfectionism are much more likely to interpret setbacks or challenges in life as indicators of failure, and are more likely to experience self-conscious emotions like humiliation, guilt, and/or shame (O'Connor & Noyce, 2008; O'Connor & O'Connor, 2003; O'Connor, Rasmussen, & Hawton, 2010). These feelings of defeat and humiliation can trigger a sense of entrapment (e.g., "I see no way out of my current situation") when an individual also experiences factors that strengthen their potency. Such factors are referred to as *threat to self moderators* in the integrated motivational-volitional model, and include variables such as impaired problem solving, coping deficits, and rumination. Feelings of entrapment, in turn, lead to suicidal ideation and intent when they are combined with cognitive–affective factors such as thwarted belongingness, perceived burdensomeness, absence of hope and optimism, and limited social support, all of which are collectively referred to as *motivational moderators*. The motivational phase corresponds to the fluid vulnerability theory's concept of the suicidal mode and its assumption that interactions among multiple domains of risk (i.e., cognitive, emotional, behavioral, physiological) facilitate the emergence of suicidal thinking and enhance the severity of suicidal crises.

The third phase of the model, the *volitional* phase, entails the transition from suicidal ideation and intent to behavior. According to the integrated motivational-volitional model, individuals will act upon their suicidal thoughts when they experience a sufficient level of *volitional moderators*, which include variables and factors that strengthen the intensity of suicidal intent or weaken the barriers that impede acting on suicidal thoughts. These volitional moderators include variables such as fearlessness about death, pain tolerance, impulsivity, access to lethal means, and rehearsal or preparatory behavior. The integrated motivational-volitional model is therefore similar to the interpersonal psychological theory in its perspective of how individuals transition from suicidal thought to action.

Similar to the interpersonal psychological theory, the integrated motivational–volitional model targets thwarted belongingness and perceived burdensomeness for clinical modification to reduce the risk of suicidal behavior. The integrated motivational-volitional model provides several additional cognitive–affective targets that are not articulated in the interpersonal psychological theory: defeat, humiliation, and entrapment. These constructs fall within the cognitive and affective domains of the suicidal mode and are modified via cognitive interventions during the second phase of BCBT. In addition to cognitive reappraisal skills training, the integrated motivational–volitional model further supports the benefits of problem solving and emotion regulation skills training, two of the central mechanisms that have been hypothesized to underlie BCBT's effects on suicidal behavior (Bryan, 2016; Bryan, Grove, & Kimbrel, 2017).

ILLUSTRATIVE CASE EXAMPLES

To help illustrate many of the concepts and principles of BCBT, we will introduce here three patients who completed BCBT, although details have been changed to protect their privacy: John, Mike, and Janice. We will return to their cases throughout this manual to demonstrate how BCBT can be successfully implemented with a diverse range of patients.

The Case of John

John is a 22-year-old Hispanic male who currently serves in the U.S. military. Approximately 1 week prior to meeting with his therapist, he had an argument with his wife while she was out of town visiting her family. During the argument, she commented that he "wasn't listening" and "wasn't being a good husband." John became angry and frustrated, noting that he "just got tired of her always saying negative things." With his wife on the phone, John went to the storage shed for their apartment and grabbed his rifle. His wife heard what he was doing and started pleading with him to stop. John ignored her and took the rifle inside the apartment, placed the bullets on the coffee table, then sat against the wall with the rifle resting on his shoulder. John's wife continued to plead with him to stop and told him that she would call a friend. John said he suddenly "snapped out of it" and told his wife to call a friend. The friend immediately rushed over and took John to a local psychiatric unit, where he was assessed but was not admitted for inpatient care. He was released early the next morning and called the clinic to set up a walk-in appointment. John has no history of psychiatric diagnoses and denies a history of suicidal thoughts and behaviors prior to this incident. He says he feels "guilty" about what he did and feels "embarrassed" that others know what happened.

The Case of Mike

Mike is a 55-year-old Caucasian male who previously worked as a law enforcement officer. Approximately 15 years ago, he was "forced out" of his position by his supervisors, whom he described as "manipulative, deceitful bastards" who "betrayed me." Since then, he has bounced from job to job, but over the past few years has settled into a part-time position as a shopping mall security guard. He describes his job as unrewarding and "humiliating" but has stayed with this position "because I have to pay the bills somehow." During the past few years, he and his wife have had an on-again, off-again relationship. They lived together for a time, but several months ago he moved out after an argument in which his wife expressed uncertainty about their future. Mike moved into the basement of his mother's house, which contributes to further embarrassment because "I'm a grown man living with his mommy." He reports drinking alcohol on a regular basis to the point of intoxication, feels like his emotions "are out of control," and "can't stand what I've become." Mike was strongly encouraged to seek out treatment by his sister when he sent her a series of text messages late one night in which he expressed severe depression and hopelessness, and reported that he was sleeping with his gun. During his initial consultation appointment, Mike was visibly uncomfortable and agitated, was tearful, and spoke with a pressured voice. When becoming tearful, he would break eye contact and his leg would begin bouncing rapidly. Mike admitted to depressed mood, anger, and severe insomnia, but when asked about recent and past suicidal thoughts and behaviors, he denied both.

The Case of Janice

Janice is a 42-year-old Caucasian female who is currently unemployed due to medical disability. She was sexually assaulted on several occasions in the past by her then-husband and was subsequently diagnosed with PTSD and borderline personality disorder. During the height of her PTSD, prior to military discharge, Janice made a near-lethal suicide attempt via medication overdose. Two years later, she made a second suicide attempt, also via medication overdose, that resulted in a coma that lasted for over a week. She has been treated with various antidepressants, mood stabilizers, and anxiolytic medications and has undergone various forms of psychotherapy during the past 5 years for PTSD, depression, anxiety, and borderline personality disorder. She was referred for treatment by her clinical social worker to address "chronic suicide risk and PTSD" following a session during which Janice admitted to her social worker that she had a suicide plan, although Janice stressed that she "has had a suicide plan for years now, so what's the big deal?" Janice reports that she thinks about suicide "constantly."

CHAPTER 3

Core Principles of Treatment
with Suicidal Patients

In 2006, the Suicide Prevention Resource Center identified 24 core clinical competencies for the assessment and management of suicide risk that were organized into seven domains: attitudes and approach, understanding suicide, collecting accurate assessment information, formulating risk, developing a treatment and services plan, managing care, and understanding legal and regulatory issues related to suicide risk. These competencies provide the foundation for the basic principles of effective care for suicidal patients. BCBT maps directly onto these core competencies and provides the structure and specific strategies that ensure the clinician meets all of the 24 competencies. This, in turn, leads to high quality and effective care. Although a full discussion of the core clinical competencies is beyond the scope of this chapter, three issues related to these core competencies warrant particular attention for the clinician using BCBT with suicidal patients: language, therapeutic alliance, and informed consent.

THE LANGUAGE OF SUICIDE

One of the primary factors contributing to our limited understanding of what works to prevent suicide attempts is inconsistency in language and terminology among researchers and clinicians. The terms used to describe suicide-related thoughts and behaviors are remarkably diverse and vary widely across settings and professions (Silverman, 2006). To highlight the magnitude of this problem, Silverman (2006) noted that at least 11 distinct definitions of *suicide* exist within the extant literature and dozens of terms for other suicide-related phenomena can be found, many of which have no formal definition. For example, the term *suicide gesture* is a term commonly used by many clinicians, although no formal definition of this term is known to exist. In the absence of a formal definition, different clinicians use this term in so many different ways that it has virtually no reliability or clinical meaningfulness (Bryan & Tomchesson, 2007). From a practical perspective, this means it is very unlikely that any two clinicians would agree upon what a suicide gesture is and what it is not. This presents a considerable challenge for the coordination of care across settings and clinicians.

From a research perspective, inconsistencies in suicide-related terminology have slowed the advancement of knowledge about suicide and interfered with the ability to identify the most effective methods for preventing suicide attempts. Consider, for example, several of the clinical trials of cognitive-behavioral therapies discussed in previous chapters. In the first randomized clinical trial of DBT, Linehan and colleagues (1991) reported a 33% decrease in the risk for *parasuicide* among patients who received the treatment. In that study, parasuicide included suicide attempts and other intentional forms of self-injury that were not intended to result in death (i.e., *nonsuicidal self-injury*, which is explicitly defined and discussed below). In the 2006 randomized clinical trial of DBT, by contrast, Linehan and colleagues considered suicide attempts separate from nonsuicidal self-injury, and reported a 50% decrease in the risk for suicide attempt among patients receiving DBT but no effect on nonsuicidal self-injury. When comparing the results of the 1991 clinical trial to the 2006 clinical trial, one possible explanation for the difference in results is that, following the conclusion of the first study, DBT was refined and improved, which yielded better outcomes (i.e., 33% reduction vs. 50% reduction). Another possible explanation is that DBT has differential effects on suicide attempt and nonsuicidal self-injury, but this was only apparent in the second trial. The combination of suicide attempts with nonsuicidal self-injury in the first trial may therefore have "diluted" the observed outcomes, such that DBT's effects on suicide attempts may have been underestimated in the first trial because suicide attempts and nonsuicidal self-injury were not considered separately. Unfortunately, there is no way to know this for sure. Our understanding of how and why DBT works is not so straightforward because these two landmark studies measured outcomes in different ways.

In light of these problems, a concerted effort to standardize language and terms for suicide-related outcomes has emerged, culminating in formal definitions for use across both research and clinical settings (Crosby, Ortega, & Melanson, 2011). These definitions have since been adopted by the Centers for Disease Control and Prevention, the Department of Defense, and the Department of Veterans Affairs and are being adopted by a growing number of researchers and clinicians. Of particular relevance for clinicians using BCBT is the distinction between suicide attempt and nonsuicidal self-injury:

- *Suicide attempt:* A nonfatal, self-directed, potentially injurious behavior with any intent to die as a result of the behavior. A suicide attempt may or may not result in injury.
- *Nonsuicidal self-injury:* Behavior that is self-directed and deliberately results in injury or the potential for injury to oneself. There is no evidence, whether implicit or explicit, of suicidal intent.

As can be seen in these definitions, suicide attempts and nonsuicidal self-injury are similar in that both are intentional and self-directed and can result in nonfatal injury. What differentiates the two behaviors is intent. Suicide attempts are motivated by the desire to die as a result of the behavior, whereas nonsuicidal self-injury is motivated by reasons other than death, the most common of which is emotion relief (Nock & Prinstein, 2005).

Although suicide attempts and nonsuicidal self-injury are similar and overlap with each other, standardized definitions provide a simple method for accurately classifying a given behavior: the presence of *any* suicidal intent. Suicidal intent is defined as any evidence, whether explicit or implicit, that the individual intended to kill him- or herself or wished to die at the time of the injury and understood the likely consequences of the behavior. For the purposes of classifying a patient's behavior, suicidal intent is therefore operationalized in a binary manner: it is either present to any degree or it is not. If suicidal intent is present to any degree, the behavior is classified as a suicide attempt, but if there is no suicidal intent at all, the behavior is classified as nonsuicidal self-injury. This provides a practical solution for clinicians working with patients who report ambiguous intent or ambivalence during an instance of self-injury (e.g., "I'm not really sure how much I wanted to die" or "I guess I sort of wanted to die a little bit"): if suicidal intent equals zero, then the behavior is classified as nonsuicidal self-injury, but if suicidal intent is greater than zero, even if only very small in value, then the behavior is classified as a suicide attempt.

Note also that the definitions of suicide attempt and nonsuicidal self-injury only require the behaviors to be *potentially* injurious; they do not require an injury to actually occur. This is perhaps most important to keep in mind for classifying suicide attempts, as many clinicians assume this behavior must result in some form of physical injury or tissue damage to be considered a suicide attempt. A patient can make a suicide attempt without sustaining an injury, however. For example, if he or she jumps into traffic but is not struck by a vehicle, they have made a suicide attempt without injury. Similarly, a patient may attempt suicide without injury by taking a nonlethal amount of medication, falling asleep, and then waking up with no physical consequences or injuries. In each of these cases, the behaviors meet definitional criteria for a suicide attempt even though no injury actually occurred because they were (1) self-directed, (2) potentially injurious, and (3) intended to result in death.

In addition to standardizing and recommending the use of certain terms to more accurately describe suicide-related outcomes, several terms are now considered unacceptable and are therefore discouraged from being used in clinical settings due to their conceptual inaccuracies and/or the presence of negative or pejorative connotations (Crosby et al., 2011). *Completed suicide* and *successful suicide* are no longer recommended because the terms imply the achievement of a desired outcome when the outcome (i.e., death) is not considered desirable. In BCBT, we would argue that there is no such thing as a "successful" suicide. The recommended terms to use instead are *suicide* or *death by suicide*. *Failed attempt* is similarly unacceptable because it implies that death is the criterion for success and reinforces the individual's perception that he or she is a failure; the term *suicide attempt* is recommended instead. *Parasuicide,* an umbrella term to refer to all forms of self-directed violence, and *suicidality,* an umbrella term to refer to the full spectrum of suicidal thoughts and behaviors, are not acceptable because they are not sufficiently specific; the terms *suicide ideation, suicide plan, suicide attempt,* and *nonsuicidal self-injury* are recommended instead, depending on the actual construct being considered. Finally, *suicide gesture* and *suicide threat* are not acceptable because these terms make a pejorative value judgment about the individual's intent and motivations.

The language that clinicians use is essential to good treatment outcomes because it ensures consistency in treatment delivery and documentation across time and across clinicians and reduces the likelihood that clinicians will use pejorative terms that could be iatrogenic and, as a result, interfere with the therapeutic alliance (Bryan & Rudd, 2006). In BCBT, clinicians should use the recommended standardized terminology and avoid using those terms that are deemed unacceptable for use.

THE THERAPEUTIC ALLIANCE

A critical but often underappreciated area of clinical competency entails clinicians' recognition of how their personal beliefs and assumptions about suicide can influence their actions and decisions during the course of treatment. Just as the patient's beliefs can influence his or her choices and behaviors, so can the clinician's beliefs and assumptions influence the decisions made and actions taken in BCBT. Thus, one domain of competency for clinicians focuses on the clinician's self-awareness of those beliefs and attitudes that can influence treatment decisions. Prior to implementing BCBT with suicidal patients, clinicians are therefore encouraged to take the time to identify their personal beliefs about suicide, a process that can be accomplished by considering questions such as:

- "Why do people die by suicide?"
- "What are my personal moral, spiritual, and/or religious beliefs about suicide?"
- "What type of person makes a suicide attempt?"
- "Can suicide be prevented?"
- "Who do I know who has been suicidal, made a suicide attempt, or died by suicide?"
- "What do I think about my own personal experiences being suicidal?"
- "How have the suicide deaths of my patients influenced my practice?"
- "What is my responsibility to my patients as a clinician?"

Although there are no clear "right" or "wrong" answers to these questions, and some questions may not be applicable to all clinicians, these questions nonetheless reflect clinician-specific factors that can influence the course and process of treatment. At a more fundamental level, the clinician's beliefs and assumptions play a central role in the ability to maintain a productive therapeutic alliance or rapport because they influence the clinician's emotional reactions to suicidal patients.

One of the most consistent research findings in psychotherapy research is that a strong therapeutic alliance is positively correlated with treatment outcome (Martin, Garske, & Davis, 2000). This has led many clinicians to assume that the therapeutic alliance is the primary, or even the *only*, treatment factor that contributes to positive treatment outcomes. This perspective implies that specific techniques and strategies conducted within the context of treatment are less important or even irrelevant for treatment outcome. Research suggests the relation of therapeutic alliance with suicide-related outcomes may be more complex than often assumed, however (Bedics, Atkins, Comtois, & Linehan, 2012; Bryan, Corso, et al., 2012). Among patients receiving brief interventions in primary care, for instance, therapeutic alliance has not been found to be associated with subsequent change in suicide ideation at all (Bryan, Corso, et al., 2012). Although the reasons for this absence of findings are not clear, one possibility is that the relation of therapeutic alliance with suicide-related outcomes depends on the type of treatment provided.

In DBT, for instance, therapeutic alliance tends to strengthen across treatment and is associated with decreased incidence of nonsuicidal self-injury; in psychoanalysis, however, therapeutic alliance initially weakens but then returns to initial levels across treatment and is actually associated with *increased* incidence of nonsuicidal self-injury (Bedics et al., 2012). When considering the two treatments together, there was no apparent relation of therapeutic alliance to nonsuicidal self-injury, but this is only because the relationship differed across the two types of treatment: a positive association in DBT but a negative association in psychoanalysis. The attempted suicide short intervention program (ASSIP), Gysin-Maillart and colleagues (2016) similarly found that stronger therapeutic alliance at the end of the first session was associated with significantly reduced suicide ideation at the 12- and 24-month follow-up assessments, but therapeutic alliance at the end of treatment was not correlated with suicide ideation. This suggests that therapeutic alliance moderates, rather than mediates, the effect of certain treatments on suicide-related outcomes. Suicide risk reductions therefore seem to require a combination of effective intervention *and* strong therapeutic alliance.

Contemporary theoretical and empirical work has conceptualized therapeutic alliance as the mutual influence of three interrelated but distinct processes: goals, tasks, and bond (Horvath & Greenberg, 1989). *Goals* refer to the extent that the patient and the clinician agree upon the overall objectives and/or purpose of the treatment. *Tasks* refer to the extent that the patient and the clinician agree upon the specific activities and techniques used within treatment to achieve these goals. Finally, *bond* refers to the extent that the patient and the clinician feel emotionally connected with each other. Because the emotional bond between patient and clinician is assumed to be associated with other critical interpersonal dynamics such as empathy and compassion, it is considered by many to be an especially central dimension of the therapeutic alliance. Being mindful of the emotions that one experiences when working with suicidal patients is therefore an important clinical competency.

Treating suicidal patients can be a stressful clinical activity that can elicit in clinicians a range of negative emotions including anxiety, fear, frustration, and anger. These emotions can potentially influence the clinician's decision making in a number of ways. Anxiety and fear, for instance, can lead the clinician to take a "better safe than sorry" approach in which a higher level of care than warranted is recommended or pursued, which could needlessly restrict the patient's autonomy and cause a disruption in the therapeutic relationship. Frustration and anger, in contrast, can lead the clinician to underestimate risk and even reject the patient. Rejection of the patient can manifest in many ways within the context of treatment, such as terminating treatment early, starting sessions late, or avoiding follow-up with patients who do not show up for their appointments. Clinicians are especially vulnerable to experiencing anger and hostility toward patients who are persistently suicidal, interpersonally difficult to work with, and/or who attempt suicide during treatment. To determine if one is vulnerable to these unhelpful reactions to suicidal patients, the clinician should take the time to consider the following questions:

- "Which patients cause me to feel stressed when I see them on my daily schedule?"
- "Which patients do I wish would receive treatment from a different clinician?"
- "Which patients annoy me or routinely cause me to have a 'bad day'?"
- "When a patient doesn't improve, what is my emotional reaction?"
- "When a patient attempts suicide during treatment, what is my initial reaction?"

Overall, emerging evidence suggests that therapeutic alliance may not be a "common factor" that cuts across all types of treatment, as is often assumed. Rather, therapeutic alliance may be intimately intertwined with the specific type of treatment provided. This provides one possible explanation for the differences in the relation of therapeutic alliance with nonsuicidal self-injury across DBT and psychoanalysis (Bedics et al., 2012). It may be that certain cognitive-behavioral therapies such as BCBT provide a framework that supports the creation and development of an effective collaborative alliance. This is likely due to the fact that cognitive-behavioral therapies like BCBT are based on a collaborative model of care that explicitly invites the patient to take an active role in the development of treatment goals and the implementation of specific strategies to achieve these goals. The collaborative approach also contributes to a strong emotional bond because it helps to resolve a conflict inherent to work with suicidal patients: the patient's primary goal to reduce psychological suffering as compared to the clinician's primary goal to prevent death by suicide. As a treatment that explicitly conceptualizes suicide as a coping strategy, BCBT circumvents this conflict and provides a framework within which the clinician and the patient can align together around the common goal of pain remediation, which lays the groundwork for the development of a nonadversarial, collaborative stance in which the clinician and patient work together as a team to target the problems that contribute to and sustain the patient's risk for suicide.

RESPECTING AND SUPPORTING PATIENT AUTONOMY

Traditional approaches to treating suicidal patients place a heavy, explicit emphasis on preventing the patient's death. This is an understandable and reasonable perspective. However, this emphasis often leads clinicians to pursue treatment options and make clinical decisions that restrict or impinge upon patients' personal autonomy and sense of control over their lives. Fear about losing their autonomy can reduce patients' motivation to fully and openly disclose inner thoughts and feelings, especially those that are of greatest concern to the clinician (e.g., suicidal thoughts and behaviors). This tension between the clinician's goal to prevent death and the patient's goal to alleviate emotional distress, potentially via the mechanism of death, can adversely impact the therapeutic alliance as well was treatment outcomes.

In BCBT, this discrepancy is addressed by adopting a general interpersonal approach that prioritizes and facilitates patient autonomy. Patients are viewed as experts on their own experience and, as such, are asked to be actively involved in all aspects of treatment planning and clinical decision making. Related to this issue, BCBT also acknowledges and embraces an uncomfortable (and unsettling) reality of clinical work with suicidal patients: the patient *can* kill him- or herself. By extension, the patient can choose to live. Indeed, BCBT is perhaps best conceptualized as a treatment that helps individuals to choose life despite adversity and stress. In order to feel empowered to choose life and to find meaning and purpose within it, patients must feel that they are in the driver's seat. If they do not perceive that they are the ones making decisions about their lives, they are unlikely to internalize new information and skills that counteract their vulnerabilities to suicide. Respecting and supporting the patient's sense of autonomy is therefore key to rapid recovery and long-term reduction in suicide risk.

INFORMED CONSENT AND LEGAL IMPLICATIONS

Less than 15% of the U.S. general population utilizes mental health services each year (Substance Abuse and Mental Health Services Administration, 2014). By comparison, over half of individuals reporting suicide ideation utilize mental health services each year (Substance Abuse and Mental Health Services Administration, 2014), and up to half of individuals who die by suicide each year are estimated to be in active mental health treatment at the time of their deaths (Fawcett, 1999), which counters the general assumption that suicide decedents were not receiving professional care or help of some kind. On the contrary, the majority of suicidal individuals do receive mental health treatment of some kind. The fact that so many individuals die by suicide while in mental health treatment does not suggest that mental health treatment *causes* suicide, however, but rather reflects the fact that individuals who seek out mental health treatment have conditions that, by default, increase their risk for suicide. Said another way, the individuals most likely to seek out mental health treatment (i.e., those with psychiatric illness and/or intense emotional distress) are also those who are most likely to die by suicide.

Suicide attempts and suicide deaths are therefore a very real potential outcome for patients receiving mental health care. Not surprisingly, the likelihood of a patient making a suicide attempt during or immediately following treatment (and by default, dying as a result of the attempt) increases with the severity and/or complexity of his or her presentation. Patients with a history of suicide attempts have the greatest risk, especially those who have made multiple suicide attempts. Few mental health clinicians discuss the realities of this risk with their patients, however, often due to concerns about patients' inability to effectively cope with the topic (VandeCreek, 2009) and/or the possibility that a conversation about the risks associated with treatment could trigger emotional distress and hopelessness (Cook, 2009). Despite these concerns, clinicians are obligated to discuss with patients both the risks and the benefits associated with treatment (Bennett et al., 2006). Pomerantz and Handelsman (2004) have suggested that patients should be informed, at a minimum, about the following issues noted below. A patient handout that covers these areas in detail can be found in Appendix A.2. This handout can be used by clinicians as a practical tool for facilitating a conversation with patients regarding the risks and benefits of BCBT.

- The name of the treatment being provided.
- How the clinician learned to administer the treatment.
- How a particular treatment compares to other treatments.
- How the treatment works.
- Treatment frequency and duration.
- The possible risks associated with the treatment.
- The proportion of patients who improve in treatment, the way(s) in which patients improve, and the source of this information.
- The proportion of patients who get worse in treatment, the way(s) in which patients get worse, and the source of this information.
- The proportion of patients who improve and the proportion who get worse without treatment and in other treatments.
- What to do if the patient feels the treatment is not working.

Information specific to BCBT with respect to each of these issues can be found in Appendix A.2.

Although frank and direct discussions regarding the potential risks (and benefits) of mental health treatment are an essential element of the informed consent process, the application of informed consent procedures to the specific issue of suicide risk has remained largely unaddressed in the literature until only recently (Rudd, Joiner, et al., 2009), which is surprising given how commonly death by suicide and suicide attempts occur in mental health treatment. For instance, an estimated 2% of patients with major depressive disorder who receive outpatient mental health treatment will die by suicide and an estimated 9% who receive inpatient treatment will die by suicide (Bostwick & Pankratz, 2001). In terms of suicide attempt rates, aggregated data across clinical trials suggest that up to 50% of patients who start treatment with active suicide ideation or a history of suicide attempts will make a suicide attempt during or immediately after treatment, although this risk is reduced by at least half among patients who received DBT (Linehan et al., 1991; Linehan, Comtois, Murray, et al., 2006), cognitive therapy (Brown, Ten Have, et al., 2005), or BCBT (Rudd et al., 2015). Taken together, these data highlight several critical points. First, suicide attempts are common among patients in mental health treatment, especially among those who have a history of suicide attempts and/or who are suicidal when they start treatment. Second, although death by suicide is much less common than suicide attempts, some patients die by suicide even when they receive mental health treatment. Third, some treatments reduce risk for suicide attempts more than other treatments.

This latter point highlights an important but underappreciated component of thorough informed consent in psychological treatments: a discussion of the risks and benefits of a particular treatment *relative to alternative treatments*. Unfortunately, too few patients are informed about the availability of treatment alternatives, let alone the comparative risks and benefits that exist among different treatment options, because most clinicians tend to focus only on the benefits (but not the risks) of the specific treatment that they offer and the risks (but not the benefits) of alternative treatments. In the case of suicidal patients, these alternative treatments include both psychotherapy and psychotropic medication options.

Informed consent is best understood as an ongoing process rather than an event. Within BCBT, informed consent begins in the first session with an initial discussion about the risks and benefits of treatment and continues across the remainder of the treatment in the form of discussions regarding the nature and form of specific interventions. For instance, early in BCBT the patient commits to certain behavioral expectations during treatment as a part of the commitment to treatment statement (described in Chapter 11). With the introduction of each new skill or concept in subsequent sessions, the clinician describes the skill and provides its rationale in detail, and allows the patient to ask questions about the skill. This process continues to the very end of BCBT when, prior to conducting the relapse prevention task, the clinician outlines the risks (i.e., emotional distress, unpleasant memories) and the benefits (i.e., acquisition of skill mastery) of this final procedure and invites the patient to raise concerns that he or she might have. Thus, although the *documentation* of informed consent is a discrete event that occurs at the outset of BCBT, the *process* of informed consent continues throughout the treatment.

Consistent with the recommendations of Rudd, Joiner, and colleagues (2009), the informed consent process in BCBT should include the following elements:

1. For patients who have made a suicide attempt in the past or who are suicidal when they start treatment, suicide risk can persist throughout treatment, although this risk tends to decrease over time. Patients who have made multiple suicide attempts are at the highest risk for making a suicide attempt while in treatment.

2. Up to half of patients who have made a suicide attempt or start treatment with suicide ideation will make a suicide attempt during treatment.

3. Fewer than 2% of patients in outpatient treatment die by suicide while in treatment. Patients who make a suicide attempt during treatment are at risk for dying by suicide.

4. Treatment will involve discussions of emotionally difficult topics that can sometimes increase a patient's distress in the short term. These periods of increased distress tend to be very brief, but they could increase the patient's desire for suicide for short periods of time. The clinician and patient will work together to help the patient get through these periods.

5. To manage the patient's risk for suicide during periods of distress, the patient and clinician will discuss and practice crisis management procedures that the patient can use to solve problems.

6. Treatment involves experimenting with new skills designed to solve problems without suicide attempts.

7. The primary goal of BCBT is the prevention of suicide attempts.

8. The risk for a suicide attempt is reduced by half among patients who receive BCBT as compared to patients who do not receive this treatment. However, patients may nonetheless prefer a different kind of treatment including other forms of psychotherapy and/or medication. For example, many patients choose to take medication in addition to receiving BCBT.

9. In order to achieve the patient's goals, the clinician and patient will need to work together using a collaborative approach to treatment.

Following appropriate informed consent procedures can have a positive influence on malpractice liability. As discussed by Berman (2006), malpractice liability largely surrounds the legal concept of the *standard of care*, which is established by experts who make determinations about whether or not the care and/or services delivered by a health care provider were reasonable and prudent. These latter descriptors generally mean that the services provided do not deviate from those provided under similar circumstances by similarly trained professionals. Negligence can be established if a clinician is determined to have breached his or her *duty of care* to the patient, which means that the clinician has assumed a responsibility to act in a manner that protects the patient from harm. Negligence can be established if a clinician acts in a way that harms the patient (i.e., an act of commission) or if a clinician fails to act in a way that could prevent harm to the patient (i.e., an act of omission).

Two factors primarily drive standard of care and negligence determinations in liability cases involving suicide deaths: *foreseeability* and *reasonable care*. Foreseeability typically refers to the nature of the clinician's assessment of the patient's risk for engaging in suicidal behavior. At the most fundamental level, foreseeability entails whether or not a particular outcome, in this case a suicide death, could have been reasonably expected based on the information available during the course of service delivery. Although foreseeability is most often associated with the requirement for clinicians to conduct and document a risk assessment that addresses each patient's risk and protective factors for suicide, foreseeability can also be addressed by an informed consent process that explicitly addresses suicide risk because it clearly delineates at the outset of treatment that suicide is a possible outcome. Because informed consent entails a process by which patients are educated about the risks and benefits of treatment as well as treatment alternatives, including no treatment at all, clinicians who explicitly incorporate suicide-focused information into their informed consent procedures can directly address issues of foreseeability both within and outside of treatment.

Including suicide risk in one's informed consent process therefore helps to demonstrate the clinician was aware that (1) suicidal behavior (and death) is an event that could possibly occur during the course of treatment, (2) the expectation of suicidal behavior is higher for some patients than others, and (3) risk for suicidal behaviors can be reduced with certain treatments. By directly addressing the risk of suicide at the outset of treatment and having a frank discussion with patients about this risk, the clinician mitigates risk for malpractice actions in the event of a patient suicide.

CHAPTER 4

Suicide Risk Assessment and Its Documentation

In many clinical settings, the clinician's first clinical contact with a suicidal patient typically involves an initial appointment. This initial appointment often entails a review of intake paperwork designed to collect relevant clinical and historical information, a review of initial screening and assessment results, a discussion about the presenting complaint, and an initial conversation about treatment goals. These data sources can provide valuable information about the patient's predispositions to suicidal behavior, such as history of trauma, family history of suicide, current and past physical and medical conditions, and previous suicidal thoughts and behaviors. No matter how an initial appointment is conducted, clinicians should integrate suicide screening and assessment methods into their routine intake procedures for all patients. Suicide risk screening and assessment is an expected practice in all mental health settings. The omission of suicide risk assessment procedures during an initial mental health appointment, even if the purpose of the visit is not to provide crisis or emergency services, falls short of the standard of care in the mental health professions. Considerations for selecting assessment instruments and tools for measuring clinically relevant indicators of suicide risk and treatment response are discussed in Chapter 5.

After the conclusion of the intake session, the clinician should document the patient's risk and protective factors and the assessed level of risk for suicide. The documentation of suicide risk should include data gained from all sources of information including, but not necessarily limited to, intake paperwork, results of psychological testing or symptom checklist, the clinical interview, and collateral sources of information.

RATIONALE

Documenting a suicide risk assessment serves both clinical and legal purposes. From a clinical perspective, the suicide risk assessment directs the clinician's decision making regarding the most appropriate level of intervention at the outset of treatment and also provides a foundation for ongoing monitoring of risk. Legally, documentation of a suicide risk assessment is a requirement for meeting the standard of care in outpatient mental health practice. As has been discussed in the previous chapter of this manual, the standard of care is a legal concept determined by statutes and judicial decisions that can vary across jurisdictions and is often influenced by determinations regarding *foreseeability* and *reasonable care* (Berman, 2006). Foreseeability refers to the steps the clinician takes to estimate the potential for an event like suicide. Clear documentation of a suicide risk assessment therefore directly addresses one of the two issues related to meeting the standard of care in outpatient mental health settings. Failure to document the results of a suicide risk assessment is often used to support the contention that the clinician failed to meet the standard of care under the assumption that "if it isn't documented, it didn't happen."

Aside from these clinical and legal purposes, documentation of a suicide risk assessment provides a method for the clinician to consolidate various sources of clinical information to guide treatment decisions over the course of BCBT. Clinical data relevant to suicide risk assessments can be organized into two empirically derived categories (Joiner, Rudd, & Rajab, 1997; Minnix, Romero, Joiner, & Weinberg, 2007): suicidal desire and resolved planning. *Suicidal desire* includes factors such as a low desire to live, strong desire to die, passive thoughts about suicide (e.g., being unlikely to remove oneself from a life-threatening situation), and few deterrents to suicide. *Resolved planning*, by contrast, entails factors such as active thoughts of suicide (e.g., considering methods for self-inflicted death), formulating a specific plan, availability and opportunity for an attempt, perceived ability or courage to make an attempt, and practicing or rehearsing of an attempt. Although both of these factors are associated with elevated suicide risk, resolved planning has a relatively stronger association with suicide and suicide attempts. The clinician should therefore pay particular attention to signs and indicators of the resolved planning factor and should weight these variables more heavily than variables from the suicidal desire factor (Bryan & Rudd, 2006; Joiner, Walker, Rudd, & Jobes, 1999). In addition to suicidal desire and resolved planning, the clinician should document risk and protective factors in several domains that map onto the suicidal mode (see Table 4.1): baseline risk factors (with particular attention to past suicide attempts), activating events, emotional and physical symptoms, suicide-specific beliefs, impulse control and behavioral dysregulation, and protective factors.

In cases where the patient has recently made a suicide attempt, the clinician should additionally document information regarding subjective and objective indicators of suicidal intent. Suicidal intent is defined as evidence, whether explicit or implicit, that the individual intended to kill him- or herself at the time of the injury and that he or she understood that death was a likely outcome of the act (Crosby et al., 2011). *Subjective intent* entails what the patient explicitly reports to the clinician regarding his or her motivations at the time of the injury (e.g., "I wanted to die" or "I didn't think it would actually hurt me"), whereas *objective intent* entails those situational, contextual, or behavioral factors present at the time of

TABLE 4.1. Domains for Documenting a Suicide Risk Assessment

Domain	Variables
Baseline risk factors	• Previous suicide attempts • Previous psychiatric diagnoses • Male gender • History of abuse or trauma • Family history of suicide (proxy for genetic risk)
Activating events	• Relationship problems • Financial problems • Legal or disciplinary problems • Acute health condition or exacerbation • Other significant loss (actual or perceived)
Symptoms (Emotional and physical)	• Depression • Guilt • Anger • Physiological agitation • Insomnia • Hallucinations • Pain
Suicide-specific beliefs	• Hopelessness • Perceived burdensomeness • Shame • Self-hatred • Isolation or thwarted belongingness • Feeling trapped
Impulse control and behavioral dysregulation	• Nonsuicidal self-injury • Substance abuse • Aggression
Protective factors	• Reasons for living • Hope • Meaning in life • Optimism • Social support

the injury that provide indirect or implicit evidence for the patient's motivations. For example, careful planning of a suicide attempt, taking steps to prevent rescue or discovery, and/or practicing the suicide attempt in advance are all objective indicators of high suicidal intent. Although subjective intent correlates strongly with emotional distress, objective intent correlates more strongly with the lethality of suicide attempts (Horesh, Levi, & Apter, 2012). Objective intent is therefore a relatively better indicator of likelihood to die by suicide and should be weighted more heavily by the clinician. By extension, subjective intent correlates with suicidal desire, whereas objective intent correlates with resolved planning. From a practical perspective, what this means is that if the patient reports holding a gun to his or her head the night before while intoxicated but is currently denying subjective suicidal intent (e.g., "I was just being drunk and stupid; I don't actually want to kill myself"), the clinician should nonetheless consider the patient to be high risk because there are clear indicators of recent objective intent and resolved planning.

By extension, the clinician should be careful not to underestimate risk among patients who deny current or recent suicide ideation, as considerable evidence suggests that the majority of individuals who make a suicide attempt or die by suicide actually *denied* suicidal ideation or intent during the most recent medical appointment immediately preceding their attempts or deaths (Busch, Fawcett, & Jacobs, 2003; Coombs et al., 1992; Hall, Platt, & Hall, 1999; Kovacs, Beck, & Weissman, 1976). Indeed, patient report of suicide ideation or intent to their health care providers does no better than chance in differentiating those patients who will die by suicide from those who will not (Poulin et al., 2014). By contrast, patient reports of agitation accurately differentiate patients who die by suicide from those who do not (Poulin et al., 2014), and endorsement of suicide-specific beliefs such as guilt, shame, and self-deprecation significantly predict future suicide attempts better than suicide ideation and history of suicide attempts (Bryan, Rudd, Wertenberger, Etienne, et al., 2014). The clinician therefore should not consider the patient who reports (or behaviorally demonstrates) physiological agitation and/or verbalizes suicidal beliefs to have low risk for suicide even if he or she denies suicide ideation or intent.

HOW TO DO IT

After the conclusion of the intake session, the clinician records the presence or absence of relevant risk and protective factors in the patient's file. Although BCBT does not require any particular documentation structure, a practical approach is to use standardized templates such as the one available in Appendix B.2, the Suicide Risk Assessment Documentation Template. Standardized templates can be used for two purposes. First, they can be used as a checklist to prompt the clinician to ask about key risk and protective factors that did not come up during the narrative assessment. For example, if a patient does not mention alcohol or substance use during the course of the narrative assessment, a quick review of this template might prompt the clinician to inquire about this, for instance, "I noticed you didn't mention anything about alcohol use during your story. I'm wondering how that might have played a role in your suicidal crisis." The second purpose of the standardized template is to help clinicians improve the thoroughness of documentation, thereby minimizing the likelihood of missing or omitting an important variable. The standardized risk assessment template not only includes a method for the clinician to note the presence or absence of key risk factors for suicide, it also provides space for the clinician to include more detailed information about the patient's risk and protective factors. Wherever possible, it is recommended that the clinician document the patient's exact language or statements. This template can be used in paper format, or it can be converted for use in electronic medical record systems. In BCBT, the clinician does not necessarily need to fill out the full risk assessment template during each follow-up appointment. However, after each follow-up appointment, the clinician documents *changes* to these risk and protective factors to document patient progress (whether improved or declined) over the course of treatment.

When documenting their suicide risk assessment, clinicians should be sure to assign an overall risk level for the patient. This risk level determination should drive the clinician's treatment decisions. Risk level assignment can be an especially challenging activity for clinicians, as there currently exist no empirically supported algorithms for assigning risk probabilities to patients. In the absence of such algorithms, expert consensus and best practice recommendations have generally recommended several key considerations (e.g., Bryan & Rudd, 2006). First, patients who have made multiple suicide attempts should be considered higher risk than patients who have made one or no suicide attempts, even when these patients are at their relative best. Second, indicators of objective intent and resolved planning should be weighted more heavily than indicators of subjective intent and suicidal desire. Third, outpatient safety is influenced by contextual demands that could vary from setting to setting. For instance, clinics with patient populations characterized by severe, persistent mental illness and limited access to care have different safety considerations than clinics with patient populations characterized by easy access and low-severity conditions. Fourth, access to firearms significantly influences the estimation of risk and outpatient safety determinations. Finally, in many settings there exists a range of intermediary levels of care between weekly outpatient psychotherapy and inpatient psychiatric care (e.g., twice-per-week outpatient sessions, phone call contacts in between sessions). Clinicians should therefore consider the possibility of increasing the intensity or "dose" of outpatient treatment in addition to psychiatric inpatient admission. A general approach to operationalizing various levels of suicide risk within BCBT, based on the number of indicators of resolved planning and suicidal desire, is summarized in Table 4.2.

Note that, consistent with general practice recommendations, a history of multiple suicide attempts affects the final estimation of suicide risk. Specifically, even when patients with a history of multiple suicide attempts report few indicators of resolved planning and suicidal desire, they are considered to have elevated suicide risk relative to patients who do not have this history. Clinicians should use a well-defined method for assigning risk levels to suicidal patients so that increases and decreases in risk can be easily tracked and monitored over the course of treatment. This assigned risk level should be clearly documented in the medical record along with a clear statement about why hospitalization is (or is not)

TABLE 4.2. Operationalization of Suicide Risk Assessment Levels, with Indicated Clinical Response

	Risk level	
Criteria	Multiple prior attempts	Zero or one prior attempt
• No resolved planning • No suicidal desire.	Low	Not elevated
• No resolved planning • Less than two suicidal desire indicators	Moderate	Low
• No resolved planning • More than two suicidal desire indicators	High	Moderate
• Any resolved planning • Less than two suicidal desire indicators	High	Moderate
• Any resolved planning • More than two suicidal desire indicators	High	High

being pursued at a particular time. This raises an important question when working with suicidal patients: *What is the threshold for hospitalizing a patient?* Unfortunately, at this time there is no clear answer to this question. In BCBT, the decision to hospitalize a patient is driven in large part by the clinician's estimation of outpatient safety. Specifically, if the parameters of outpatient treatment cannot be sufficiently changed to maintain safety (e.g., increased session frequency, restricted access to firearms), hospitalization may be indicated among high-risk patients. If these parameters can be sufficiently changed, however, outpatient treatment can be maintained even with high-risk patients.

DOCUMENTATION FOR THE ILLUSTRATIVE CASE EXAMPLES

Examples of documentation for John, Mike, and Janice are provided in Table 4.3. In these sample notes, we provide sample text based on notes utilizing a narrative-based documentation method rather than the fill-in-the-blank templates discussed previously, as this is a commonly used strategy for documenting suicide risk by many clinicians. Sample notes are provided from the first contact with each patient, as well as one follow-up contact. In each note, the clinician lists risk and protective factors and refers to other sources of information where appropriate and available. Note, as well, how the clinician documents improvements as well as worsening in risk over time and provides a brief statement that clarifies his or her decision making regarding outpatient treatment versus inpatient treatment. Note, also, how the clinician regularly differentiates between different dimensions of risk, especially subjective versus objective suicidal intent.

TABLE 4.3. Sample Suicide Risk Assessment Text in the Notes from Three BCBT Case Examples

Session No.	Sample text
	John
Intake	Risk factors for suicide include male gender, marital strain, depression, anger, and guilt. No history of psychiatric diagnoses, suicidal thoughts, or suicide attempts. Recent interrupted suicide attempt involving personally owned firearm with minimal advance planning, high objective intent, and high subjective intent. No evidence of hallucinations, psychotic symptoms, or substance abuse. Firearm in home has been temporarily removed by friend. Additional risk and protective factors are noted in intake paperwork. Collaboratively developed a crisis response plan with the patient, who was engaged in the process and indicated high likelihood of use. Based on this combination of risk and protective factors, overall risk for suicide is assessed to be moderate. Outpatient safety is judged to be sufficient at this time. Inpatient hospitalization is not indicated at this time.
3	Depression and guilt continue to improve. Patient denies new suicidal thoughts or urges, and no evidence of preparatory or rehearsal behaviors. No other changes in risk or protective factors. Based on this combination of risk and protective factors, overall risk for suicide is assessed to have decreased to low risk level. Outpatient safety is judged to be sufficient at this time. Inpatient hospitalization is not indicated at this time.

(continued)

TABLE 4.3. *(continued)*

Session No.	Sample text

Mike

Session No.	Sample text
Intake	Risk factors for suicide include male gender, middle-aged, relationship problems, anger, depression, self-criticism, and "feeling out of control." Patient reports heavy alcohol consumption. Suicidal beliefs include hopelessness and self-hatred ("I can't stand what I've become"). Elevated level of physiological agitation and self-reported insomnia. Reports firearms located at home, but these have been "locked away" by his sister. Denied suicidal thoughts or intent, and a history of suicidal behavior. Despite this denial, suicide risk was assessed as high, so a crisis response plan was collaboratively developed with the patient, who indicated high perceived efficacy and ability to use. Based on this combination of risk and protective factors, overall risk for suicide is assessed to be high. However, outpatient safety is judged to be sufficient and inpatient hospitalization is not indicated at this time.
2	Patient reported no alcohol use since last session. Anger and depression have improved slightly due to use of crisis response plan. Patient reports crisis response plan also helps him to feel more in control of his emotions. No change in any other risk factors. Patient still denies suicidal thoughts and intent. Based on this combination of risk and protective factors, overall risk for suicide continues to be assessed as high. Outpatient safety is still judged to be sufficient at this time and inpatient hospitalization is not indicated.

Janice

Session No.	Sample text
Intake	Risk factors for suicide include history of PTSD, borderline personality disorder, and a history of multiple suicide attempts via medication overdose. In both attempts, patient had very high levels of subjective and objective intent, which included taking steps to prevent rescue. Patient reports she "has had a suicide plan for years now, so what's the big deal?" but denies subjective suicidal intent at this time. Thinks about suicide "constantly." Denies alcohol consumption or firearms at home. Collaboratively developed a crisis response plan with the patient, who indicated high perceived efficacy and ability to use. Based on this combination of risk and protective factors, overall risk for suicide is assessed to be moderate. Outpatient safety is judged to be sufficient at this time; inpatient hospitalization is not indicated.
4	Despite steady declines in risk factors over the course of treatment, patient reported a suicide attempt via medication overdose within the past week. In contrast to previous suicide attempts, the recent attempt had moderate subjective suicidal intent and low objective intent. Depression, insomnia, suicidal beliefs, and intensity of suicidal ideation are increased. Reviewed patient's crisis response plan together and identified strategies for improving its effectiveness and her motivation to use the plan during periods of crisis. Since this suicide attempt has occurred, patient's overall level of distress has declined, as has her subjective suicidal intent. Overall risk for suicide is increased to high. Patient indicated she is willing and able to increase outpatient session frequency until risk has returned to moderate level. In light of this change in outpatient intensity, hospitalization is not recommended at this time, although risk levels will be reassessed on a more frequent basis to reevaluate this treatment option.

TIPS AND ADVICE FOR
SUICIDE RISK ASSESSMENT DOCUMENTATION

1. **Use intake paperwork and assessment scales to your advantage.** Clinicians should take advantage of data available from intake paperwork, symptom scales, and other such sources of information to complement their suicide risk assessments. These sources of data can be integrated into documentation.

2. **Differentiate between subjective and objective suicidal intent.** When assessing and documenting information about suicidal intent, clinicians often think about subjective suicidal intent only. As was discussed earlier in this chapter, however, suicidal intent is comprised of subjective and objective dimensions, the latter of which is a stronger correlate of current and future suicide risk. Clinicians should therefore pay attention to these two separate dimensions of suicide risk and make decisions accordingly. Furthermore, their documentation should reflect these two separate dimensions of intent.

3. **Use checklists and templates to minimize inadvertent omissions.** Arguably the greatest practical value of checklists and templates is their capacity to help clinicians minimize oversights and/or omissions in suicide risk assessment and documentation. Within the context of BCBT, checklists can be used to complement the narrative assessment. Specifically, clinicians who use checklists can quickly reference them at the conclusion of a narrative assessment to determine if any important risk or protective variables were not mentioned. When this happens, clinicians can gently prompt patients to provide additional information about these variables by asking them how they fit into the story.

CHAPTER 5

Monitoring Treatment Progress

A common question that many clinicians have when learning and implementing BCBT is how to best track and monitor patient outcomes, especially with respect to fluctuations in suicide risk. Monitoring of suicide risk and patient progress is an essential component of BCBT and may be one of the elements that contributes to its efficacy for preventing suicidal behavior. Indeed, the tracking of treatment response with standardized assessment scales has repeatedly been shown to enhance clinical outcomes in psychotherapy in general when these outcome measures are shared with both the patient and the clinician (e.g., Crits-Christoph et al., 2012; Harmon et al., 2007; W. Simon et al., 2013; Slade, Lambert, Harmon, Smart, & Bailey, 2008). In a meta-analysis of six clinical trials comparing psychological treatments with patient tracking and feedback systems to psychological treatments without such systems, results indicated that tracking and feedback systems had an especially powerful effect on those patients who were predicted at the outset to be treatment failures. In this high-risk subgroup of patients, tracking and feedback systems reduced the rate of clinical deterioration by half and nearly doubled the rate of patients showing positive outcomes (Shimokawa, Lambert, & Smart, 2010). Results further showed that tracking and feedback systems could help patients showing signs of clinical deterioration and/or slower-than-expected response to "catch up" by the end of treatment.

These patterns have been found across diverse clinical settings (e.g., outpatient mental health, inpatient psychiatric units) and are successful even in settings where clinicians were not previously using such systems and/or are skeptical about using tracking and feedback systems. Furthermore, the benefits of tracking and feedback systems appear to hinge on clinician receipt of feedback; tracking patient progress without providing feedback to the clinician does not provide the same benefits for patients who are slow treatment responders or nonresponders (Lambert et al., 2001). Feedback and tracking systems therefore appear to enhance treatment outcomes by facilitating recovery among those patients who are the least likely to improve because it allows clinicians and patients to identify suboptimal treatment response early in the course of care and to take appropriate corrective actions (Lambert, 2013).

In our initial study of BCBT (Rudd et al., 2015), clinicians assessed a number of relevant clinical variables at each session and used these data to guide clinical decision making. In light of the known benefits of tracking and feedback systems, it is possible that part of BCBT's effect on reducing suicidal behavior is attributable in part to the use of a tracking and feedback system. Although no BCBT-specific tracking and feedback system has yet been developed, we have found that the assessment of several constructs and variables is especially helpful: suicide ideation, subjective sleep quality, suicidal beliefs, alcohol use, and general symptomatic distress. These particular constructs were selected for our tracking and feedback system for several reasons. First, these variables reflect well-established risk factors for suicide. As such, they provide a basis for continually tracking and monitoring fluctuations in suicide risk over the course of treatment, an important data source for making informed clinical decisions and, as will be discussed in greater depth below, addressing legal requirements related to the standard of care. Second, several of these variables (i.e., suicidal beliefs, alcohol use) have been shown to differentiate between suicidal thoughts and suicidal behaviors. As discussed previously in this manual, BCBT was developed to address several core mechanisms believed to underlie the transition from suicidal thought to action: emotion regulation, cognitive appraisal style, and problem solving. Suicide-specific beliefs that capture the patient's subjective appraisal of these core mechanisms have been shown to differentiate patients who think about suicide from those who have attempted suicide, and they predict future suicide attempts better than suicide ideation and other indicators of psychological or emotional distress (Bryan, Rudd, Wertenberger, Young-McCaughon, & Peterson, 2014). Alcohol use has similarly been shown to differentiate between suicidal thoughts and actions (Kessler et al., 1999; Nock et al., 2008; May & Klonsky, 2016) and to facilitate the transition from suicidal thought to action (Bagge, Conner, Reed, Dawkins, & Murray, 2015; Bryan, Garland, & Rudd, 2016), probably because alcohol use often functions as a coping strategy to alleviate or escape from emotional distress, similar to suicidal behavior. Fluctuations in alcohol use during the course of treatment might therefore serve as a useful indicator of emotion regulation and likelihood for engaging in suicidal behavior.

In addition to these core variables, clinicians may also consider selecting other patient-specific outcomes that align with the patient's treatment goals. In BCBT, outcome and progress variables are assessed at each session. Upon arriving for their appointment, patients are asked to complete the assessments in the waiting room via paper-and-pencil survey or an electronic data collection system. The assessment typically takes only 5–10 minutes for patients to complete. Scores are then reviewed by the clinician and patient together at the start of each session, with particular attention being paid to how change since the previous session is related to specific interventions and the patient's implementation of new behavioral skills. In this way, progress monitoring can be used to monitor fluctuations in suicide risk (both positive and negative) while reinforcing treatment adherence.

METHODS AND STRATEGIES FOR MONITORING PATIENT OUTCOMES

A wide array of assessment scales and tools have been developed and can be used by clinicians to track patient progress. Because no studies have yet been conducted that support the superiority of any particular scale or tool over others, clinicians have some flexibility in selecting and creating a tracking and feedback system that is practical and suited to the needs of their clinical practice. In general, however, we recommend that clinicians select assessments that have strong psychometric properties and have garnered empirical support as useful measures of the construct of interest. Several examples of assessment methods and strategies are listed in Table 5.1 and described below.

The most efficient method for tracking patient progress on a session-to-session basis is to select a scale including items that directly assess multiple constructs of interest. For example, many depression scales such as the Beck Depression Inventory–2nd Edition (BDI-II; Beck, Steer, & Brown, 1996) and the Patient Health Questionnaire–9 (PHQ-9; Kroenke, Spitzer, & Williams, 2001) are not only validated measures of general symptom distress, they also include items that directly measure sleep quality as well as suicide ideation, the latter of which have been shown to be significant predictors of suicide death and suicide attempts (Green et al., 2015; Simon et al., 2013). General symptom scales such as

TABLE 5.1. Sample Scales for Tracking Patient Progress in BCBT

Measure	No. of items	Suicide ideation	Sleep quality	Suicidal beliefs	Alcohol use	Symptom distress
Beck Depression Inventory–II	21	X	X			X
Patient Health Questionnaire–9	9	X	X			X
Outcomes Questionnaire–45	45	X	X		X	X
Behavioral Health Measure–20	20	X	X		X	X
Scale for Suicide Ideation	19	X				
Depression Symptom Index— Suicidality Subscale	4	X				
Insomnia Severity Index	7		X			
Medical Outcomes Study Sleep Scale	12		X			
Pittsburgh Sleep Quality Index	19		X			
Alcohol Use Disorders Identification Test	10/3[a]				X	
Interpersonal Needs Questionnaire	15			X		
Suicide Cognitions Scale	18/9[a]			X		

The table has a spanning header "Outcomes assessed" above the columns Suicide ideation, Sleep quality, Suicidal beliefs, Alcohol use, Symptom distress.

[a]Number of items for the full scale and shortened scale.

the Outcomes Questionnaire–45 (OQ-45; Lambert et al., 2004) and the Behavioral Health Measure–20 (BHM-20; Bryan, Kopta, & Lowes, 2012; Kopta & Lowry, 2002) similarly assess symptom distress, sleep quality, and suicide ideation. These scales' ability to predict suicidal behaviors has yet to be empirically examined, although the BHM-20 has been shown to significantly increase the detection of suicidal patients in practices that do not use tracking and feedback systems (Bryan, Corso, Rudd, & Cordero, 2008). As compared to depression scales, general symptom scales often assess a wider range of symptoms and risk factors (e.g., alcohol use, relationship problems) that can enable the clinician to consider a broader spectrum of variables that are relevant to monitoring suicide risk.

In some cases, clinicians might choose to use measures developed for the explicit purpose of assessing suicidal thoughts, intentions, and behaviors such as the 19-item Scale for Suicide Ideation (SSI; Beck & Steer, 1991), which has very strong psychometric properties and well-established predictive validity (Beck, Brown, & Steer, 1997; Beck, Kovacs, & Weissman, 1979; Brown, Beck, Steer, & Grisham, 2000), or the four-item suicidality subscale of the Depressive Symptom Index (DSI-SS; Joiner, Pfaff, Acres, 2002). Such measures have the benefit of assessing multiple dimensions of suicidal thoughts and suicide-related behaviors, which can provide a more nuanced understanding of risk fluctuations. For example, factor analyses of the SSI have shown that it is comprised of several subscales (e.g., Beck et al., 1979, 1997) that are differentially correlated with suicidal behavior (Joiner et al., 2003).

Construct-specific measures of sleep quality and alcohol use can similarly provide more detailed understanding of these constructs than are obtained from general symptom scales. A number of brief scales exist to measure each. With regard to sleep quality, the seven-item Insomnia Severity Index (ISI; Bastien, Vallieres, & Morin, 2000), the 12-item Medical Outcomes Study sleep scale (Stewart, Ware, Brook, & Davies, 1978), and the 19-item Pittsburgh Sleep Quality Index (PSQI; Buysse, Reynolds, Monk, Berman, & Kupfer, 1989) are reliable and valid measures that are widely used in clinical practice. In terms of alcohol use, the most widely used measure is arguably the 10-item Alcohol Use Disorders Identification Test (AUDIT; Saunders, Aasland, Babor, De la Fuente, & Grant, 1993), which assesses alcohol consumption, drinking behaviors, and alcohol-related problems and has considerable empirical support as an indicator of problematic and disordered alcohol use (Allen, Litten, Fertig, & Babor, 1997). A shortened, three-item version of the scale (the AUDIT-C) has also been developed and demonstrated similar psychometric properties as the full scale (Bush, Kivlahan, McDonell, Fihn, & Bradley, 1998).

The assessment and measurement of suicidal beliefs is a rather recent development that has demonstrated considerable clinical utility. Two scales in particular, the Interpersonal Needs Questionnaire (INQ; Van Orden, Cukrowicz, Witte, & Joiner, 2012) and the Suicide Cognitions Scale (SCS; Bryan, Rudd, Wertenberger, Young-McCaughon, & Peterson, 2014), have been created to measure different types of suicidal beliefs. Based on the interpersonal-psychological theory of suicide (Joiner, 2005), the INQ was designed to assess perceived burdensomeness and thwarted belongingness, two of the theory's primary constructs that have been shown in numerous studies to be strongly correlated with suicidal thoughts and behaviors. Multiple versions of the scale (10-, 12-, 15-, 18-, and 25-item versions) have been used over the years, which has created considerable confusion among researchers and clinicians. Although all versions demonstrate acceptable reliability and validity, the 10- and 15-item versions have demonstrated the relative strongest psychometric properties and validity, which has led researchers to recommend the use of one of these two versions (Hill et al., 2015). In contrast to the INQ, the 18-item SCS was based on the fluid vulnerability theory (Rudd, 2006) that underlies the conceptual basis for BCBT. Initial factor analyses of the SCS suggested it was comprised of two factors, unlovability and unbearability (Bryan, Rudd, Wertenberger, Young-McCaughon, & Peterson, 2014), but subsequent work has indicated that a third factor, unsolvability, provides somewhat better fit than the two-factor solution (Bryan, Kanzler, et al., 2016; Ellis & Rufino, 2015). The SCS therefore measures perceptions that one is hopelessly defective and flawed (unlovability) and unable to tolerate seemingly overwhelming pain (unbearability), and that one's problems have no solution (unsolvability). More recent work suggests the SCS can be reduced to nine items (three items per subscale) without sacrificing reliability, validity, or clinical utility (Bryan, Kanzler, et al., 2016). Within BCBT, measures of suicidal beliefs can help clinicians and patients track a central mechanism of action, thereby providing critical information for determining a patient's underlying vulnerability to suicidal behavior. These scales can be especially beneficial during the second phase of BCBT by helping clinicians and patients focus on especially strong or pernicious suicidal beliefs.

LEGAL IMPLICATIONS

As discussed in Chapter 4, standard of care and negligence determinations in liability cases involving suicide deaths are driven primarily by considerations regarding foreseeability and reasonable care. Whereas foreseeability typically refers to the clinician's assessment of the patient's risk for engaging in suicidal behavior, reasonable care typically refers to the clinician's use of a systematic approach for treatment planning that does not depart significantly from what a typical clinician would do under similar circumstances (Berman, 2006). Tracking and feedback systems such as those described in this chapter not only provide a foundation for improving the effectiveness and quality of clinical care, they also address both foreseeability and reasonable care. With respect to foreseeability, tracking and feedback systems that are used on a session-to-session basis provide a clear and direct method for clinicians to demonstrate that they were monitoring fluctuations in a patient's suicide risk. These fluctuations should, in turn, drive clinician decision making and contribute to appropriate adjustments to the treatment plan (i.e., increasing session frequency, selecting interventions that target relevant risk variables).

If, for example, a patient reports significant increases in suicidal ideation, symptom distress, and alcohol use since the last session, a clinician may choose to reevaluate the efficacy of the patient's crisis response plan or choose to revisit an emotion regulation skill that the patient has not been using with regularity. Such information can also be used to document the clinician's decision making with respect to level of care, specifically their decision-making process surrounding inpatient psychiatric hospitalization. Making (and documenting) treatment decisions based on tracking and feedback systems therefore demonstrates a systematic approach to decision making that speaks directly to the issue of reasonable care.

The importance of documenting assessment results as well as documenting how these results influenced clinical decision making cannot be stressed enough within the context of medical malpractice. In many cases, the absence of documentation is often presumed to indicate the absence of a particular action or decision. Practically speaking, a suicide risk assessment that was not documented is presumed to have not occurred at all. Clinicians should therefore be sure to develop a system for documenting the results of session-to-session monitoring of outcomes and documenting how those results influenced their treatment decisions. A relatively simple and straightforward method for accomplishing this task is to record the patient's assessment scores in the medical record and then providing an "update" to the patient's risk assessment that is based on these scores as well as any other sources of information obtained during the session.

Illustrative Case Example

Consider, for example, our hypothetical patient Janice. Janice's scores during the first four sessions of BCBT are presented in Table 5.2. Janice showed some initial improvement across multiple outcome metrics: depression, suicide ideation, suicidal beliefs, and sleep quality. In light of these scores, the clinician's plan at the end of the third session was to proceed to a new intervention, relaxation skills training, during the fourth session. During the fourth session, Janice filled out the forms a usual. The clinician gathered these scales and asked Janice how she had been doing since the last session. Janice stated that she had been "doing OK," which seemed to contradict her symptom scores, all of which had reversed directions. The clinician called attention to this change and asked Janice what had happened since the previous session that might account for this change despite her subjective report that she had been "OK." Janice explained that she and her spouse had a significant conflict that resulted in her moving out of the home 2 days before and making a suicide attempt. Following that incident, Janice had been sleeping very little, was experiencing uncontrollable worry, and felt highly agitated. She also reported that her suicidal thoughts had increased in frequency and intensity, especially at night when alone. In light of this information, the clinician asked about Janice's use of her crisis response plan, mindfulness skills, and survival kit, but Janice said she had not been using any of those skills despite finding them beneficial previously.

TABLE 5.2. Janice's Symptom Scores during the First Four Sessions of BCBT

Session No.	Interventions	BDI-II total score	BDI-II suicide item	SCS total score	ISI total score
1	Narrative assessment, crisis response plan, and treatment planning	51	1	48	26
2	Commitment to treatment and mindfulness skills	38	1	47	24
3	Survival kit	28	0	39	20
4	Narrative assessment and crisis response plan	48	2	47	29

The clinician and Janice decided together to review and practice these skills and to develop a new plan for practicing them on a regular basis. By the end of the session, Janice reported that she felt much calmer than at the beginning of the session and felt comfortable with her new crisis response plan and skills practice schedule. Because Janice's risk factors had increased so much, the clinician assessed her risk as being higher than the previous session, but not so high that inpatient hospitalization was warranted. The clinician therefore asked if Janice would be willing to schedule the next session for 2 days later instead of next week to check in and modify the plan again if needed. Janice agreed that this would be helpful. After she left, the clinician documented her assessment scores, the content of their session, and his decision to increase the frequency of outpatient sessions in light of increased suicide risk. The clinician also noted that although suicide risk had clearly increased, it did not increase to a level that would necessitate inpatient hospitalization.

The use of a tracking and feedback system therefore enabled the clinician to identify a sudden turn for the worse despite Janice's subjective report of "doing OK." In light of these data, the clinician appropriately reassessed Janice's risk for suicide. These two actions directly address the concept of foreseeability. Next, the clinician modified the treatment plan in response to the reassessment of Janice's risk level, specifically by forgoing the previous plan to introduce a new skill and choosing instead to review previously learned skills, of which the most important was the crisis response plan. The clinician also decided to target the issue that was most directly and proximally related to Janice's increase in suicide risk: use of her behavioral skills and crisis response plan. Finally, the clinician decided to intensify Janice's level of care by scheduling the next session much sooner than typical: 2 days later instead of 1 week later. These three decisions directly address the concept of reasonable care.

Summary

Regular assessment and monitoring of clinical outcomes in BCBT can enable the clinician to provide targeted interventions that facilitate the patient's recovery process and reduce the risk of malpractice litigation. Though the exact ways in which tracking and feedback systems contribute to improved clinical outcomes are not fully understood, research conducted in general psychotherapy settings suggests that progress monitoring likely enhances outcomes for those patients who are most likely to attempt suicide. Session-by-session tracking is therefore considered an important part of BCBT.

ADDRESSING SUICIDE ATTEMPTS AND HOSPITALIZATION DURING TREATMENT

Janice's case highlights an important issue when using BCBT or any other treatment for high-risk patients: responding appropriately to suicidal behavior and psychiatric hospitalizations during the course of treatment. BCBT has been shown to significantly reduce patients' risk for making suicide attempts during and after treatment, but this risk is not completely eliminated. Suicide attempts can therefore be expected to occur among patients receiving

BCBT. Results across clinical trials conducted with suicidal individuals indicate that up to half of patients who are actively suicidal and/or have recently made a suicide attempt at the start of treatment will make a suicide attempt during treatment (Rudd, Joiner, et al., 2009), although in BCBT and other similar cognitive-behavioral treatments, fewer than 25% of patients make a suicide attempt (Brown, Ten Have, et al., 2005; Linehan, Comtois, Murray, et al., 2006; Rudd et al., 2015). If a patient makes a suicide attempt during treatment, he or she is very likely to attempt suicide a second time during treatment (Rudd, Joiner, et al., 2009). Research further suggests that a patient is most likely to make a suicide attempt during the first 6 months of starting treatment, which generally corresponds to the active treatment phase. For example, Rudd and colleagues (2015) reported that approximately 7% of patients receiving BCBT made a suicide attempt within the first 6 months of starting treatment, representing half of all the patients in BCBT who would eventually make a suicide attempt. Similar results were reported by Brown, Ten Have, and colleagues (2005): 14% of patients in cognitive therapy, somewhat more than half the patients in this treatment who attempted suicide, made their first suicide attempt during the first 6 months of treatment. On average, clinicians treating acutely suicidal patients with BCBT can therefore estimate that up to one in six patients will make a suicide attempt *during* BCBT, and another one in six will make a suicide attempt within 18 months of starting BCBT.

According to the fluid vulnerability theory, suicide risk can persist for some patients *despite* treatment. It is therefore unrealistic to assume that no patients will ever make a suicide attempt during BCBT. Suicide attempts that occur during treatment do not necessarily reflect failure on the part of the clinician; rather, they reflect the chronic and persisting nature of suicide risk over time. Treating suicidal patients is inherently "risky business," and sometimes patients will make suicide attempts even when the clinician administers BCBT appropriately. Suicide attempts during treatment also do not reflect failure on the part of the patient, although patients who attempt suicide while in treatment often perceive it as such. Being hospitalized during the course of BCBT can similarly be experienced by the patient as a personal failure. Because the shame and embarrassment that often accompany the patient's suicide attempt or hospitalization can sustain an active suicidal mode, the clinician must be prepared to respond appropriately.

Because suicide attempts are fundamentally conceptualized to be the result of skill deficiencies, attempts that occur during treatment are viewed as opportunities for learning and skills practice rather than being viewed as failures. Of note, a suicide attempt that occurs within the first 3 to 6 months of starting BCBT is assumed to be the result of lingering vulnerabilities that have not yet been sufficiently targeted or reduced. When a patient makes a suicide attempt within the first few months of treatment, for instance, it is typically because the patient has not yet received a sufficient "dose" of treatment and has not yet had enough practice with new skills to offset his or her underlying baseline risk factors. From a skills training perspective, we would not be surprised if someone "slips up" or reverts to old habits soon after being introduced to a new concept or alternative behavior; clinicians should therefore expect that patients will sometimes slip into old behavioral patterns, which can include suicide attempts, during the course of BCBT.

When a patient reports a suicide attempt made during treatment, the clinician should conduct a narrative assessment of the new suicide attempt, just as he or she did in the first session of BCBT. However, the clinician should also be sure to elicit specific information about the patient's use of the crisis response plan and other newly learned coping skills during the suicidal crisis. The purpose of conducting a narrative assessment focused on the new suicide attempt is several-fold. First, the narrative assessment enables the clinician and the patient to understand the structural components of the suicidal crisis (i.e., the suicidal mode) and the context within which the suicide attempt occurred, which may point to a need to make adjustments or refinements to the case conceptualization and treatment plan. Second, the narrative assessment enables the clinician and the patient to evaluate the effectiveness of the crisis response plan and/or the patient's mastery of learned skills. In some cases, certain strategies may be less effective than initially believed; these strategies may need to be removed or refined. In other cases, the patient may not have used a strategy optimally (e.g., discontinuing the strategy too early); additional skills training would therefore be warranted. The narrative assessment therefore helps to diagnose "what went wrong" and, by extension, what modifications need to be made to address this problem. Finally, the narrative assessment provides an opportunity for the clinician and patient to determine "what went right." Because suicidal patients often have negative cognitive biases, they tend to view their suicide attempts as evidence that the treatment "doesn't work." It is much more often the case that the patient successfully utilized one or more strategies during the crisis, but the strategies were not yet sufficiently developed to offset his or her baseline risk factors. In such cases, the clinician can use the information gained from the narrative assessment to help the patient reframe his or her perspective in a manner that is more conducive to progress, growth, and health. For instance, the patient may have successfully coped with a problem for several hours prior to making the suicide attempt, whereas in the past he or she would not have endured for this long. Once the new narrative assessment is complete, BCBT continues where it left off.

A similar approach is taken when patients are hospitalized during the course of BCBT. Hospitalization is often experienced by patients as a shameful or embarrassing event that reflects their inherent incompetence (e.g., "I can't handle my own problems without being locked up"). Although BCBT aims to avoid or reduce the need for inpatient hospitalization, a patient who, in lieu of making a suicide attempt, seeks out professional assistance during a crisis and is hospitalized as a result has followed the steps outlined in his or her crisis response plan. Following a patient's discharge from inpatient hospitalization, the clinician should therefore conduct a narrative assessment to understand the circumstances and experiences associated with the event and respond accordingly. Similar to responding to a suicide attempt, BCBT picks up where it left off prior to the hospitalization with the recognition that some content may need to be revisited and/or revised. Many of these points are highlighted by Janice's case, which is described here in greater detail.

Illustrative Case Example

After making some good progress early in BCBT, Janice made another suicide attempt via overdose between the third and fourth sessions. As noted previously, Janice initially did not disclose this suicide attempt to her clinician, but the elevated scores on her symptom scales prompted the clinician to inquire about recent events and changes. When asked about her sudden worsening, Janice apologized profusely to the clinician for "screwing up yet again" and "failing." The clinician subsequently conducted a new narrative assessment, during which Janice stated that she became upset and, when she had the thought "You should just kill yourself," she pulled out her crisis response plan and followed its steps: practicing mindfulness for 10 minutes, going for a 10-minute walk, and calling her friend to talk, although her friend was not available. Janice was still feeling "miserable" and "worthless" after doing these activities, and when her friend did not answer the phone she also started feeling "all alone in the world." At that point, she went to her medicine cabinet and grabbed what few sleeping pills remained (a total of six pills). She swallowed them with a glass of wine and eventually fell asleep, then woke up the next day "feeling like I had the worst hangover ever." Upon completing her story, Janice expressed concern that the crisis response plan "can't help me; I'm a failure." The clinician asked Janice to think back to her first attempted overdose and to estimate how much time passed between her decision to kill herself and the actual suicide attempt itself. Janice estimated that only "a minute or two" passed between her decision to act and her first overdose. The clinician then pointed out that during this most recent suicidal crisis, approximately 30 minutes passed between Janice's decision to act (i.e., the thought, "You should just kill yourself") and the overdose itself, and suggested that this served as evidence that Janice was "about 30 times better at managing emotions now than at the start of treatment." This, in turn, suggested the crisis response plan was improving Janice's ability to tolerate distress, although this recent suicide attempt suggested that additional practice was needed.

Using the narrative assessment, both the clinician and Janice were able to recognize those areas where the crisis response plan was helping (i.e., improving distress tolerance) and those areas where additional work was needed (i.e., practicing skills to develop even greater distress tolerance). Perhaps of greatest significance, the clinician was able to use the narrative assessment to help Janice reconsider her recent crisis as an indication of the considerable growth and progress she has made in treatment, rather than being a sign of failure. Thus, despite the fact that Janice had made a suicide attempt, she also came to realize that she was "heading in the right direction," which "makes me feel hopeful."

Summary

In summary, suicide attempts and hospitalizations that occur during the course of BCBT are conceptualized as a manifestation of the patient's chronic, underlying risk for suicide, which continues to persist during treatment. When suicide attempts and hospitalizations occur, the clinician and patient should collaboratively seek to understand the circumstances surrounding and context within which these events occurred, which may point to needed adjustments in the case conceptualization and treatment plan but are just as likely (if not more likely) to reveal indicators of improvement and growth on behalf of the patient. Once these adjustments are identified, the clinician and patient resume BCBT where the treatment left off, recognizing that some previously covered material may need to be readdressed.

CHAPTER 6

An Overview of
Brief Cognitive-Behavioral Therapy

BCBT is structured using a phased approach that sequentially orders interventions that correspond to clinical priorities and the natural process of suicide risk over time. This sequence begins within the first few minutes of the first session of BCBT, during which a detailed narrative assessment of the patient's suicidal crisis is obtained. This initial assessment provides an understanding of the unique factors and circumstances surrounding the patient's clinical needs, thereby setting the stage for the remainder of treatment. Because many patients initiate BCBT in the midst of an acute crisis or the residual stages of an acute suicidal crisis (e.g., discharge from inpatient hospitalization following a recent suicide attempt), the first phase of treatment, which is typically four sessions in duration, is focused on deactivation of the suicidal mode and symptom stabilization via emotion regulation skills training. Once the suicidal mode has been resolved and the patient has returned to his or her baseline risk level, BCBT transitions to the second phase of treatment, which is typically five sessions in duration. In this second phase of treatment, BCBT focuses on the suicidal belief system that underlies long-term vulnerability to suicidal crises. This middle section of BCBT is therefore aimed at modifying baseline cognitive risk factors for suicide. In the third and final phase of BCBT, which typically lasts two sessions in duration, the focus shifts to skills integration and rehearsal. The final sessions of BCBT are therefore aimed at relapse prevention. All of the procedures and interventions used in BCBT are listed in Table 6.1, by phase, along with the specific domains of the suicidal mode that are targeted by each.

From start to end, BCBT is sequenced in a manner that begins with assessment and case conceptualization, transitions to the targeting of behavioral and cognitive baseline risk factors, and concludes with relapse prevention. To illustrate this sequence, the

TABLE 6.1. List of Intervention Procedures Used in BCBT, Organized by the Phase in Which They Are First Introduced, with the Suicidal Mode Domains Targeted by Each

Phase	Behavior	Emotion	Cognition	Physical
Phase One				
Crisis response plan	X	X	X	X
Means restriction counseling	X			
Sleep stimulus control				X
Relaxation skills training	X	X		X
Mindfulness skills training	X	X	X	
Reasons for living list/survival kit		X	X	
Phase Two				
ABC Worksheet			X	
Challenging Questions Worksheet			X	
Problematic Patterns of Thinking Worksheet			X	
Activity planning	X			
Coping cards	X		X	
Phase Three				
Relapse prevention task	X	X	X	X

session-by-session structure of BCBT for John, Mike, and Janice are displayed in Table 6.2 and referenced throughout the subsequent discussion.

THE FIRST SESSION

The first session of BCBT serves several key purposes including risk assessment, case conceptualization, and crisis response planning. Tragically, many suicidal patients report negative experiences and dissatisfaction with the mental health care they have received in the past. One of the most frequently reported experiences is the perception that their health care providers and clinicians did not listen to them or spend enough time with them to truly help. Suicidal individuals often feel that health care providers were rushed or in a hurry, and, in the words of one BCBT patient, "were only interested in filling out their forms." Health care providers are often experienced as rude and brusque, as if they had been inconvenienced by the suicidal patient. Negative health care experiences are especially common for patients who have made multiple suicide attempts. Consistent with these reports, such patients are often described by health care providers as "attention seeking," "manipulative," or other similar disparaging terms. These negative experiences shape patients' expectations of future treatment providers and the treatment process, including BCBT. Other patients report considerable anxiety and fear about the treatment process, especially if this is the first time they have engaged with the mental health care system. Because these patients do not know what to expect from treatment, their impressions are frequently shaped by popular culture (e.g., movies, television shows) and the reports of others.

Because these negative experiences are so common among suicidal patients, the "opening move" of BCBT is designed to allow the patient sufficient opportunity to explain the circumstances surrounding the suicidal crisis and to describe his or her subjective experience of it. Thus, within the first few minutes of the first session of BCBT, the clinician conducts a *narrative assessment*, which is described in detail in Chapter 8. In the narrative assessment, the clinician invites the patient to "tell the story" of his or her suicidal crisis in the patient's own words. In contrast to the typical risk assessment interview format that is largely clinician driven and intended for information-gathering purposes, the narrative assessment allows the patient to provide an account of his or her subjective experience of

TABLE 6.2. Session-by-Session Flow of BCBT for Three Patients, with Primary Interventions and Procedures Highlighted

Session No.	John	Mike	Janice
Pretreatment	• Intake	• Narrative assessment • Crisis response plan • Means safety plan	• Intake
1	• Narrative assessment • Crisis response plan • Means safety plan	• Crisis response plan • Means safety plan • Treatment planning	• Narrative assessment • Crisis response plan • Treatment planning
2	• Treatment planning • Commitment to treatment • Relaxation skills	• Commitment to treatment • Mindfulness skills	• Commitment to treatment • Mindfulness skills
3	• Means safety plan • Crisis support plan • Reasons for living list	• Sleep stimulus control	• Survival kit
4	• Sleep stimulus control	• Reasons for living list	• Narrative assessment • Crisis response plan
5	• Mindfulness skills	• Mindfulness skills	• Relaxation skills
6	• ABC Worksheet	• ABC Worksheet	• ABC Worksheet
7	• Challenging Questions Worksheet	• ABC Worksheet	• Challenging Questions Worksheet
8	• Activity planning	• Challenging Questions Worksheet	• Activity planning
9	• Coping cards	• Activity planning	• Patterns of Problematic Thinking Worksheet
10	• Patterns of Problematic Thinking Worksheet	• Coping cards	• Coping cards
11	• Relapse prevention task	• Relapse prevention task	• Relapse prevention task
12	• Relapse prevention task	—	• Relapse prevention task

the suicidal crisis. For many patients, this is the first time they have been allowed to share their experience without feeling rushed or dismissed by a health care provider. The narrative assessment in particular, and the first session of BCBT more generally, is therefore critical for building rapport with the patient. The narrative assessment also provides the information needed to gain an understanding of the patient's unique needs, an essential step for case conceptualization and subsequent treatment planning. The first session concludes with the central intervention of BCBT: the *crisis response plan,* which teaches patients how to identify an impending crisis and provides a step-by-step checklist of "what to do" when this occurs. By the end of the first session, patients have (1) discussed and agreed to the structure and process of BCBT, (2) gained an understanding of the factors that contributed to and sustain their suicidal crises, and (3) developed the first plan for more effectively managing their emotional distress and suicidal crises. As noted by one patient following her first session of BCBT, "This is the first time someone's really listened to me, and it's the first time I actually understand what's happening to me. It's like the light bulb is finally turned on."

Illustrative Case Examples

As can be seen in Table 6.2, in all three cases the first clinical contact included a narrative assessment and crisis response plan. Although this was accomplished during the first session of BCBT for John and Janice, in Mike's case these procedures were completed during the pretreatment intake session. The decision was made during the pretreatment intake to move rapidly into a narrative assessment and crisis response plan due to Mike's many risk factors and high agitation during his initial presentation. Of note, Mike *denied* suicidal thoughts during his intake session (and all subsequent sessions). Despite his denial of explicit suicidal intent, the clinician nonetheless assessed his risk for suicide as being high and decided against waiting any longer to complete a narrative assessment and formulate a crisis response plan with Mike. As will be discussed in greater detail later in this manual, the narrative assessment and crisis response plan serve as the backbone for BCBT and can be effectively accomplished in most health care settings, including settings characterized by time limits and rapid decision making (e.g., emergency departments, primary care).

SESSIONS 2 THROUGH 5:
TARGETING BASELINE BEHAVIORAL RISK FACTORS

The first phase of BCBT, which typically spans the second through fifth sessions, focuses on the deactivation of the suicidal mode. At the outset of treatment, most patients have recently experienced an acute suicidal crisis and/or made a suicide attempt and are still experiencing high levels of symptom distress, although they may no longer be at the peak of their acute crisis. Thus, this first phase of treatment is when patients are most vulnerable and likely to make a suicide attempt. The earliest sessions of BCBT are therefore aimed at symptom stabilization and reduction of acute risk, both of which are accomplished by modifying baseline behavioral risk factors for suicide. The clinician's primary tasks for Phase One are to develop a treatment plan, elicit commitment to treatment, teach emotion regulation skills, and refine the crisis response plan.

Consistent with these tasks, interventions in this early stage of treatment are primarily comprised of safety-promoting measures and behaviorally oriented skills training activities designed to build competency in several key areas: distress tolerance, emotion regulation, and self-management. Explicit discussions about the patient's access to potentially lethal means for suicide, especially firearms, occur very early in the first phase of BCBT within the context of means safety counseling and the crisis support plan (described in Chapter 12), procedures that can be used to engage family members, friends, and other supportive individuals in the treatment process. The first phase of treatment also targets the patient's behavioral predispositions for experiencing suicidal episodes and making suicide attempts by directly targeting symptoms associated with increased risk for suicidal thoughts and behaviors. For example, sleep hygiene and stimulus control concepts are introduced in order to address sleep disturbance (described in Chapter 13); relaxation skills are practiced to manage physiological arousal associated with the stress response, and mindfulness skills are practiced to manage rumination, worry, and cognitive reactivity (described in Chapter 14). In addition, the patient is taught how to elicit positive emotional states and how to remember why he or she wants to continue living using the reasons for living list, which entails a handwritten list summarizing the patient's most positive life experiences, and the survival kit, which provides physical reminders of positive experiences from the patient's life (described in Chapter 15). By the end of the first phase of BCBT, the patient has (1) learned new behavioral skills for managing emotional distress and (2) started to experience symptom relief. In the words of one patient, the first phase of BCBT is focused on "learning how not to kill yourself when you feel like killing yourself."

Illustrative Case Examples

Turning to our three cases studies (Table 6.1), we see that Sessions 2 through 5 emphasize behavioral skills training across all patients. Note, however, how the specific procedures used do not necessarily follow a prescribed order or sequence in all cases. Specifically, although all three patients received common interventions and procedures (e.g., all three underwent mindfulness skills training, completed either the reasons for living list or survival kit, and received sleep stimulus control training), clinicians are allowed some flexibility in determining the specific sequence with which these BCBT interventions are introduced. Finally, note as well that some procedures are repeated across multiple sessions, allowing the patient to strengthen skills that may need additional practice or refinement beyond what can be accomplished in a single session. BCBT therefore provides a "menu" of core procedures from which clinicians can choose, with the specific sequence being driven in large part by the specific needs of the patient. In the case of Janice, the narrative assessment and crisis response plan are repeated during the fourth session. This is because Janice made a suicide attempt between the third and the fourth sessions. As will be discussed later in this manual, when a patient makes a suicide attempt during the course of BCBT (or has a severe suicidal crisis or is admitted for psychiatric inpatient care), clinicians conduct a new narrative assessment at the next session and review the crisis response plan to make changes and/or refinements. Clinicians then continue with BCBT rather than starting over.

SESSIONS 6 THROUGH 10:
TARGETING BASELINE COGNITIVE RISK FACTORS

As the patient begins to demonstrate the ability to effectively use emotion regulation skills, symptoms generally remit and/or stabilize. As this initial skill mastery emerges, BCBT transitions to the second phase of treatment, which is focused on undermining the suicidal belief system, thereby reducing long-term vulnerability to suicidal mode activation. These gains in effective self-management and self-regulation positively impact the patient's sense of competency and self-efficacy. Because most patients are feeling better at this point in treatment, both in terms of their emotional distress and their sense of self, many patients will drop out of treatment or suggest that treatment be discontinued. Discontinuation of BCBT at this stage is not recommended, however, as the patient's cognitive predispositions have not yet been adequately targeted. When this situation arises, the clinician should review the structure of BCBT and the notion of cognitive predispositions to risk as conceptualized by the suicidal mode. Thus, although progress has certainly been made during the first phase of BCBT, during the second phase the primary focus of intervention is the patient's cognitive predispositions for suicide, or the suicidal belief system. The clinician's primary tasks for Phase Two are therefore to reinforce the use of emotion regulation strategies, teach cognitive reappraisal skills, and reinforce engagement in meaningful and pleasurable activities.

Although the second phase of BCBT is focused primarily on cognitive reappraisal, patients should continue to practice the skills learned in the first phase. At the beginning of each session, the clinician therefore continues to ask patients if they have used the crisis response plan since the previous session. If they state that they used the crisis response plan, the clinician asks them to describe the situation and circumstances that led them to use it, and the specific strategies used. If patients state that they did *not* use the crisis response plan, the clinician asks them how they effectively managed stressful situations such that the crisis response plan was not needed. This reinforces the effective use of emotion regulation, problem solving, and crisis management skills and bolsters the patient's sense of self-efficacy.

Interventions in the second phase are specifically designed to develop the patient's cognitive reappraisal skills. First, the patient learns to use the ABC Worksheet to learn how one's thoughts and beliefs influence the emotions one experiences in response to triggering situations (described in Chapter 16). Once this foundational skill is acquired, the patient is taught how to critically evaluate the helpfulness and usefulness of their beliefs with the Challenging Questions Worksheet (described in Chapter 17) and how to recognize and label different types of unhelpful beliefs with the Patterns of Problematic Thinking Worksheet (described in Chapter 18). In addition, the patient's sense of personal meaning in life, connectedness with others, and experience of positive emotional states is developed using activity planning and coping cards, which entails the scheduling of enjoyable activities (described in Chapter 19). By the end of the second phase of BCBT, the patient has (1) learned new ways for thinking about him- or herself, the world, and others and (2) started to acquire a new self-image and general cognitive style that reduces the likelihood of future suicidal mode activation in response to life stress. Although the patient will continue to experience stress in life, he or she is better positioned to respond to this stress in a more adaptive and functional way. For instance, one patient who completed BCBT and was sexually assaulted several months afterwards reported to her clinician, "I won't lie: I thought about killing myself after this happened to me, but then I remembered what we talked about, and I realized that this wasn't my fault and I'll make it through OK, even though it'll be tough. I'm going to be OK."

Illustrative Case Examples

All three of our sample cases begin the second phase of treatment with the ABC Worksheet. As is discussed in a later chapter, we have learned that the ABC Worksheet is especially well suited for the start of the second phase of BCBT. Similar to the first phase of BCBT, all three cases receive the same interventions and procedures, although their specific sequencing varies based on their unique needs.

SESSIONS 11 AND 12: RELAPSE PREVENTION

In the third phase of BCBT, relapse prevention becomes the focus. In this final stage of BCBT, the primary objective is to ensure the patient is sufficiently competent in using learned skills to effectively manage emotional crises without making a suicide attempt or using other maladaptive behaviors associated with the suicidal mode (e.g., substance use, nonsuicidal self-injury). This process is accomplished with the relapse prevention task, an imagery task in which the patient visualizes him- or herself experiencing suicidal crises and effectively resolving them (described in Chapter 20). During this final procedure, the patient is asked to imagine two different types of suicidal crises: the suicidal crisis that immediately preceded the start of BCBT and a hypothetical future crisis. The patient then imagines him- or herself successfully resolving the crises by using one or more skills learned in BCBT. This imagery task is repeated multiple times, each iteration becoming progressively more difficult, thereby requiring the demonstration of effective problem solving and sufficient cognitive flexibility. Although the third phase of BCBT usually only lasts two sessions, additional sessions are added if the patient is unable to complete the relapse prevention task with sufficient competence. During these additional sessions, the clinician and the patient continue skills training and testing skills mastery via the relapse prevention task. The third phase of treatment is therefore akin to a "final exam" that the patient takes until he or she receives a passing grade. By the end of the third phase, which coincides with completion of BCBT, the patient has demonstrated skills mastery specific to the prevention of suicide attempts. BCBT was therefore developed as a competency-based approach to treatment progress and treatment completion.

Illustrative Case Examples

In the final phase of BCBT, all three of our case-example patients participated in the relapse prevention task. Whereas John and Janice completed two full sessions of the relapse prevention task, Mike participated in only a single session. During Session 11, Mike completed several iterations of the relapse prevention task with considerable skill. He then rescheduled Session 12 several times. When the clinician finally reached him by phone, Mike explained that he had found a new job and did not want to ask for time off to attend another session. Because he successfully completed the relapse prevention task in the previous session, Mike had demonstrated sufficient skill mastery and competency, thereby meeting the BCBT criteria for treatment completion. These criteria are discussed in the next section.

THE GENERAL STRUCTURE OF BRIEF COGNITIVE-BEHAVIORAL THERAPY SESSIONS

BCBT is most effective when its sessions are structured and this structure is supported and followed by the clinician. The first session of BCBT is the most structured and scripted of the treatment due to the number of procedures that must be completed. Though the content of BCBT's subsequent sessions are more variable due to the clinician's ability to tailor the specific sequence of interventions and procedures to the patient's unique needs, the flow of each session generally follows this sequence:

- **Assess the patient's use of his or her crisis response plan.** The clinician opens each session by asking if patients have used their crisis response plan since the last session. If so, the clinician asks them to describe the situation and to review their use of crisis response plan steps. If not, the clinician asks them to review the crisis response plan's items. During this review, the clinician reinforces effective skills use and helps to troubleshoot any challenges with or barriers to effective skills use.

- **Introduce a new skill or intervention.** Whenever the clinician introduces a new skill, he or she clearly articulates how each intervention fits with each individual patient's unique case. This personalizes the intervention and increases the patient's willingness to use the skill in his or her life.

- **Verbally describe the skill.** The clinician describes the skills and then invites the patient to ask any questions that he or she might have about it. This provides patients with an idea of what to expect when they practice the skill, consistent with the principle of informed consent.

- **Demonstrate the skill and allow the patient to practice the skill in session.** The clinician guides the patient to use the skill in session. This enables the patient to gain first-hand experience with the skill and to have any questions answered immediately, thereby increasing the likelihood of effective utilization between sessions.

- **Review the patient's experience with practicing the skill.** The clinician asks the patient to discuss what he or she noticed while practicing the skill, what changed as a result of the skill, and what his or her impressions or opinions of the skill are. This heightens the patient's awareness of the skill's utility and enables the clinician to identify and correct any problems with skill use.

- **Identify and problem-solve potential barriers to skill use in daily life.** The clinician and patient consider likely barriers to skill utilization and then develop strategies for getting around these barriers. This increases the likelihood of effective skill use between sessions and teaches basic problem-solving skills.

- **Assess the patient's motivation to use the skill.** The clinician asks the patient to rate the likelihood that he or she will use the skill between sessions on a scale from 0 (not at all likely to use) to 10 (definitely will use). If the patient provides a rating lower than 7, the clinician and patient discuss likely barriers to and then modify the intervention in a way that achieves a higher rating. This increases the likelihood of effective skill use between sessions and teaches basic problem solving skills.

- **Finalize a plan for practicing the skill between sessions.** The clinician and patient collaboratively establish a schedule for the patient to practice the new skill between sessions. The practice plan should be as specific as possible to maximize the likelihood of use by the patient. This facilitates skill acquisition and mastery.

- **Enter a lesson learned into the treatment log.** At the end of every session the clinician asks the patient to identify a "lesson learned" for the session. The "lesson learned" entails the session's main theme or the primary piece of information that patient acquired during the session. Patients write the lesson learned from each session in their treatment log, using their own words. Sample lessons learned include (1) "The crisis plan helps me figure out what to do when I'm upset"; (2) Breathing exercises help me calm down"; (3) "I'm being too hard on myself"; and (4) "Maybe things will be OK after all."

DEFINING TREATMENT COMPLETION
IN BRIEF COGNITIVE-BEHAVIORAL THERAPY

Although treatment completion, often referred to as *termination* in the psychotherapeutic disciplines, is considered an essential element of mental health care, surprisingly little attention has been given to defining when a patient should be considered "done" with treatment. In some therapeutic traditions, treatment completion assumes there will be no further contact at all between the clinician and the patient at any point in the future (Budman & Gurman, 2002). Other therapeutic traditions such as cognitive-behavioral models tend to be less absolute in defining completion, however, and often assume that patients can return for additional treatment at a later date if so needed. Although plenty of guidance is available to clinicians about *how* to complete treatment, there is almost no guidance regarding *when* treatment should be considered complete (Bryan, Gartner, et al., 2012). This poses a critical challenge for the care of suicidal patients: premature treatment completion could leave patients vulnerable to an especially adverse and potentially life-threatening outcome: suicide attempts.

There is no single approach or method for defining treatment completion, although treatment completion is often determined using one or more of three general approaches that are not mutually exclusive (Bryan, Gartner, et al., 2012): clinician judgment, patient outcomes, and number of sessions attended. The *clinician judgment* approach is based largely on the clinician's assessment of the patient's progress in treatment, such that treatment is not considered complete until the clinician determines this to be the case. The criteria by which the clinician makes this decision differ from patient to patient because they are based on each patient's case conceptualization and unique needs. The *patient outcomes* approach, in contrast, is based largely on the magnitude of patient change across treatment, which is typically indicated by some form of objective measure that was (ideally) selected at the outset of treatment. For example, the patient's symptom severity might be tracked over treatment using a self-report checklist until scores fall below a specified threshold, at which time the patient is considered to be recovered. The third approach, *number of sessions,* is usually based on empirical findings (e.g., results of randomized clinical trials) suggesting that a certain "dose" of therapy is sufficient for recovery in a predetermined proportion of patients. Using this approach, treatment completion is defined by overall session attendance: for example, attending at least 75% of the planned sessions. In some cases, economic factors (e.g., limited finances by the patient, third-party payer restrictions) also drive clinicians and patients to use the number of sessions as the primary determination of treatment completion.

Each approach has unique strengths and weaknesses that are relevant to the treatment of suicidal patients. For instance, some patients are inherently more complex and challenging than others, and some patients do not respond to treatment as quickly as others. Defining treatment completion based solely on the number of sessions attended could therefore be problematic for patients who remain highly symptomatic or unimproved by the time they reach the predetermined total number of sessions. In cases like this, the clinician judgment and patient outcomes approaches hold clear advantages. The clinician judgment approach is limited, however, by the fact that clinicians are notoriously bad at making decisions in general based solely on subjective or "clinical" experience (Dawes, Faust, & Meehl, 1989; Grove, 2005), a finding that applies to the prediction of suicide attempts (Cha, Najmi, Park, Finn, & Nock, 2010; Nock et al., 2010). The patient outcomes approach also has important limitations that are due in large part to the methods currently used to assess clinical outcomes, the most common of which are patient self-report symptom scales. As discussed previously, psychiatric symptom severity and even suicide ideation tend to be very poor indicators of clinical outcome with suicidal patients. Defining treatment completion based on these particular patient outcomes may therefore less than ideal for patients at risk for making suicide attempts.

In BCBT, treatment is considered complete when the patient demonstrates the ability to effectively use emotion regulation, problem solving, and cognitive reappraisal skills within the specific context of emotional and suicidal crises, a criterion that is assessed with the relapse prevention task. At its core, this *competency-based approach* to determining treatment completion is consistent with the patient outcome approach in that progress is determined by the magnitude of patient change across treatment. However, the patient outcomes of interest are those that are hypothesized by the fluid vulnerability theory to be directly and proximally related to the mechanisms that underlie risk for making suicide attempts: baseline cognitive and behavioral risk factors. BCBT is therefore considered complete only when the patient can clearly *show* that he or she is able to effectively use skills to manage crises and prevent suicide attempts. To this end, treatment completion is established in part by clinician judgment, since the clinician plays a significant role in determining whether or not the patient is "competent" in using self-management skills. If the clinician determines that a patient has not yet acquired sufficient competence, then additional sessions are added until this criterion is achieved.

At first glance this might seem to suggest that treatment completion in BCBT is not influenced by the number of sessions approach, but this is not entirely the case. A common "turning point" in treatment occurs during the transition from the first to second phase of BCBT, typically around the fifth session. At this transition point, many patients will stop attending treatment or suggest that treatment is complete because they have generally returned to their baseline risk levels and are no longer in crisis; however, ending BCBT at this point is premature for most, if not all, suicidal patients because there has not yet been sufficient time to address their cognitive predispositions. Although completion of BCBT is not defined by a minimum number of sessions attended, in general BCBT should not be considered complete before the end of the second phase. This consideration is therefore similar to the number of sessions approach to defining treatment completion.

To minimize the potential for error that accompanies subjective decision making, BCBT employs reliability checks to ensure fidelity to the protocol. As noted previously, fidelity monitoring checklists are included in Appendix B.1 of this treatment manual and are used to ensure that clinicians are administering BCBT in a reliable and consistent manner across patients. Treatments delivered with higher fidelity by clinicians obtain better outcomes (Bond, Becker, & Drake, 2011), which may be due to reduced clinician bias or subjectivity with regard to determining progress (or lack thereof) in treatment. Because clinicians are vulnerable to making determinations about treatment completion based on their personal emotional reactions to patients, fidelity is especially important when treating particularly challenging or difficult cases that elicit strong negative reactions, as suicidal patients sometimes do. In BCBT, patient competencies are assessed throughout the entire course of treatment, not just in its final phase. From a practical perspective, what this means is that clinicians should not transition from the first to second phase of BCBT with a patient who is unable to effectively use a crisis response plan and/or self-management skills, as this is an indication that the patient's behavioral predispositions to suicide have not yet been sufficiently reduced. Self-management is an important competency for the patient to have prior to cognitive work focused on the suicidal belief system because the recall of suicide-specific beliefs can elicit very strong negative emotions and maladaptive behavioral responses. In sum, a patient is unlikely to be ready to successfully complete the relapse prevention task if he or she has not yet demonstrated the ability to effectively regulate emotions, solve problems, and reappraise maladaptive thoughts and beliefs. Maintaining a competency-based approach to assessing patient progress across the entire course of BCBT ensures that patients make steady progress in treatment and are well prepared for the final sessions as well as life after treatment.

CONTRAINDICATIONS FOR BRIEF COGNITIVE-BEHAVIORAL THERAPY

BCBT is appropriate for use with a wide range of patients who span the full continuum of risk and present with a diversity of clinical conditions. With regard to suicide risk level, we have used BCBT effectively with patients who have recently made a suicide attempt and/ or were recently discharged from inpatient psychiatric hospitalization, as well as patients who have experienced suicidal thoughts but have not yet engaged in suicidal behavior. We have even used BCBT with patients reporting morbid thoughts without suicidal intent (e.g., "I wish I weren't around anymore") as a preventative intervention. As noted in Chapter 1, BCBT reduces suicide attempt rates across patients with a variety of diagnoses, even those with diagnosed with borderline personality disorder, a condition that is often assumed to require long-term, multimodal treatment.

Although BCBT is effective and appropriate for use with a wide range of patients, a handful of conditions contraindicate the initiation of outpatient BCBT: acute mania, acute psychosis, and the need for medical detoxification. If a patient is experiencing an acute psychotic and/or manic episode that sufficiently compromises his or her mental status and safety, clinicians should prioritize the stabilization of these mental states before initiating BCBT. Such stabilization will typically necessitate the involvement of psychopharmaco-logic intervention. For patients experiencing severe withdrawal symptoms secondary to a substance use disorder, clinicians should prioritize medical detoxification. Once a patient's psychotic episode, manic episode, or physiological withdrawal symptoms has been stabi-lized, BCBT can be safely initiated. These conditions should be integrated into the suicidal mode and targeted within BCBT accordingly. For example, a patient experiencing com-mand hallucinations may conceptualize this symptom within the physical domain (because the voices are experienced as a sensory experience). The clinician may choose to select the ABC Worksheet to help teach the patient how to respond to the voices in an alternative way.

ADDRESSING SUBSTANCE USE

Substance use disorders are common among suicidal patients and represent one of the strongest risk factors for death by suicide (Inskip, Harris, & Barraclough, 1998; Price, Risk, Haden, Lewis, & Spitznagel, 2004; Wilcox, Conner, & Caine, 2004). Substance use of any severity level is associated with increased risk for suicide attempts beyond the effects of other psychiatric conditions (Borges, Walters, & Kessler, 2000), suggesting it facilitates the transition from suicidal thoughts to behavior. As such, substance use often needs to be directly targeted as a part of treatment with suicidal patients. Risk for suicide attempts is especially increased among patients with comorbid substance use and mood disorders, the latter of which are especially common among suicidal individuals. Patients for whom the onset of a depressive disorder occurred prior to the onset of the substance use disorder tend to report higher levels of suicidal intent (Aharonovich, Liu, Nunes, & Hasin, 2002), which may be due to the fact that substance use serves as an avoidance-based coping strategy for reducing or numbing emotional distress, a function that parallels the motivations underlying suicide ideation and suicide attempts.

Because substance use frequently serves as a coping strategy for suicidal patients, it is conceptualized in BCBT as part of the behavioral domain of the suicidal mode. For those with chronic substance use problems, it is also conceptualized as a baseline behavioral risk factor. As a maladaptive coping strategy, substance use is typically targeted during the course of BCBT by adapting BCBT's procedures and interventions accordingly. For example, the crisis response plan may include "craving for alcohol" as a warning sign, whereas relaxation skills might be taught and used to manage the emotional distress that sustains the patient's cravings. Mindfulness training may be especially helpful in light of evidence that this intervention effectively modifies the cognitive, affective, and physiological mechanisms that contribute to substance dependence (Garland, Gaylord, Boettiger, & Howard, 2010). Furthermore, coping cards focused on cognitive reappraisal of substance-related thoughts (e.g., "I must have a drink now") can help the patient to better manage the cravings that facilitate suicidal crises. BCBT therefore targets substance use directly as a behavioral component of suicide risk.

Clinicians should be especially mindful of patients who experience acute depression during periods of abstinence, as clinicians may mistakenly assume that such patients are at relatively decreased risk for suicide. On the contrary, depression during periods of abstinence is actually associated with multiple suicide attempts (Aharonovich et al., 2002), suggesting it may be an indicator of future recurrence of suicidal behavior. Substance use also appears to affect the trajectory of suicidal crises over time. For instance, patients with comorbid PTSD and substance dependence experience slower resolution of their suicidal crises over time (Price et al., 2004), which may necessitate a greater number of BCBT sessions and/or more frequent visits. Substance use is also associated with increased risk for "unplanned" suicide attempts (Borges et al., 2000), a finding that aligns with many patients' expressed motivations to use substances in order to facilitate their capacity to make a suicide attempt or reduce barriers to this action (e.g., "I never wouldn't been able to do it if I had been sober"). Other research suggests that alcohol facilitates or "speeds up" the transition from suicidal impulse to action (Bryan, Garland, et al., 2016).

In terms of treatment outcomes for suicidal patients with substance use disorders, a recent study testing the efficacy of a 12-month cognitive-behavioral therapy for suicidal adolescents diagnosed with a substance use disorder found that patients who received this therapy were less likely to make a suicide attempt during the 18-month follow-up period than patients who received usual care (Esposito-Smythers, Spirito, Kahler, Hunt, & Monti, 2011). A separate study of suicidal patients diagnosed with substance use disorders found that greater participation in substance use disorder treatment was associated with an approximately 50% reduction in suicide attempts during the next year (Ilgen, Harris, Moos, & Tiet, 2007). Results of a secondary analysis from our own clinical trial suggest that the risk for suicide attempt may be reduced among patients diagnosed with a substance use disorder who receive BCBT. Specifically, among the 21 participants who met criteria for a substance use disorder at intake, 21% of those receiving BCBT as compared to 47% of those receiving treatment as usual made a suicide attempt during the 2-year follow-up. This lends some support to the notion that BCBT may be effective for preventing suicide attempts among suicidal patients with substance use disorders. Overall, studies that examine treatment efficacy among suicidal patients with substance use disorders remain sparse, but emerging evidence suggests that substance use and suicide risk should be treated concurrently as opposed to one condition at a time.

Illustrative Cases Examples

Substance abuse was an issue of particular concern for Mike, who reported heavy alcohol consumption on a regular basis. In Mike's own words: "I drink when I get upset to turn my mind off and get to sleep. The problem is that I make the decision to drink as soon as I get off work, so I end up drinking for hours at a time and get way more drunk than I need to, at which point I become a total jerk and just make things worse for myself." Mike's alcohol consumption was included as a behavioral feature of his suicidal mode, and was included on his treatment plan as a treatment target. Because his alcohol consumption functioned as a stress management technique, Mike was taught mindfulness skills very early in the course of BCBT as an alternative strategy for managing emotional distress.

PSYCHOTROPIC MEDICATION

The majority of suicidal patients who begin psychological treatments for suicide risk will be taking psychotropic medications of some kind, the most common of which are antidepressants (Brown, Ten Have, et al., 2005; Linehan, Comtois, Murray, et al., 2006; Rudd et al., 2015). Although the majority of suicidal patients are taking psychotropic medications at the start of treatment, there remains little scientific evidence supporting the use of psychotropic medication as a stand-alone treatment modality for suicide risk. Exhaustive scientific reviews conducted by the U.K. National Institute for Health and Clinical Excellence (2012) and the U.S. National Action Alliance for Suicide Prevention (2012) concluded that psychotropic medications do not play a direct role in the management of suicide risk, but confirmed that they have an important role to play in the management of psychiatric symptoms often associated with suicide risk, such as depression and anxiety. One notable exception to these findings is the antipsychotic drug clozapine, which has been found to reduce suicide attempts by 50% among individuals with psychotic disorders as compared to patients who received olanzapine, a different type of antipsychotic drug (7.7% in clozapine vs. 13.8% in olanzapine; Meltzer et al., 2003). Lithium has also received considerable attention as a medication with possible "antisuicide" effects among patients with diagnosed with bipolar disorder (Cipriani, Pretty, Hawton, & Geddes, 2005). However, other researchers have questioned the reliability and validity of these conclusions in light of the fact that studies supporting an antisuicide effect of lithium have largely been comprised of secondary analyses from randomized controlled trials, naturalistic studies, meta-analyses, and open-label medication trials, all of which entail designs that could bias the prescribing practices of prescribing physicians (Oquendo et al., 2011). For example, clinicians may be less likely to prescribe lithium to patients who are judged to be high risk for suicide due to lithium's high lethality profile when taken in excess. As discussed by Oquendo and colleagues (2011), the apparent "antisuicide effect" attributed to lithium could actually be due to a relic of the decision-making process used by physicians, who are less likely to prescribe lithium to those patients who are most likely to make a suicide attempt. Indeed, recent research has failed to support the effectiveness of lithium for preventing suicide attempts as compared to valproate, a newer-generation mood stabilizer that is not believed to have an antisuicide effect despite being widely used to treat bipolar disorder (Oquendo et al., 2011). These results call into question the relative efficacy of lithium as a stand-alone treatment for the prevention of suicide attempts as compared to other commonly used medications for bipolar disorder.

Unfortunately, no studies have yet been conducted to determine if certain combinations of medications and cognitive-behavioral therapy yield better outcomes than cognitive-behavioral therapy alone, although combination treatment is undoubtedly the most common treatment package that suicidal patients receive. Because psychotropic medication use typically has not been described with considerable detail in clinical trials of cognitive-behavioral therapy, details about how and under what conditions medications are used effectively in conjunction with cognitive-behavioral therapy remain relatively unknown, although there is general consensus that medications play an important role in the short-term stabilization of acute psychiatric symptoms that contribute to risk for suicide attempts. Clinicians should be mindful of the potential for overdose, however, and work closely with prescribing professionals to limit the patient's access to potentially lethal amounts of medications, especially medications with known synergistic effects and/or narrow therapeutic windows.

Understanding the Black-Box Warning Label for Antidepressants and Mood Stabilizers

In 2004 the U.S. Food and Drug Administration (FDA) placed a black box warning label on all antidepressant drugs, including selective serotonin reuptake inhibitors (SSRIs), the most widely prescribed psychotropic drug class in the United States, in light of concerns about increased risk for suicide ideation and suicide attempts in children and adolescents up to the age of 18 years who were prescribed these medications. The warning label was subsequently updated in 2007 to extend the warning to all patients up to 24 years of age, and in 2009 the warning label was extended again to the antiepileptic class of medications commonly referred to as "mood stabilizers." During the past decade there has been considerable discussion and debate in the scientific community and the general public about the black-box warning label's impact on mental health treatment, especially among patients with elevated risk for suicide (Rudd, Cordero, & Bryan, 2009).

Although the original intent of the warning label was to alert patients and clinicians of possible iatrogenic effects of these medications in the form of increased suicide ideation and suicide attempts associated with antidepressant and antiepileptic use, the result has been considerable confusion and misconception about the benefits and risks associated with these medications. For example, although the black-box warning label included information about the benefits of antidepressants among older adults ages 65 years and above (i.e., *decreased* suicide rates), very few health care providers or patients are aware of this benefit.

Similarly, very few patients and health care providers know that *no deaths* occurred in any of the FDA's clinical trials that prompted the original black-box warning label for antidepressants. In one survey of primary care providers, more than 90% incorrectly believed there were suicide deaths in the aggregated FDA pediatric trials (Cordero, Rudd, Bryan, & Corso, 2008). This finding is especially troubling in light of the fact that 90% of these same prescribers indicated they regularly provide supplemental information about the risks associated with antidepressants because of the FDA black-box warning label, and the fact that over three-quarters of the antidepressants used in the United States are prescribed by primary care providers. Taken together, these data suggest that the vast majority of patients who discuss psychotropic medication with their providers are likely receiving inaccurate information. Because there is little reason to suspect that mental health clinicians are more knowledgeable than primary care providers about this issue, it seems reasonable to assume that most consumers of mental health care in the United States are receiving incorrect information about psychotropic medication as a treatment option.

Misconceptions about medication-related risk for suicide attempts are also likely due to the general tendency to emphasize the acute dimension of risk and overlook the critical role that baseline risk plays in conceptualizing and understanding suicide risk over time. Two studies illustrate this limitation very well. In the first study, risk for suicide attempt among 120,000 patients who were prescribed antidepressants across three outpatient settings (i.e., primary care, outpatient psychotherapy, and outpatient psychiatry) was analyzed during the year before and the year after the antidepressant prescription (Simon & Savarino, 2007). Consistent with general concerns about antidepressants "causing" increased suicide risk, the first month after receiving antidepressant prescriptions was the relative highest-risk month during the subsequent year. However, when also considering the year *prior* to receiving the antidepressant prescription, the highest-risk month was the month *immediately preceding* the antidepressant prescription. Antidepressants were therefore most often started *after* the patient's highest risk period, suggesting that patients are prescribed antidepressants as a treatment for their suicide risk as opposed to becoming suicidal as a result of the antidepressants. A similar pattern has been reported among patients treated with antiepileptic medications (Pugh et al., 2013). In their study of over 90,000 patients, Pugh and colleagues (2013) demonstrated that the highest-risk period for suicide ideation and suicide attempts among patients who received antiepileptic drugs was during the month immediately before they received the prescription. Pugh and colleagues additionally showed that patients who received antiepileptic drugs were more likely to make suicide attempts both before *and* after receiving these drugs, suggesting that patients who are prescribed antiepileptics are at elevated risk for suicide attempts regardless of the medication they receive. From the perspective of the fluid vulnerability theory, patients who are prescribed psychotropic medication have higher baseline risk. Due to the chronic and enduring nature of their elevated baseline risk, these patients are more likely to be prescribed psychotropic medications in general. Taken together, these findings suggest that antidepressants and antiepileptics probably do not *cause* suicide attempts; rather, those patients who are most likely to make suicide attempts are also more likely to be treated with psychotropic medications because they have skills deficits that lead to the emergence of psychiatric distress.

Although scientific evidence suggests that psychotropic medications likely do not cause suicide, clinicians should nonetheless monitor patients for potential side effects that may indicate increased risk such as psychomotor agitation, physiological restlessness, and racing thoughts. Each of these symptoms are associated with short-term increases in suicide risk, especially when they occur within the context of a depressive episode (Akiskal & Benazzi, 2005; Benazzi, 2005; Judd et al., 2012; Rihmer & Pestality, 1999). Irritability and psychomotor agitation, in particular, reliably differentiate mixed depressive from unipolar depressive episodes, suggesting these two symptoms may serve as useful "red flags" for clinicians (Benazzi & Akiskal, 2006). Depressed patients who report or manifest these symptoms should therefore be evaluated for the possibility of unrecognized mixed or hypomanic episodes, which may require augmentation medication therapy with benzodiazepines, mood stabilizers, or antipsychotics (Rihmer & Akiskal, 2006). Regardless of the final psychiatric diagnosis, clinicians should continue to monitor patient risk for suicide and clinical status over the course of BCBT and encourage their patients to take medications as prescribed.

FOUNDATIONAL KNOWLEDGE FOR BRIEF COGNITIVE-BEHAVIORAL THERAPY

Although there are no "prerequisites" for learning BCBT, we have found that clinicians who possess certain skill sets and competencies learn the treatment much faster and implement the protocol with greater fidelity. These foundational principles are beyond the scope of this treatment manual to discuss in general but are summarized here to aid clinicians in conducting a self-assessment of their own knowledge and competencies. Clinicians who have limited experience with the following areas of clinical practice should seek out additional training prior to implementing BCBT with their patients:

1. **Training and supervision in cognitive-behavioral case conceptualization.** Cognitive-behavioral therapy is more than just a collection of procedures and interventions; rather, it is a conceptual framework by which a clinician understands his or her patients and approaches the treatment process. Clinicians who have received training and supervision in case conceptualization from a cognitive-behavioral perspective tend to adhere to and demonstrate greater fidelity to the BCBT protocol and implement the treatment with greater precision and effect. Specifically, clinicians whose training enables them to articulate *why* and *how* certain procedures and interventions would benefit a suicidal patient tend to be the most effective.

2. **Training in basic learning theory.** Suicidal behavior functions primarily as a coping strategy to reduce or escape from emotional distress but responds to other environmental contingencies as well. Knowledge of basic learning theory and experience in using this model to inform clinical practice can help clinicians to target suicidal behaviors and the variables that sustain them with greater precision.

3. **Training and supervision in motivational interviewing.** An important part of BCBT is motivating patients to change when they may be reluctant or uncertain about the change process. Clinicians who have received training in motivational interviewing and

have experience using its general principles with patients tend to have a more effective interpersonal style with patients and find it easier to address their patients' ambivalence.

SUMMARY

BCBT specifies for the clinician an outline of procedures and interventions to choose from that fit with the specific deficits presented by each individual patient. This allows for the considerable structure of a manualized treatment to be balanced with flexibility: by selecting skills that best fit with the patient's unique needs, especially his or her needs surrounding emotion dysregulation and cognitive inflexibility, the clinician can optimally sequence procedures while also maintaining high fidelity to the underlying treatment model. Clinician fidelity, in turn, leads to greater consistency in outcomes across high-risk patients. BCBT therefore provides a practical model for tailoring treatment to each patient's unique needs while ensuring reliable treatment delivery.

PART II

THE FIRST SESSION

CHAPTER 7

Describing the Structure of Brief Cognitive-Behavioral Therapy

BCBT begins with the clinician providing a brief overview of the structure and flow of the treatment. This discussion reviews several issues already addressed as a part of the initial informed consent discussion (cf. Rudd, Joiner, et al., 2009):

1. The name of the therapy (i.e., brief cognitive-behavioral therapy, or BCBT).
2. How the therapy works (i.e., session structure, phases of therapy).
3. Possible risks associated with the therapy (i.e., confidentiality limitations).
4. How long the therapy will take (i.e., approximately 12 sessions).

The clinician should be sure to explain the treatment using simple and easy-to-understand language, and should invite the patient to provide feedback, seek clarification, and ask questions throughout the process.

RATIONALE

Explaining the structure of the cognitive-behavioral therapy session not only socializes patients to the treatment process, it also provides a framework for organizing their psychological turmoil. The predictability of each session helps suicidal patients with markedly chaotic lives to gain a sense of mastery and control over their lives, especially when confronting or talking about emotionally upsetting or difficult topics. The session structure also provides the patient with a template for prioritizing problems and issues, an essential skill for effective problem solving and crisis management. Finally, the early emphasis on the time-limited and skills-oriented nature of BCBT fosters hope for recovery. Many suicidal patients have participated in a diverse range of therapies and treatments, few (if any) of which have been as highly focused and active as BCBT. Hopelessness and skepticism about treatment are therefore common. Education about BCBT directly targets this hopelessness and motivates the patient to increase their commitment to treatment.

HOW TO DO IT

Step 1: Describe the Cognitive-Behavioral Session Structure

The clinician explains the primary components of each cognitive-behavioral session structure, which includes (1) a mood check, (2) setting an agenda, (3) reviewing use of the crisis response plan, (4) reviewing skills practice since the previous session, (5) introducing a new skill and practicing in session, and (6) assigning between-session skills practice.

SAMPLE CLINICIAN SCRIPT

Before we get started, I'd like to take a few minutes to explain how this treatment is structured so you have a better idea of what you can expect while we work together over the next few months. Is that OK with you?

First, I'd like to talk about how we'll structure each appointment. Each time we meet, we'll do a mood check and then set an agenda, just like we did today. We'll set an agenda each time so we make sure we prioritize the most important topics and then write it down so we don't get too far off topic. A big part of this treatment will be practicing new skills in your daily life between our sessions, so at the beginning of each session we'll also make sure that we talk about how your practice went. That way you can let me know what works for you and what doesn't work for you and we can make adjustments as we go. After we review what you've already learned and practiced, in each session we'll then talk about a new skill or idea and then practice it together so you can learn how to do it. Once you have a pretty good grasp of that new skill, we'll develop a schedule for you to practice the skill in between each session. We'll then wrap up and come up with what we call a "lesson learned" for the session. The lesson learned for each session will be the most important concept or the main idea of the session. We'll keep track of these lessons learned and write them down in a little notebook called a "treatment log," which we'll talk about in more detail a little bit later today.

So, in summary, every time we'll meet I'll ask about your mood, then we'll set an agenda, then we'll talk about the skills you've been practicing since our last appointment, then we'll talk about a new skill and practice it together, then make a plan for you to practice, and then wrap up by identifying the most helpful or important part of the appointment. Does that make sense to you?

What questions do you have about how each appointment will be structured?

Step 2: Describe the Phased Structure of Treatment

The clinician next provides an overview of the 12-session BCBT treatment structure and describes each of the three phases of treatment.

SAMPLE CLINICIAN SCRIPT

Now that we've talked about how we'll structure each session, let's talk a little bit about the bigger picture of this treatment. This particular treatment is called brief cognitive-behavioral therapy because it typically lasts only 12 sessions in duration. If we meet once a week every week, that means we can anticipate finishing this treatment in about 3 months. Some people finish the treatment in fewer than 12 sessions and others finish the treatment in more than 12 sessions, but 12 is the average, so that's what we'll plan for.

This treatment is split up into three phases. The first phase will last for five sessions and will focus on teaching you new skills to better manage emergencies and crises. The second phase is also five sessions long, but in this next part of treatment we will focus on how your assumptions and beliefs about yourself and the world may be causing and maintaining problems for you in life. We'll also focus on learning new, more helpful ways to think about stressful events so you can be more successful in life. In the third and final phase, which will last for two sessions, we'll do what's called a relapse prevention task. The relapse prevention task is an activity designed to put everything together, sort of like a final exam.

What questions do you have about the overall flow and design of the treatment from start to finish? Could you summarize for me how this treatment is structured so I can be sure that I explained things clearly?

Step 3: Discuss Confidentiality and Limits to Confidentiality

The clinician reviews privacy and confidentiality policies, and clarifies the conditions under which confidentiality may be breached.

SAMPLE CLINICIAN SCRIPT

The next thing I'd like to talk about is confidentiality. I want you to understand that what you and I talk about will remain confidential unless you give me permission to share information about your treatment with anyone else. If situations like this arise, we'll talk together first to clarify what I can and cannot say to someone else, so that we are in agreement about what I have permission to talk about and what is off limits. Because you have recently made a suicide attempt [or experienced a severe suicidal crisis[we should talk about an important limitation to confidentiality that we may face at some point. If I assess you to be at severe or imminent risk for suicide and do not feel that your safety can be adequately maintained on an outpatient basis, I may be required to contact someone who can assist us in securing your safety. Wherever possible, you and I will discuss this option before I contact anyone, so that you are fully informed and aware of what is happening, and can be a part of the process for ensuring your safety. There may be situations where it is not possible for me to discuss this option in advance, such as when you don't show up for an appointment. In a situation like this, I will contact those individuals whom you have provided permission for me to contact to see if they know where you are and if you are doing OK. In situations like this, I'll be sure to limit what I tell others to only that information that is essential to ensure your safety. If I ever have to do this, I'll also make sure that I inform you immediately and that you and I talk about it as soon as possible.

I think this is an important issue to understand, so I want to pause here to see what questions you might have about confidentiality and limits to confidentiality.

Step 4: Inform about the Potential Role of Family Members

The clinician informs the patient that he or she can choose to bring in a family member or supportive other to attend one or two treatment sessions to assist with the treatment process.

SAMPLE CLINICIAN SCRIPT

The last thing I want to talk about before we get started is the possibility of having a family member or another supportive person attend one or two sessions early in the treatment to assist with the treatment process. If this is something you'd be interested in, we could plan to have a family member come to an appointment with you around the third or fourth session. This is not a requirement, but it is an option that some patients have found helpful. We'll talk about this option in greater detail in a few weeks, but I wanted to give you a heads up about it from the start.

Step 5: Assess Comprehension and Invite Questions

The clinician asks if the patient understands the information about BCBT and then invites the patient to share any thoughts or reactions that he or she might have about BCBT.

SAMPLE CLINICIAN SCRIPT

That's everything I wanted to cover at the outset of treatment. I know that was a lot of information, so what questions do you have about anything we've talked about? Do you have any thoughts or general reactions about treatment structure, confidentiality, or bringing in a family member?

TIPS AND ADVICE FOR
DESCRIBING BRIEF COGNITIVE-BEHAVIORAL THERAPY

1. Model the cognitive-behavioral therapy session structure. Consistent with the general cognitive-behavioral therapy model, clinicians should emphasize the importance of session structure from the very beginning of BCBT. Even though it is the first session, clinicians should conduct a check-in and set an agenda should before moving into their description of BCBT. This helps to socialize the patient from the outset and also helps to support fidelity to the model on the part of the clinician.

2. Remember that BCBT is an individual therapy. Although family members are invited to attend some BCBT sessions, clinicians should remember that BCBT was not designed or tested as a family (or couple) therapy. Considerable evidence supports the efficacy of treatments that contain strong individual therapy components, but little to no evidence exists (yet) supporting family- or couple-oriented components. Clinicians are therefore encouraged to maintain the individual therapy perspective even when family members attend BCBT sessions.

CHAPTER 8

The Narrative Assessment

After providing an overview of BCBT and describing the treatment's structure, the clinician conducts a narrative assessment of the index suicidal crisis. The index suicidal crisis refers to the recent suicidal episode (which may or may not include a suicide attempt) that was most directly related to the patient seeking out or initiating the current course of treatment. For example, if the patient is initiating outpatient treatment following a discharge from inpatient psychiatric hospitalization subsequent to a suicide attempt, the clinician would focus the narrative assessment on the suicide attempt prompting the hospitalization. Alternatively, if the patient is resuming outpatient treatment due to the recurrence of a major depressive episode marked by severe suicide ideation and planning, the clinician would focus the narrative assessment on a recent suicidal crisis, typically the one identified by the patient as the "worst" crisis (i.e., the time during which he or she most intensely wanted to die by suicide). In the narrative assessment, the clinician seeks to obtain a detailed understanding of the contextual circumstances, thoughts, behaviors, feelings, and physical sensations associated with the index suicidal crisis. The clinician therefore seeks to identify in detail the sequence of events leading up to and following the suicidal crisis. The information gained from this narrative assessment serves as the basis for the suicide risk assessment, the case conceptualization, and the overall treatment plan.

RATIONALE

As the first major activity within BCBT, the narrative assessment serves several purposes. First, it is an alliance-building strategy. Suicidal individuals often feel that they have never really been "listened to," even by health care providers and mental health professionals. For many patients, the narrative assessment is the first time they have been asked to tell the story of their suffering in their own words and at their own pace. By actively listening and asking clarifying questions regarding the sequence of events that led up to and surrounded the patient's suicidal episode, the clinician communicates interest and the desire to help. The second purpose of the narrative assessment is to obtain the information needed to form an accurate case conceptualization: the context and circumstances surrounding the suicidal episode, the "major players" involved, the patient's preferred coping strategies and behavioral responses, and the thoughts, feelings, and physiological experiences associated with the active suicidal mode. The third and final purpose of the narrative assessment is to obtain the information needed to assess the patient's risk for suicide and to document this risk assessment accordingly.

The narrative assessment approach differs markedly from the traditional suicide risk assessment interview format used by many clinicians. In a traditional suicide risk assessment interview, the clinician typically asks a series of questions regarding the presence (or absence) and nature of the patient's suicide risk and protective factors. Underlying this approach is an assumption that the patient is willing to disclose the requested information and is doing so with a high degree of accuracy. The process is largely, if not entirely, driven by the clinician, whereas the patient plays a relatively passive role. Depending on the work setting, the structure and flow of the suicide risk assessment interview is dictated by agency checklists and/or forms, which are required to be filled out by the clinician afterwards. Because these forms and checklists must be completed to meet agency procedural requirements, clinicians often fill in the forms during the interview. In these cases, agency forms often determine the specific sequence of interview questions because clinicians start at the top of the form and work their way down.

In contrast to the interview-based approach to suicide risk assessment, the narrative assessment approach invites the suicidal patient to "tell the story" of his or her suicide attempt or suicidal crisis. To conduct a narrative assessment, the clinician asks the patient to recount the chain of events leading up to the index suicidal crisis, which might also include a suicide attempt. The clinician initiates this process by asking the patient to tell the story of his or her suicidal crisis, "wherever the story begins." The clinician then assists the patient in eliciting details about the internal experiences (e.g., thoughts, emotions, physical sensations) and external cues (e.g., sights, sounds, contextual circumstances) associated with the crisis and concludes by validating the patient's experience.

As compared to the traditional interview format, the narrative assessment facilitates the emergence of unique interpersonal processes that are conducive to treatment. First, the narrative assessment is associated with greater synchrony in emotional states between the clinician and the patient as compared to the traditional interview. Affective synchrony is the degree to which the suicidal patient and the clinician match each other with respect to level of affective arousal and expression, which can be measured via a variety of methods. Voice pitch is an especially practical and noninvasive one. Recent research indicates that synchronization of voice pitch between an acutely suicidal patient and his or her clinician serves as an objective marker of patient-rated empathy and emotional bonding (Bryan et al., 2017). The concept of affective synchrony is depicted in Figure 8.1. In this figure, the fundamental frequencies of two separate, acutely suicidal patients (represented by the dashed lines) and their clinicians (represented by the solid lines) are plotted on a moment-to-moment basis during an initial clinical encounter. Note that on the left-hand side, the

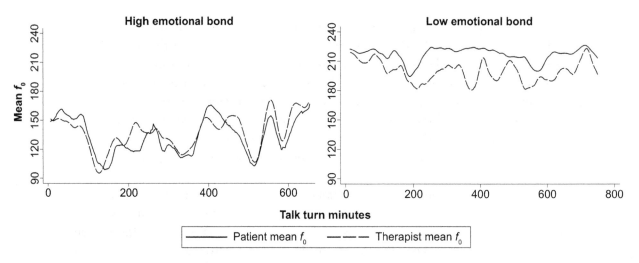

FIGURE 8.1. Two sample cases demonstrating synchrony of emotional states among acutely suicidal patients and their clinicians. The figure on the left depicts high synchrony and is characteristic of the narrative assessment process, whereas the figure on the right depicts low synchrony and is characteristic of the traditional suicide risk interview. f_0, fundamental frequency.

patient and clinician show similar levels of affective arousal and tend to track each other over the course of the session, which signals emotional synchronization. On the right-hand side, the patient and clinician initially show some signs of synchronization, but this does not endure for very long. This signals a lack of synchronization. Narrative assessments are more likely to be characterized by emotional synchrony, akin to the figure on the left, whereas interview assessments are more likely to be characterized by a lack of synchrony, akin to the figure on the right (Bryan et al., 2017).

A second way in which the narrative assessment positively impacts the treatment process is affective co-regulation. Affective regulation refers to the process by which an individual influences his or her own emotional state over time, specifically by calming him- or herself down. Affective *co*-regulation is similar, but entails an interpersonal process by which an individual influences the emotional state of another individual over time, specifically by calming the other person down. The narrative assessment is characterized by two interdependent affective co-regulation processes: the clinician influencing the suicidal patient's emotional state and, in return, the suicidal patient influencing the clinician's emotional state (Bryan et al., 2017). The narrative assessment therefore entails an interpersonal process by which the patient and clinician effectively calm each other down during the encounter. The traditional interview approach, by contrast, is not characterized by this process to the same degree.

Finally, the narrative assessment is characterized by less complex speech than the traditional suicide risk assessment interview (Nasir, Baucom, Bryan, Narayanan, & Georgiou, 2017), which suggests that patients and clinicians use simpler and more accessible language during the narrative assessment. Because speech complexity is correlated with empathy, this pattern aligns with previously noted findings regarding affective synchrony.

As the patient relates the story of his or her suicidal crisis, the clinician organizes the reported risk and protective factors into the suicidal mode framework. This facilitates the

TABLE 8.1. Suicide Risk and Protective Factors, by Suicidal Mode Domain

Domain	Variables
Activating events	• Relationship problems • Financial problems • Legal or disciplinary problems • Acute health condition or exacerbation • Other significant loss (actual or perceived)
Emotional	• Depression • Guilt • Anger • Anxiety • Numbness • Shame
Physical	• Physiological agitation • Insomnia • Hallucinations • Pain
Cognitive	• Hopelessness • Perceived burdensomeness • Self-hatred • Thwarted belongingness • Feeling trapped • Reasons for living • Meaning in life/purpose • Optimism • Hope
Behavioral	• Previous suicide attempts • Nonsuicidal self-injury • Substance abuse • Aggression • Social withdrawal • Avoiding others

case conceptualization process and prepares the clinician to discuss his or her case conceptualization with the patient, an activity that occurs immediately after the narrative assessment is complete. Table 8.1 lists key risk and protective factors and shows how they can be organized within the suicidal mode.

HOW TO DO IT

Step 1: Invite the Patient to Tell His or Her Story of the Index Suicidal Episode

The clinician begins the narrative assessment by asking the patient to tell the story of his or her most recent suicidal crisis.

SAMPLE CLINICIAN SCRIPT

I'd like to learn more about the details of what happened to you when you last experienced that intense desire to kill yourself [or made a suicide attempt]. Could you tell me the story of your suicidal crisis [or suicide attempt]? [If the patient asks where he or she should begin:] Wherever the story begins.

Step 2: Assist the Patient in Identifying and Describing the Sequence of Events

The clinician ensures that the patient identifies those thoughts, emotions, physical experiences, and behaviors associated with the index suicidal episode, and encourages the patient to continue moving through the narrative account by encouraging the patient to elaborate further or to provide more details. If the patient does not provide this information on his or her own, the clinician prompts the patient accordingly to obtain a clear moment-by-moment account of the steps that led up to the suicidal episode.

SAMPLE CLINICIAN SCRIPT

[Sample prompts to elicit the patient's narrative account of the suicidal crisis:]

And then what happened?
What happened next?
Did anything happen right before that?
How did you get to be in that place?
What, specifically, was going through your mind at that moment?
What was the emotion you felt at that moment?
Where did you feel that sensation in your body?
Describe what the room that you were in looked like.
What did you see?
What did that person specifically say to you? What were his/her exact words?
At what point did you decide to make the suicide attempt?

Step 3: Provide Emotional Validation

Upon concluding the narrative assessment, the clinician acknowledges that telling the story may have been emotionally difficult and thanks the patient for sharing the story. The clinician concludes by allowing the patient one more chance to share any additional information or details about his or her story.

SAMPLE CLINICIAN SCRIPT

Thank you for being willing to share your story with me; I'm sure it wasn't easy. Is there any other part of the story that needs to be told, or any other information that you think I may need to know?

ILLUSTRATIVE CASE EXAMPLES

The narrative assessment differs considerably from the more traditional interview-based approach to assessment. As a result, patients initially may not provide many details about the index suicidal crisis. In our experience, this most frequently occurs with patients who have been in treatment previously and/or experienced multiple instances of suicidal thoughts and behaviors. Because this patient subgroup has been socialized into providing brief answers to relatively closed-ended questions, clinicians may need to encourage patients to expand upon their stories and/or ask more clarifying questions. To demonstrate the process of the narrative assessment, partial transcripts from our three case studies are provided.

The Case of John

John's case demonstrates a common issue during the narrative assessment: confusion on the part of the patient about what the clinician is asking for. As noted above, patients are rarely asked to describe their suicidal crises as a "story," so clarification by the clinician may be needed. Note how John's clinician clarifies the task by providing a description of stories in general and then ties the notion of storytelling to John's suicidal crisis. Once John starts telling his story, the clinician asks clarifying questions at key moments to elicit details about John's thoughts and emotions, then encourages John to continue his story:

CLINICIAN: John, we've talked a little bit about what happened last week when you came close to killing yourself but stopped yourself at the last minute. I'd like to spend some time learning more about what happened that day, so that we have a better sense of how you got to that point. I'm wondering, would you be willing to share the story of the day that you almost killed yourself?

JOHN: Yeah. I mean, I guess so. I'm not really sure what you mean.

CLINICIAN: Well, if you think about what a story is, it typically involves a description of a series of events, from beginning to end. Stories have a beginning, a middle, and an end. The beginning of a story usually sets the stage for what's going to happen so that we have a sense of who's involved and what's going on. The middle of the story is usually when we learn how the events unfold over time, and the end of the story is when we learn how things resolve or wrap up. My guess is that there's a beginning, a middle, and an end to your story of almost killing yourself. If you were think about that day from this perspective, how would you tell your story?

JOHN: Yeah, I see. Well, I guess to understand the start of the story you have to know some of the background about my wife's family. They're really critical of her, always telling her she does things wrong and stuff. Whenever she talks to them, especially her dad, she ends up feeling depressed and stuff afterwards, so I've told her that she should stop talking to them so often. Well, when she was planning her trip to visit them, I told her that she shouldn't go because I knew they would treat her bad and then she'd be upset the whole time, but she wouldn't listen to me and just kept saying that that wouldn't happen. Well, she goes to visit them last week and, as expected, her dad was treating her really bad, putting her down and telling her she's a screw-up and stuff. So when she called me she was in tears and all upset, like I knew she would be. I was talking with her and telling her not to listen to her dad because he's always telling her negative things and putting her down, and telling her that her dad's just a total jerk. That's when she said that I wasn't listening to her.

CLINICIAN: When she said that, what did you say to yourself? What went through your mind?

JOHN: Well, I said to myself, "That's not true." I also thought it was unfair for her to say that because I told her this was going to happen and was trying to avoid this very situation, but she didn't listen to me again.

CLINICIAN: So it sounds like you were frustrated? Annoyed? Angry?

JOHN: I don't know if I'd say angry, but I was definitely frustrated.

CLINICIAN: OK, so you don't think this is fair, you're thinking that she didn't listen to your advice, and now you're feeling frustrated?

JOHN: Yeah.

CLINICIAN: OK, then what happened?

John continued to describe the chronology of his conversation with his wife, which quickly devolved into an argument, and the sequence of events leading up to his aborted suicide attempt. As he relayed the story, John's clinician periodically asked questions to identify his thoughts, emotions, and other internal experiences (e.g., physical sensations) using an approach similar to that employed in the partial transcript above.

The Case of Mike

Although Mike denied a history of suicidal thoughts and behaviors, his clinician nonetheless assessed his risk for suicide to be high; BCBT was therefore initiated. Due to his denial of suicidal thoughts and behaviors, there was no index suicidal episode to describe. The clinician therefore conducted a narrative assessment of a recent episode characterized by acute and intense emotional distress:

CLINICIAN: You described your emotions as "out of control."

MIKE: Yeah, sometimes I just feel like they overwhelm me, like I'm losing it or something, you know?

CLINICIAN: Yeah, I get that. How often would you say this happens?

MIKE: Seems like all the time now.

CLINICIAN: Daily?

MIKE: No, not that often. I guess more like once a week, maybe twice a week. It used to be every few months at most, but now it's every week at least.

CLINICIAN: I'd like to learn a bit more from you about these "out-of-control" times. Has there been a time in the past month when you felt more out of control than others?

MIKE: Yeah, probably 2 weeks ago. My wife and I really got into it and I got really pissed off and started drinking a lot. I don't even remember a lot about that night, but my wife says I was being a real jerk and I broke some beer bottles and stuff. That's probably the worst it's been.

CLINICIAN: OK. Let's talk about that night. I'd like to know how you got to that point, the things that led up to it and such. Would you be willing to tell me that story?

MIKE: Yeah, sure. I guess that night really started that morning when I woke up, and things just sort of escalated over the day.

Although Mike had denied past suicidal thoughts and behaviors, the clinician nonetheless conducted a narrative assessment focused on a recent incident during which he experienced intense emotional arousal and felt "out of control." The reason for conducting a narrative assessment under these conditions is that suicidal thoughts and behaviors are very likely to emerge in the future during such peaks in emotional distress. By identifying the sequence of events that lead up to these emotional crises, the clinician and patient could potentially prevent the later emergence of suicidal thoughts and behaviors. Another possibility is that Mike *has* experienced suicidal thoughts but is not comfortable disclosing these thoughts to the clinician. Under such circumstances, the narrative assessment could serve as a tool that promotes eventual disclosure. Even if such disclosure never occurs, the narrative assessment can nonetheless help him to recognize the factors that lead up to and surround suicidal crises, thereby enabling him to more effectively employ self-regulatory strategies in the future.

The Case of Janice

Janice's most recent suicide attempt was more than 2 years in the past. Since then, she has experienced "constant" suicidal thoughts that mirror her previous two suicide attempts, both of which involved medication overdoses. In cases characterized by multiple suicide attempts and recurrent suicidal thoughts and planning, the clinician could focus the narrative assessment on a past suicide attempt or a recent suicidal episode characterized by heightened suicidal intent and emotional distres. Because Janice denied experiencing a recent "crisis" and also described the content of her suicidal thoughts as being similar to her previous suicide attempts (i.e., medication overdose), the clinician decided to focus the narrative assessment on her most recent suicide attempt. Below is a partial transcript that demonstrates how the clinician can elicit details about the patient's suicidal experience while also facilitating the patient's description of the sequence of events involved in the suicidal episode:

CLINICIAN: Would you be willing to tell me the story of your second suicide attempt? The one that happened just a couple years ago?

JANICE: Yeah. That one started about a week before I actually made the attempt. My supervisor was really being a jerk, just on my ass for every little thing, like I couldn't do anything right, which was a complete 180 for him. Just the week before I was his superstar, so to speak, and he was putting me up for awards and recognition and all that. Then all of a sudden it all changed, and I couldn't do anything right. Going to work that week was just miserable. Every morning I would wake up and feel more and more dread. I would have this emptiness in my stomach and I didn't want to eat at all. I had to force myself to go in every morning because I just didn't want to see him or be there.

CLINICIAN: So for about a week before your attempt, things were getting really stressful at work, you weren't eating, you felt an emptiness in your stomach, and you didn't want to go to work.

JANICE: Yeah.

CLINICIAN: What sorts of things were you telling yourself during that week? Like what was going through your mind?

JANICE: That I'm a failure and an idiot, that I can't do anything right, that I don't want to have to deal with this anymore. I knew that I wasn't actually doing anything wrong, it's just that he was being such a jerk it was like I couldn't help myself.

CLINICIAN: OK, so you also started thinking you were a failure, an idiot, and that you didn't want to have to deal with all that anymore. That makes sense.

JANICE: Yeah.

CLINICIAN: OK, so then what happened?

JANICE: Well, my supervisor was just on me all day. I just couldn't get away from him so finally I just said to myself, That's it, I'm done, and I just went home. I left work early and went home. And so I was there at home by myself, and I remember being in the family room and just kind of looking around at everything, and thinking about how I just didn't want to deal with this anymore, how I was just tired and couldn't do it anymore.

CLINICIAN: Mm-hmm. Do you mind if I ask what emotion you were feeling at that moment?

JANICE: Numb. I was just numb. I think I had sort of checked out at that point because I wasn't angry or sad or anything. I was just standing there, feeling empty.

CLINICIAN: OK. Then what happened?

JANICE: Well, that's when I decided to just do it, so I went to the bathroom to see what pills I have. I don't think I really intended to do it right then, but I went to go count the pills and to get things ready. Like, I think I had made up my mind but I wasn't going to do it right then. I wanted to do it at night because I knew my daughter was stopping by that evening and I wanted to wait until after she had left. I didn't want her to come in and see me or something.

CLINICIAN: So you made the decision then but waited because you knew your daughter was coming by to visit?

JANICE: Yeah, and I figured she'd either find me dead or I would be close to dead, in which case she could call the ambulance and they might get in the way.

CLINICIAN: OK, I see. So you were worried that your daughter could potentially disrupt your plans?

JANICE: Yeah.

CLINICIAN: So then what happened?

In this manner, Janice continued to relay the story of her second suicide attempt, and the clinician periodically jumped in to clarify a point or to ask a follow-up question intended to elicit more information about the contextual factors, thoughts, emotions, and other internal experiences that surrounded Janice's suicidal crisis.

TIPS AND ADVICE FOR
THE NARRATIVE ASSESSMENT

1. **Leave some stones unturned.** The narrative assessment is *not* a general biopsychosocial interview, which is typically completed during an initial intake appointment before the start of BCBT. Thus, the clinician should avoid probing or asking about life events or experiences that are not directly or proximally related to the index suicidal episode. If, for example, the patient mentions child abuse or other traumatic experiences, take note of this but do not interrupt the flow of the patient's story to pursue more details about these experiences. The primary objective of the narrative assessment is to understand the contextual factors that surround the patient's suicidal thoughts and behaviors, not to obtain a detailed history of the patient's life.

2. **Help patients to stay on track.** If the patient gets "off track" by talking about other life events, problems, or situations that do not appear to be proximally related to the index suicidal episodes, the clinician can redirect the patient by asking the patient to explain how the current topic is related to the index suicidal episode. For example, during the narrative assessment the patient may begin to talk about memories of child abuse which might be related to the index suicidal episode (e.g., the patient's memories or flashbacks of the abuse trigger suicidal thoughts) but also might not be (e.g., the patient's recounting of child abuse was a tangential distraction). In this situation, the clinician might ask, "Just so I'm clear, when you made the suicide attempt last week were you thinking about being abused as a child? Or were these memories of child abuse involved in your suicide attempt in another way?" If the patient indicates that the child abuse was not directly involved in the index suicidal episode, the clinician can then ask the patient to resume the story from where he or she left off: "Oh that makes sense. So you were saying that on the day of your suicide attempt . . ." This strategy can help to redirect patients in a gentle and respectful way that minimizes the likelihood that they will feel interrupted or invalidated.

3. **Distinguish between proximal and distal variables.** Related to the previous point, when conducting the narrative assessment, the clinician should be cautious about assuming that certain events or topics are directly or proximally related to the index suicidal crisis. Trauma exposure, for instance, is an important risk factor for suicide, but this does not mean that the patient's most recent suicide attempt was directly related to a particular trauma. For example, although combat exposure (especially exposure to killing) is associated with increased risk for suicide ideation, suicide attempts, and death by suicide among military personnel and veterans (Bryan, Griffith et al., 2015), very few military personnel report thinking about combat-related memories on the day of their suicide

attempts (Bryan & Rudd, 2012). Combat exposure may therefore serve as a predisposing vulnerability for suicide, but it may not be a trigger.

4. Conceptualize as you go. In addition to its utility as a rapport-building strategy and suicide risk assessment process, the narrative assessment enables the clinician to gather the information needed to "fill in" the various domains of the suicidal mode so that an accurate case conceptualization can be formulated. As the patient relays his or her story, the clinician can organize the patient's risk and protective factors into the various domains of the suicidal mode. This will not only set up the clinician for the next step of the first session—the case conceptualization—it will also help him or her to start thinking about potential strategies for the crisis response plan.

5. Take your time. Because of elevated anxiety and/or situational pressures, clinicians initially push through the narrative assessment process at a faster than ideal pace. Clinicians who work in fast-paced settings characterized by rapid triage and decision making (e.g., emergency departments, primary care clinics, mobile crisis response teams) are especially vulnerable to this tendency. Most clinicians are able to complete the narrative assessment in 10–15 minutes on average. Although this may be longer than the traditional suicide risk assessment interview approach, clinicians who slow down and take their time during the narrative assessment often report that they obtain better, more nuanced information from their patients. Several additional minutes often pay large dividends.

CHAPTER 9

The Treatment Log
and the Case Conceptualization

The treatment log is a small, handheld notebook approximately 3″ × 4″ in size (slightly smaller than an index card) that is given to the patient so that he or she can take notes and keep track of "lessons learned" at the end of each session. For instance, patients may write something about the effectiveness of an intervention (e.g., "breathing exercises help me calm down"), or they may write a positive reappraisal or thought about themselves (e.g., "I'm not such a bad person after all"). The treatment log is given to the patient by the clinician; the patient is not asked to buy a notebook him- or herself because the act of giving the notebook to the patient appears to increase the emotional salience and meaningfulness of the treatment log. This in turn increases the overall effectiveness of the treatment log and reduces the likelihood that it will be lost or misplaced. Because it is intended to be highly transportable for easy access and reference by the patient, the treatment log should be small enough to fit into a pocket, purse, or backpack (see Figure 9.1). The small size of the treatment log also enables the patient to use the book with greater discretion and privacy.

The treatment log is introduced to the patient during the first session of BCBT as part of the case conceptualization, which serves as the working model for understanding each patient's case. The case conceptualization, which is based on the concept of the suicidal mode, helps the patient to understand why he or she got to the point of contemplating or attempting suicide and helps the clinician to develop a targeted treatment plan. The case conceptualization flows directly from the narrative assessment and serves to organize the many features of the patient's suicidal crisis into a simple and easy-to-understand framework: the suicidal mode. Upon providing the patient with a treatment log, the clinician invites the patient to draw a copy of his or her personal suicidal mode. This drawing can be referenced throughout the rest of BCBT as new procedures and interventions are introduced.

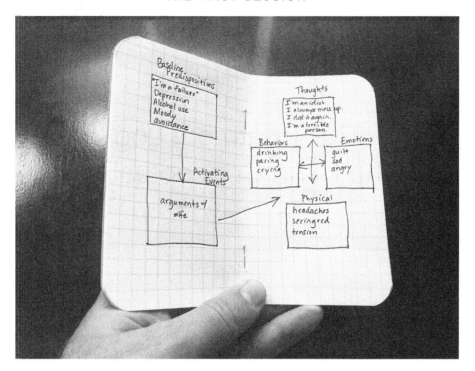

FIGURE 9.1. Sample treatment log for Mike.

RATIONALE

The primary purpose of the treatment log is to create a written record of "what works" for the patient. The treatment log helps the patient to gain a perspective on health, identify patterns in behaviors and life situations, track effective emotion regulation and problem-solving strategies, and track success across treatment. As the patient acquires new lessons learned over the course of BCBT, the treatment log becomes an evolving record of progress, growth, and hope. After the conclusion of BCBT, the patient can reference the treatment log whenever needed to help solve problems and/or remind him or her about how a situation or problem was successfully resolved or coped with during treatment. At the time of treatment completion, the treatment log therefore becomes a customized relapse prevention plan. The treatment log should not be conceptualized as or understood to be a journal or diary within which the patient records all thoughts, feelings, and life situations, however. Journals and diaries are often used to track negative life experiences, problems, and emotions on a daily basis to provide content for therapy sessions. Tracking negative life experiences can actually facilitate hopelessness among suicidal patients, however, because it serves as a written record of adversity, failure, and despair. In contrast to a journal or diary, the treatment log only includes entries that record growth, development, success, and empowerment; it therefore serves to facilitate the recovery process.

As discussed in Chapter 1, effective treatments for preventing suicide attempts are based on a straightforward, easy-to-understand model of suicide that integrates situational stressors, thoughts, feelings, and behaviors. Within BCBT, the suicidal mode serves as the conceptual model for explaining why the patient experienced a suicidal episode or made a suicide attempt, and why the clinician is selecting specific interventions in a particular sequence. The case conceptualization therefore serves as the foundation for the treatment plan, with all subsequent interventions being logically selected from this mutually agreed-upon model for "what is wrong" and "what needs to be done about it."

HOW TO DO IT

The treatment log is first presented to the patient after the narrative assessment has been completed. When introducing the treatment log, the clinician briefly describes its purpose and then asks the patient to bring the log to every session. At the end of each session, the clinician asks the patient to identify a "lesson learned" from the current session and then directs the patient to write this lesson into his or her treatment log. The treatment log is referenced throughout BCBT and plays an important role in the relapse prevention task during the final phase of treatment. The first use of the treatment log within BCBT is for the purpose of case conceptualization, which is completed collaboratively by the clinician and patient.

To facilitate this process, the clinician draws the various domains of the suicidal mode on a whiteboard (or a piece of paper) so the patient can see a visual representation of the case conceptualization as he or she is verbally describing it. The clinician begins the case conceptualization by describing the concept of the suicidal mode. The clinician then asks the patient to help conceptualize the case by "filling in the boxes" of the patient's unique suicidal mode. As the clinician and patient review each domain of the suicidal mode together, the clinician adds relevant patient-specific information to the image on the whiteboard, thereby providing a personalized "map" of the patient's suicidal crisis. During this process, the clinician facilitates patient engagement in the task by inviting the patient to make additions or recommend changes to the suicidal mode. Upon completion of the case conceptualization, the clinician invites the patient to draw a copy of his or her customized suicidal mode in the treatment log so it can be referenced again at a later date.

Step 1: Introduce the Treatment Log

The clinician provides the patient with a treatment log and explains its purpose.

SAMPLE CLINICIAN SCRIPT

One thing that may be a little different about this particular therapy as compared to other therapies is the use of a treatment log. Let me give you one and explain what it is.

As we go through this treatment together, there will be important pieces of information or concepts that we'll want to make sure we remember. We'll keep track of the most important lessons learned in therapy by writing them down in this treatment log, sort of like how you take notes in class to remember important information that the teacher presents. At the end of each session, you and I are going to identify the main "lesson learned" for that day and then write it in the treatment log. In some sessions your lesson learned might be about how to do a new skill or strategy that we practice. For example, when we practice breathing exercises together you might decide that the lesson learned from that particular session is that breathing exercises help you to calm down. In other sessions your lesson learned might be a positive reminder or "pep talk" of sorts for yourself. For example, when we start talking about how you view yourself as a person, you might decide that the lesson learned from that particular session is that you're being too hard on or too unfair to yourself.

Over the course of treatment, as you start to accumulate a lot of these lessons learned, the treatment log will sort of become a way for you to keep track of what is helpful for solving problems and managing distress in life. It will also become a way to track your growth and progress in treatment. Once we're done with treatment, you'll be able to take this treatment log with you and reference it whenever you need a refresher about how to handle certain situations or use a particular skill. It can therefore serve as your long-term plan for success in the future. Does all of this make sense?

Step 2: Enhance Motivation to Keep the Treatment Log

The clinician engages in motivational enhancement strategies to increase the likelihood that the patient will use the treatment log and keep track of it. To accomplish this, the clinician and patient collaboratively develop a plan regarding where the treatment log will be maintained in between sessions.

SAMPLE CLINICIAN SCRIPT

Because we'll be adding to this treatment log every time we meet, it'll be important for you to bring it with you to every session. Would you be willing to bring this in every time we meet so we can review it and also add to it?

Let's talk about where you might keep this treatment log so that you can use it when you need it but also so that you remember to bring it to your appointments with me. Many patients find it's helpful to keep their treatment log in a place that is relatively easy to access during the day. For example, some people keep it in their back pocket or their purse, and others keep it in the glove box of their car or their backpack.

What are your thoughts about where you might keep your treatment log so you can use it and also remember to bring it with you to therapy?

Step 3: Identify Lessons Learned at the End of Each Session (All BCBT Sessions)

At the conclusion of every BCBT session, the clinician asks the patient to summarize the content of the current session and to identify a "lesson learned." The clinician invites the patient to write this lesson learned in his or her treatment log.

> **SAMPLE CLINICIAN SCRIPT**
>
> We've talked about a lot today. Of all the things that we've discussed and practiced, what would you say is the biggest "lesson learned"? What did you find to be most helpful or useful? What was the most important piece of information or knowledge you gained today?

Step 4: Review Lessons Learned at the Start of Each Follow-Up Session (All BCBT Sessions)

At every follow-up appointment, the clinician asks the patient if he or she brought the treatment log to the session and asks the patient to review the lesson learned from the previous session. This provides a bridge from the previous session to the current session.

> **SAMPLE CLINICIAN SCRIPT**
>
> Let's take a moment to review where we left off when we last met. Did you bring your treatment log with you? What was your lesson learned from the last session?

Step 5: Introduce the Concept of the Suicidal Mode

The clinician introduces the concept of the suicidal mode and provides a brief description. The clinician then invites the patient to draw a picture of his or her individualized suicidal mode in the treatment log for later reference.

> **SAMPLE CLINICIAN SCRIPT**
>
> Now that we've spent some time talking about what happened on the day of your suicidal crisis, I think I have a much better understanding of how you got to the place where making a suicide attempt probably seemed like a reasonable option to you. In this treatment, we find it is useful to organize such stories in a way that can guide what we do together. That way the treatment makes sense for both of us and makes sure we prioritize issues appropriately. To do this, we use a very simple model for understanding suicide risk called the suicidal mode.
>
> The suicidal mode is sort of a framework for putting together all of the information and issues that led up to your suicidal crisis and perhaps even made things worse during that crisis. The suicidal mode has several parts that apply to you. Let's talk about each of those parts one at a time. As we talk about each part, I'll draw it here on the board so we can more easily see how things go together. As we're working on this, I'd like for you to draw a copy of this model in the treatment log I just gave to you so you can keep a record of this and then we can look at it whenever we need to during treatment.

Step 6: Review Baseline Risk Factors

The clinician explains how certain genetic, biological, and historical factors (e.g., family history, gender, race, trauma exposure, past suicide attempts, previous psychiatric history) can increase the patient's baseline likelihood for experiencing a suicidal episode or making a suicide attempt in the future. The clinician and patient then collaboratively identify the patient's baseline risk factors.

SAMPLE CLINICIAN SCRIPT

The first part of the suicidal mode is what we call baseline risk factors. Baseline risk factors are things about you or things that have happened to you that increase your likelihood of becoming suicidal. Some examples include having other family members who have died by suicide, having a history of mental illness, having a history of trauma or abuse, or having made previous suicide attempts. Baseline risk factors don't necessarily cause you to think about suicide or make a suicide attempt, but they make it more likely that you will have these thoughts. Based on what you've told me about yourself, it sounds like you have the following baseline risk factors for making a suicide attempt. . . . [The clinician lists the patient's predispositions on the whiteboard.]

TROUBLESHOOTING TIPS

What if the patient disagrees? If the patient disagrees with the clinician about any suggested risk factors, the clinician should ask the patient to elaborate on his or her perspective. For example:

It sounds like you see things differently. How would you describe it?

Again, baseline risk factors just increase the likelihood that you will experience a suicidal crisis or make a suicide attempt during your life, but they don't necessarily cause you to think about suicide or make the suicide attempt by itself. Can you think of any other baseline risk factors that we haven't listed yet that might increase the likelihood of you becoming suicidal?

Step 7: Review Activating Events

The clinician explains how stressful situations or problems in life can activate emotional distress and trigger a suicidal episode. The clinician distinguishes between external activating events (e.g., relationship problems, financial strain, legal or disciplinary issues) and internal activation (i.e., traumatic memories, negative mood states, self-defeating statements) and notes that either could activate a suicidal crisis. The clinician and patient then collaboratively identify the patient's activating events.

SAMPLE CLINICIAN SCRIPT

The next part of the suicidal mode is what we call activating events. Activating events are stressful situations or problems that you experience in life that activate a suicidal crisis. Activating events can usually be categorized into one of two groups: external and internal.

External triggers are stressful situations that happen in your life such as a relationship problem, financial hardship, or legal or disciplinary problems. Internal triggers, by contrast, are mental or physical experiences that occur inside of you, like depression, worrying about a problem in life, or thinking about bad things that might happen to you.

In many cases suicidal crises are triggered by life events, but other times they are triggered by some sort of feeling or experience inside of you that is not necessarily tied to any life event. Based on the story you just told me, it sounds like your activating events included. . . . [*The clinician lists the patient's triggers on the whiteboard.*]

Do you have any other external or internal activating events for crises, even if they didn't occur on the day of your most recent suicidal crisis?

In order to understand why you experienced a suicidal crisis on that day, we have to consider both your baseline risk factors and your activating events together. A person will become actively suicidal only when they have a sufficiently stressful activating event and a sufficient number of baseline risk factors. In other words, an activating event will activate your suicidal crisis only if you are vulnerable. This is why one person can become suicidal after a particular stressor but another person doesn't become suicidal when they experience the very same thing: it depends on what the stressor is and how you've learned to respond to such stressors. Does that make sense?

When you are vulnerable to suicide and then you experience a major activating event, an active suicidal crisis occurs. This crisis is what we call the suicidal mode. The suicidal mode is made up of four areas: behavioral, physical, emotional, and cognitive.

Step 8: Review the Behavioral Domain

The clinician explains how the actions that patients take leading up to or in response to a stressful event can influence how they feel and the decisions they make. The clinician differentiates between behaviors that facilitate suicidal episodes (e.g., social isolation, substance use, nonsuicidal self-injury, preparatory behaviors) and behaviors that prevent or resolve suicidal episodes (e.g., engagement in meaningful activities, exercise, spending time with friends and family). The clinician and patient then collaboratively identify the patient's suicide-related behaviors.

SAMPLE CLINICIAN SCRIPT

Let's start with the behavioral domain. These are the things you do and the decisions you make when emotionally upset and feeling suicidal. As you were telling me the story of your suicidal crisis, you said that you did the following things leading up to and during your crisis. . . . [*The clinician lists the patient's behaviors on the whiteboard.*]

These behaviors sustained your emotional distress and made it more likely that you would attempt suicide. Are there any other behaviors that you are aware of that seem to backfire on you or make things worse when you are upset?

Step 9: Review the Physiological Domain

The clinician explains how physiological arousal and emotional arousal are interrelated, how emotional distress can trigger physical problems (e.g., muscle tension, headaches, sleep problems), and how physical problems can likewise heighten emotional distress. The clinician and patient then collaboratively identify the patient's physiological indicators of emotional arousal and any somatic issues that trigger or maintain emotional distress.

> **SAMPLE CLINICIAN SCRIPT**
>
> Next is the physical domain. When we are emotionally upset we often experience physical problems or issues like insomnia, headaches, muscle tension, pain, and difficulty concentrating. These physical symptoms can make us feel even worse than we did before. When you experienced your suicidal crisis you mentioned experiencing the following physical sensations and problems. . . . *[The clinician lists the patient's physical symptoms on the whiteboard.]*
>
> Have you ever experienced or noticed any other physical symptoms when you are upset?

Step 10: Review the Emotional Domain

The clinician explains how emotional experiences can bias one's perceptions about the self and one's situation, and how emotions can motivate the patient to make certain decisions or engage in certain behaviors in order to avoid or otherwise reduce emotional distress (e.g., substance use, nonsuicidal self-injury, social withdrawal, suicide attempts). The clinician and patient then collaboratively identify those emotional states that are most commonly experienced during the patient's suicidal crises (e.g., depression, guilt, anxiety, anger).

> **SAMPLE CLINICIAN SCRIPT**
>
> Next is the emotional domain, which typically includes negative emotions and feelings about ourselves or life, such as depression, sadness, fear, or guilt. Because these emotions are often very painful to experience, we are motivated to avoid them or get rid of them, which can lead us to make decisions or engage in certain behaviors that may not be in our best interest and may actually increase our distress. You mentioned feeling the following emotions during your suicidal crisis. . . . *[The clinician lists the patient's emotions on the whiteboard.]*
>
> Emotions like these can not only cause us to think about suicide, they can also sustain our suicidal crises over time. Do you ever experience any other emotions when you feel suicidal?

Step 11: Review the Cognitive Domain

The clinician explains how one's beliefs and assumptions about the self, others, and the world can influence the emotions one feels and the actions one takes in response to life circumstances or stressful events. The clinician distinguishes between internalized beliefs or schemas that have persisted over time and serve as cognitive predispositions (e.g., "Something is wrong with me"; "I'm a failure") and those automatic thoughts that arise in response to life stressors (e.g., "This is unfair"; "Here we go again"). The clinician and patient then collaboratively identify those core suicidal beliefs that are underlie the patient's vulnerability to experiencing suicidal crises.

SAMPLE CLINICIAN SCRIPT

The final domain of the suicidal mode is the cognitive domain. The cognitive domain includes our self-perceptions as well as our beliefs and assumptions about the world and others. If we have very negative or critical perceptions of ourselves, we are much more likely to think about suicide. Likewise, if we assume that a situation is hopeless or that we are unable to fix a problem, then we tend to stay emotionally upset for a much longer period of time. We can therefore differentiate between core beliefs and automatic thoughts.

Core beliefs include those self-perceptions and assumptions that persist over time. Our core beliefs usually take the form of "I am . . ." statements and entail a judgment of some kind. These perceptions influence how we understand what is happening to us. If, for instance, I believe that I'm a failure, I'm likely to think that bad luck is due to my incompetence. By contrast, if I believe that I'm a capable and intelligent person, I'm likely to see bad luck as just that: bad luck. How we see ourselves therefore serves as a predisposition for becoming suicidal.

Automatic thoughts are a little different. Automatic thoughts are the things we say to ourselves in reaction to life events; they are therefore situationally based. For example, we might say things like "This is unfair" or "Here we go again." These thoughts reflect our understanding of what is happening to us at that moment in time and influence how we feel and how we will respond to the situation. Our thoughts therefore shape our actions and feelings.

You've made a number of statements that suggest you see yourself in a particularly negative light. In addition, during your suicidal crisis you had a number of thoughts that probably contributed to your emotions. For example, you've said the following. . . . *[The clinician lists the patient's suicidal beliefs on the whiteboard.]*

These beliefs and perceptions make it harder for you to effectively solve problems and make it easier for you to become suicidal. When you are in an active suicidal crisis, these beliefs also make it harder for you to recover or feel better quickly. Are there any other negative or judgmental things you've said to yourself over the years that we haven't discussed here?

Step 12: Assess the Patient's Comprehension

After each of the individual components of the suicidal mode has been explained and personalized with the patient's case-specific information, the clinician asks the patient to summarize the information contained within his or her suicidal mode and then asks if the patient feels that this model accurately reflects his or her suicidal episode. If not, the clinician invites the patient to make corrections or adjustments to the conceptualization to more accurately capture the patient's vulnerabilities, stressors, and personal responses.

> ### SAMPLE CLINICIAN SCRIPT
>
> Would you say that this is a reasonably accurate way of understanding how you became suicidal and what happened to you during your last suicidal crisis? Would you say that this summarizes your experience of being suicidal? Are there any areas that you think need to be changed or adjusted?
>
> I'd like for you to summarize what we have just discussed. Using your own words, how would you explain the suicidal mode and how would you describe the various components of the suicidal mode as they apply to your life?

Step 13: Reinforce the Use of the Treatment Log

The clinician highlights the value of maintaining a copy of the patient's personalized suicidal mode in his or her treatment log for later reference and notes that the clinician and patient will refer back to this model multiple times throughout the course of treatment to ensure that the selected interventions and strategies are relevant to the patient's unique needs and goals.

> ### SAMPLE CLINICIAN SCRIPT
>
> Now that you have a written record of this in your treatment log, we'll be able to refer back to this model each time we meet. That way we can make sure that any new strategies we want to try out make sense for what's been going on in your life. Having easy access to this picture of your suicidal mode will also help us keep track of your progress in treatment. Likewise, after we have completed treatment, you can pull out this treatment log again anytime you need help figuring out what sorts of things in life help you to solve problems and what sorts of things in life sustain your problems or make them worse.

ILLUSTRATIVE CASE EXAMPLE

An example of how an index narrative assessment can be translated into a customized case conceptualization is provided by the case of Mike. Mike's case conceptualization is summarized in Figure 9.2. As can be seen, Mike's conceptualization includes relevant baseline risk factors as well as the acute manifestations of his most recent emotional crisis. This conceptualization serves as the foundation for subsequent interventions. Partial transcripts from his narrative assessment are excerpted to demonstrate how the information obtained from that procedure can be used to guide the case conceptualization.

Two weeks prior, Mike and his partner got into another argument about his drinking, during which his partner suddenly asked him to leave the apartment. Mike noted that this argument was "just like the other fights that ended my previous marriages." During his narrative assessment, Mike reported that his self-perception of being "out of control" were influenced in part by his wife, who frequently uses the phrases "out of control" and

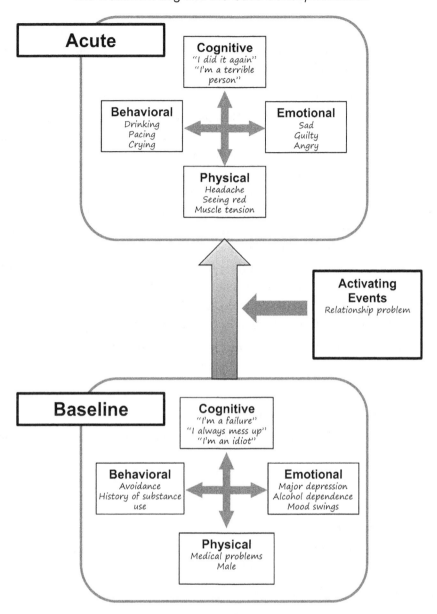

FIGURE 9.2. Case conceptualization for Mike.

"emotionally unavailable" during their arguments. She has also complained about his heavy alcohol use.

CLINICIAN: OK. Let's talk about that night. Could you tell me the story about that night? I'd like to know how you got to that point, the things that led up to it, and so on. Would you be willing to tell me that story?

MIKE: Yeah, sure. I guess that night really started that morning when I woke up, and things just sort of escalated over the day. I had a really bad headache because I had been drinking the night before and was not in a good mood when I woke up. My wife wasn't in a good mood that morning either because of my drinking. She was giving me the silent treatment and wasn't exactly being the most charitable to me.

CLINICIAN: What do you mean?

MIKE: Well, she wasn't exactly trying to be quiet or anything. She was banging cabinet doors, pots and pans, and that kind of stuff, because she knew I had a headache and she was trying to make it worse and stuff. I was already feeling terrible as it was, so her deliberately being awful to me just made me more and more mad. So finally I just blew up and told her that she doesn't have to make all that noise getting ready in the morning because I realized I shouldn't have been drinking again and I knew she was mad without her acting like that. She said she was tired of me drinking all the time and losing control of myself. I told her I knew she didn't want me drinking and that I don't drink all that often, and she said that the problem isn't that I drink often, but when I do drink I get out of control and that it's just that I don't want to face my problems. She's always saying that to me, how I'm out of control and I don't deal with problems. It's like she's my mother or something like that, scolding me and such.

CLINICIAN: I see. So it sounds like what you're saying there is that when she tells you that you're out of control and don't want to face your problems, you feel guilt or shame?

MIKE: I don't know.

CLINICIAN: Do you maybe feel a different emotion?

MIKE: I guess shame is right. I feel like a little kid or something, instead of the grown man that I am.

CLINICIAN: OK, so you're feeling angry and ashamed at this point in the story?

MIKE: Yeah.

CLINICIAN: OK, so what happened next?

MIKE: I got defensive and argued with her. I mean, I know that she's kind of right in a way, but that just makes me more pissed off.

CLINICIAN: What is she kind of right about?

MIKE: That I drink when I get upset instead of facing my problems.

CLINICIAN: Oh, OK. So there's something about that that you think may be true about yourself.

MIKE: Yeah, but I get so pissed when she's the one who says it. It's like I know it already, I don't need you treating me like some kid and making me feel like an idiot.

CLINICIAN: Yeah, I get that. So on that morning is this sort of what was going through your mind at that point?

MIKE: Yeah, I was thinking it, but I didn't say it out loud or anything. When I get in that mindset, I don't want to give her any ammunition, you know?

CLINICIAN: Mm-hmm. So then what happened?

MIKE: Well, things just kept escalating and getting worse, so I just told her that since I was such a big screw-up I'd leave her so she didn't have to deal with me anymore. She said that was fine with her, so we stopped talking at that point. She just kept getting ready for work and I got ready for work, and I packed up a bag of clothes so I could spend the night at my mom's. I've stayed there before in the past, so I figured I would just do that again. So I went to work and was just pissed all day, and just kept thinking about the argument and how I really did screw up again, and how I always seem to screw up. I just stayed away from everyone at work because I would just start crying all of a sudden and I didn't want anyone to see me doing that. When I got off my shift I went to my mom's house and had dinner. I tried to go to bed early, but I just couldn't shut off my mind. It was like my thoughts were uncontrollable.

CLINICIAN: What were you thinking about?

MIKE: How I'm such an idiot, I've screwed up again. I started worrying about my wife leaving me because I'm a such a terrible person. I just kept thinking about her leaving me and getting all worried. I couldn't control it and started feeling bad about what I had done. I got angry at myself because I can't control my drinking and started feeling sad about being alone.

CLINICIAN: What happened next?

MIKE: I got this really bad headache. Not like a hangover headache, though, an anger headache. I got really tense and started pacing around the bedroom and crying. I was trying not to cry, but I just couldn't control it. I'm such an idiot I can't even stop crying. I'm like a little baby. When I get upset like that I start seeing red, so I went to my mom's fridge and grabbed a beer. I didn't want to drink because that's the problem, you know? But I just kind of felt like what's the point by then? It kind of didn't matter anymore because I had already screwed everything up so bad.

CLINICIAN: How many beers did you drink?

MIKE: Not that many. Well, I guess not as much as I would have. That's only because my mom doesn't keep a lot of beer in her house, so maybe I had like four or five. I was just walking around basement of her house, back and forth. I couldn't stop thinking about the argument and how I had screwed up. I was replaying that argument over and over in my head and just getting more and more angry. When I drank the last beer and went back to grab another one but the fridge was empty, I just sort of snapped or something. I just felt terrible because I realized then that I had drank all my mom's beer in like 30 minutes or something like that, and I just started thinking to myself how I should just do it.

CLINICIAN: Do what?

MIKE: (*Looks away, starting to cry.*) Nothing.

CLINICIAN: When you say that you started thinking about how you should do it, what does "it" refer to?

MIKE: I wasn't thinking about killing myself. I know that's what you're getting at. That's not what it was though.

CLINICIAN: OK. If it wasn't suicide, then, what was it?

MIKE: I don't know.

CLINICIAN: OK, fair enough. So you're looking in the fridge and you're telling yourself that you should just do it. What happens next?

MIKE: Well, I started crying really hard and I texted my wife. I don't know why I did. I guess I was drunk enough at that point that I just didn't care anymore, so I texted her and told her that I loved her.

CLINICIAN: And then what happened?

MIKE: She didn't text back right away, which really made me cry and stuff, but after 10 minutes or so she texted back that she loves me, too, and that she's going to bed and hoped I was going to bed soon, too.

CLINICIAN: And then what happened?

MIKE: Well, that just made me feel a lot better. It was such a relief. It was obvious she was still mad at me but her texting back to say she loved me and that she hoped I was going to bed really meant a lot. I started calming down after that.

Note how many of the details provided by Mike during his narrative assessment are incorporated into his case conceptualization in Figure 9.2. Additional details and information obtained from his intake paperwork and other portions of his intake assessment are also integrated into this model. Perhaps most important in the narrative assessment, however, is a critical dislosure that Make eventually makes: having thoughts that he should "just do it." Although Mike quickly denies that this statement refers to suicide, the context surrounding this incident strongly implies that he was likely considering suicide to some degree. Because Mike seems unwilling to acknowledge this possibility, however, the clinician chooses to continue the narrative assessment, thereby avoiding a possible power struggle. By remaining focused on the task, the clinician is able to learn about how this incident resolved.

TIPS AND ADVICE FOR
THE TREATMENT LOG AND THE CASE CONCEPTUALIZATION

1. Give the patient a treatment log. Providing a treatment log rather than asking patients to go purchase one on their own works better for several reasons. First, it eliminates several potential barriers including insufficient finacial resources ("I can't afford it"), time constraints ("I don't have time to go get one"), and motivational issues ("I forgot to get one"). Second, providing a treatment log to patients seems to increase its meaningfulness relative to a treatment log that was purchased or obtained on their own.

2. Provide options. Although a relatively small matter, we have found that providing patients with several treatment log options from which they can choose further heightens its perceived meaningfulness and utility. Options can be as simple as providing a variety of colors or cover page designs to choose from. The provision of choice enables patients to "customize" or "personalize" their selection, which seems to enhance its value.

3. **Draw a picture of the suicidal mode during the case conceptualization.** Drawing a picture of the suicidal mode on a whiteboard or other surface helps patients (and clinicians) to visualize how various risk and protective factors influence each other. Patients often report that this helps them understand their situation, and clinicians often report that this helps them think about risk level and treatment planning.

4. **Ask patients for their feedback while creating the suicidal mode.** When discussing the suicidal mode, clinicians should check in with their patients on a regular basis to assess accuracy and buy-in, and to engage them in the process. This reduces the likelihood of misunderstandings that could stall or delay the treatment process later on and helps establish a collaborative working relationship.

CHAPTER 10

The Crisis Response Plan

The crisis response plan is the final required component of the first session of BCBT. The crisis response plan is a collaboratively developed written plan that the patient can follow during suicidal crises or periods of emotional distress that precede the onset of an acute suicidal crisis. In essence, the crisis response plan entails a written checklist of "what to do" when in crisis, and is comprised of behavioral alternatives to making a suicide attempt. The crisis response plan includes five components: (1) identifying personal warning signs indicating the possible onset of a suicidal crisis; (2) identifying self-management skills or strategies that can distract the patient from the situation or help him or her cope with it effectively; (3) identifying reasons for living; (4) identifying supportive friends or family members who can be contacted to obtain social support and assistance; and (5) identifying professional sources of support and help such as mental health providers, crisis hotlines, and emergency services (i.e., 911).

RATIONALE

The primary purpose of the crisis response plan is to aid the patient's decision-making process during acute periods of emotional distress and impaired problem solving. Relative to individuals who have not been suicidal, even those with major depression, suicidal individuals experience considerable difficulty in generating potential solutions to their problems (Williams, Barnhofer, Crane, & Beck, 2005). This deficit in problem solving is likely related to the attentional bias that suicidal individuals have toward death- and suicide-related information, which includes negative emotional states and negative expectations for the future. During a crisis, the patient's cognitive predispositions are activated, such that suicidal individuals tend to overestimate the likelihood of negative events occurring for them in the future (MacLeod, Rose, & Williams, 1993). The crisis response plan serves as a decisional aid that outlines a sequence of steps to take during a crisis, thereby counteracting the collapse in problem solving that occurs during acute crises. In essence, the crisis response plan outlines alternatives to making a suicide attempt when the patient most wants to make one.

As a suicide prevention procedure, various iterations of the crisis response plan have been used in a wide range of treatments with established efficacy for reducing suicidal behavior: DBT, cognitive therapy for suicide prevention, the attempted suicide short intervention program, and BCBT. Because of its simplicity, the crisis response plan has been extracted from BCBT for use in a wide range of settings including emergency departments, primary care clinics, inpatient psychiatric units, and outpatient mental health settings. Results of a recently completed randomized clinical trial support the effectiveness of the crisis response plan for the prevention of suicide attempts when used as a stand-alone risk management procedure (Bryan et al., 2017). In this study, two versions of the crisis response plan were examined and compared to treatment as usual, which entailed supportive listening, provision of professional crisis resources, and a verbal contract for safety. Both versions of the crisis response plan included the following four components: (1) identifying personal warning signs, (2) identifying self-management skills, (3) identifying supportive friends or family members, and (4) identifying professional crisis services. One version of the crisis response plan also included a fifth element: identifying personal reasons for living. Although the two versions of the crisis response plan did not differ from each other with respect to suicide attempt rates or suicide ideation during follow-up, they significantly outperformed treatment as usual on both metrics. Specifically, acutely suicidal participants who received a crisis response plan were 76% less likely to make a suicide attempt during the next 6 months, and they showed faster and larger declines in suicide ideation during the 6-month follow-up period. Participants who received a crisis response plan also had significantly fewer days of inpatient psychiatric hospitalization.

Our subsequent research suggests that, in addition to its long-term benefits regarding suicidal thoughts and behaviors, crisis response planning also shows immediate effects on suicidal individuals' emotional state. When assessed immediately before and after their interventions, which spanned approximately 20–30 minutes, participants who received either of the two crisis response plans showed significant declines in several negative affective states including depression, anxiety, perceived burdensomeness, and suicidal desire. In contrast, participants who received a contract for safety showed no change in emotional state afterward. Furthermore, participants who received the version of the crisis response plan that included the extra component (a discussion of their reasons for living) also showed a significant increase in hope and calmness and a significantly larger decline in perceived burdensomeness than participants in the crisis response plan condition without this extra component. Taken together, these findings indicate that crisis response planning (1) reduces suicide attempts, (2) rapidly resolves suicidal crises, (3) immediately reduces negative emotional states, and (4) immediately increases positive emotional states, but only if the patient is asked to talk about his or her reasons for living. The crisis response plan is therefore an especially potent ingredient of BCBT that serves as the platform for all subsequent interventions.

In a separate study conducted in emergency departments, the safety planning intervention (Stanley & Brown, 2008), a procedure that is similar in design to the crisis response plan, combined with follow-up phone calls was similarly associated with reduced rates of suicidal behavior as compared to treatment as usual (Miller et al., 2017), although the magnitude of effect (20% reduction) was much smaller in size than what has been seen with the crisis response plan and other interventions that integrate the crisis response plan. In this study, the safety planning intervention was self-administered by the patient rather than being developed collaboratively with a health care provider; was created using preprinted, fill-in-the-blank forms rather than being handwritten on an index card; and included a section focused on means restriction (Boudreaux et al., 2013). These differences suggest that, aside from its content, the process by which a crisis response plan is developed might influence its efficacy.

HOW TO DO IT

When creating a crisis response plan with patients, clinicians should adopt a guiding approach in which they assist patients in identifying their own solutions and strategies. By taking this approach, clinicians can increase the likelihood that patients will use the crisis response plan during periods of intense emotional distress. Because the crisis response plan serves as the platform for all subsequent interventions in BCBT, clinicians and patients should conceptualize the crisis response plan as a "living document" that will be amended and modified over the course of treatment, as that they continuously improve upon it together.

At the beginning of every follow-up session, the clinician should ask the patient if he or she has used the crisis response plan since the previous session. If yes, the clinician then asks the patient to describe the circumstances that led to the use of the crisis response plan, and how the crisis response plan was used. Successful use of the crisis response plan should be reinforced by the clinician, whereas barriers or obstacles to effective use of the crisis response plan (including failure to use it) should be collaboratively problem-solved. The clinician should thereby differentiate between those self-management skills that are not practical or helpful and those that simply require refinement and/or more practice. For example, if a patient reports that his or her use of a relaxation skill "didn't work," the clinician should first seek to determine if this is instead due to the patient not fully understanding how to use relaxation effectively and/or not practicing the skill enough for it to be beneficial. Skills that are not practical or helpful should be removed from the crisis response plan. Skills that are challenging or confusing should be practiced further before being removed from the crisis response plan, however.

A general template for the crisis response plan is provided in Appendix B.3. Clinicians have found that hanging a copy of this template on their wall or keeping a copy in an easily accessible location (e.g., a desk drawer) helps them to ensure fidelity when creating a plan with a patient. Of note, the template helps to reduce anxiety because it reduces the tendency for clinicians to worry about forgetting a component. This, in turn, helps them to focus more on the process of crisis response planning, which typically contributes to higher-quality patient encounters.

Step 1: Introduce the Crisis Response Plan

The clinician first provides a brief description of the crisis response plan and the rationale for its use.

SAMPLE CLINICIAN SCRIPT

Based on what you were telling me before, the pain that you experience when you are suicidal feels unbearable and like it will never end. Under those circumstances, many people find it hard to focus and to make decisions effectively. Would you say that's true for you as well?

TROUBLESHOOTING TIP

What if the patient disagrees? If patients disagree with this perspective or otherwise indicates that it does not apply to them, the clinician should invite them to provide their perspective. For example:

How does intense stress affect your decision-making ability?

Based on the response to this question, use the patient's language to illustrate how emotional distress can impact decision making.

Because it's so hard to make decisions when we're that upset, it can be helpful to have a plan laid out in advance to help get us through the crisis, sort of like a contingency plan or an emergency response plan that we have to prepare for disasters or other major, unexpected issues in life. Have you ever made an emergency plan or a contingency plan for your family or work? Could you describe what those plans were like?

As you noted, most emergency plans have very clear checklists of what to do when the problem arises. Basically, a good plan lists very simple instructions for what to do in response to the situation. We can create a similar crisis response plan for managing our own personal crises in life. Before we wrap up today, I'd like for us to create a crisis response plan for you. Would you be willing to do that? Let's write down the plan on this index card, so that you can keep it in your pocket or purse or somewhere else that's easy to access.

Step 2: Identify Personal Warning Signs

The clinician asks the patient to think about his or her personal indicators for emotional distress and crises. In most cases, these personal warning signs have already been described by the patient during the narrative assessment of the index suicidal crisis. Common warning signs are listed in Appendix B.4. If the patient is struggling to identify his or her personal warning signs, the clinician provides the patient with a list of warning signs to prompt or cue the patient's memory.

SAMPLE CLINICIAN SCRIPT

The first step for creating a good crisis response plan is knowing when we need to actually use the plan. If we don't know when to pull out the plan, we probably won't use it very effectively. If we were to pick some warning signs or red flags for an impending crisis in your life, what would those warning signs be? In other words, how do you know when you're getting upset and may need to use this plan? Let's write one or two of those warning signs down on the top of your index card.

Step 3: Identify Self-Management Strategies

The clinician asks the patient to identify activities or strategies that can either distract the patient from the situation or reduce his or her distress. A useful strategy is to ask the patient what activities helped to relieve stress in the past, even if he or she is no longer using them. If the patient is struggling to identify self-management strategies, the clinician provides the patient with a list of possible strategies similar to Appendix B.5 to prompt or cue the patient's memory. When identifying self-management strategies, the clinician ensures that the patient is able to effectively use the strategy and is specific about how long or under which circumstances he or she will use the self-management strategy.

SAMPLE CLINICIAN SCRIPT

Now that we know when to use this plan, let's write down some strategies you can use to manage your stress or distract you from the problem temporarily. What are some things that help you to feel less stressed or more relaxed? What are some things you used to do that helped you to feel less stressed or more relaxed, even if you don't do those things anymore? Let's write one or two of those strategies down underneath your warning signs.

How long do you think you would be able to do each of these things? Let's write down how long you'll do each of those strategies as well.

Step 4: Identify Supportive Friends or Family Members

The clinician asks the patient to identify the names and phone numbers of individuals who are supportive and/or who help the patient to feel better when distressed. The clinician directs the patient to write down both the name and phone number for the supportive person even if this information is stored in the patient's cell phone (or in another location). The clinician emphasizes that the patient is not required to tell the supportive other that he or she is in a crisis; rather, the patient can simply call this person as a distraction or to otherwise obtain support without disclosing his or her suicidal thoughts.

SAMPLE CLINICIAN SCRIPT

Sometimes we're in situations where using these strategies isn't very realistic, such as when we're at work or when there's bad weather. Other times we use these skills but we still feel upset. It's therefore good to have an alternative or backup plan, such as reaching out to a friend, family member, or another supportive person who can help us to feel better. We don't necessarily have to tell this person that we're upset or in crisis or thinking about killing ourselves; sometimes just talking with them is enough to calm us down or feel better.

Who is a person in your life who helps you feel better when you're upset or helps take your mind off of things? Let's write his or her name and phone number down next on this list, so that they're listed right there in an easy-to-access place when you need them.

Step 5: List Sources of Professional Help

The clinician lists his or her name and phone number, along with the contact information for any other mental health or medical professionals. The clinician should be very specific regarding reasonable expectations for answering phones and returning calls. For example, if he or she is unlikely to answer the phone during office hours, the patient should be instructed to leave a voice message along with the expected time to wait for a return phone call (e.g., at lunchtime or the end of the business day). The clinician should also provide the phone number for the National Lifeline (1-800-273-TALK). Finally, the patient should include going to the emergency department and calling 911 as the final steps.

> **SAMPLE CLINICIAN SCRIPT**
>
> It's also good to make sure you have easy access to professional help when your crises are especially bad or these other strategies aren't working. So let's put my name and phone number next on the list. Now one thing to keep in mind is that I don't always answer my phone because I'm helping other patients or am doing other things. Although I might not answer right away when you call, I will call you back as soon as possible, so you'll have to leave a voice mail for me. Let's add that information here after my name and number: "leave a voice message with my name, phone number, and time."
>
> I check my voice mail at the end of each day, so if you call and leave a message I'll be able to call you back in the afternoon. Sometimes I can call back sooner if a patient doesn't show up or I have an open schedule, but it'll definitely be by the end of the day. Do you have any concerns about that?
>
> Since I might not be able to answer the phone right away when you call, I want to make sure you have someone you can talk to immediately if you need assistance. Here is the phone number for the National Lifeline, which is a toll-free phone number you can call to speak with someone right away about what's bothering you: 1-800-273-TALK. You can call them 24/7 and on holidays, and someone will pick up.
>
> When all else fails, you can always go to the emergency department or call 911 for emergency assistance. Although it's unlikely that you'll need to get to this step, we should write it down anyway because it's better safe than sorry, and it's been a helpful "last step" for a number of my patients. Go ahead and write down "go to emergency department" and "call 911" as the final steps.

Step 6: Review the Plan and Elicit Patient Buy-In

Upon completion of the crisis response plan, the clinician asks the patient to verbally review each of the steps. This facilitates mental rehearsal and practice of the crisis response plan and also provides a means for determining if the patient understands how to use the crisis response plan. If the patient is unclear about how to use any portion of the crisis response plan, the clinician reviews this information again. The clinician wraps up this intervention by asking the patient to rate his or her likelihood of using the crisis response plan on a scale ranging from 0 to 10, with 0 indicating "not at all likely" and 10 indicating "very likely."

SAMPLE CLINICIAN SCRIPT

OK, so let's review these steps together. When will you know when to use this plan? And when you experience those warning signs, what will you do first? And if those strategies don't work or can't be used, what else could you do? And what if you need to speak with a professional? What are your options there?

　　　Very good. Does this plan make sense, or do you have any questions about what to do and how to do it?

　　　[After finishing the plan:] On a scale of 0 to 10, with 0 being "not at all" and 10 being "definitely," what would you say is the likelihood that you will use this crisis response plan when you're upset?

　　　[If the rating is lower than 7 out of 10:] Is there any part of this plan that reduces your likelihood for using it? What could we change about this plan to make it more likely that you would use it?

TROUBLESHOOTING TIP

What if the patient says there is nothing that will make the plan more useful? If the clinician employs a collaborative approach to the creation of a crisis response plan, this situation is exceedingly unlikely to happen because the clinician checks in with the patient at each step to ensure understanding and buy-in. At this point of the crisis response plan, a patient providing a low rating of motivation and stating that "nothing" will make the plan more useful suggests the possibility of severe hopelessness and cognitive rigidity. The clinician can address this issue by calling attention to the seeming discrepancy between the patient's earlier indications that certain strategies were practical and useful, as compared to his or her current assertion that nothing will work. For example:

> I'll admit I'm a bit confused at the moment. As we were putting this plan together, you indicated that many of these strategies have worked for you before and would likely be helpful again, but now you're saying that these same strategies won't work. Can you help me understand?

For patients who express severe hopelessness (e.g., "I just don't think anything's going to help"), clinicians should target motivation by asking patients if they would be willing to try these strategies for a brief period of time only rather than an indefinite period of time. For example:

> Given how things have been going in life lately, I can see why you might be skeptical about this. I wonder if you would be open to trying this out for a week to see how it goes, and then we can determine if this is something we want to keep doing or if we want to make some sort of change. Would you be willing to try this out for just a week?

Step 7: Review and Revise the Crisis Response Plan during Each Follow-Up (All BCBT Sessions)

During each follow-up session, new self-management and coping skills (discussed in later chapters) are added to the plan. In the event that a patient loses, misplaces, or throws away his or her crisis response plan, the clinician assists the patient in creating a new plan in session.

Did you use your crisis response plan at all since we last met?

> [If yes:] Tell me what happened and how you used it.
>
> [If no:] Tell me what you would've done if you had needed it.

ILLUSTRATIVE CASE EXAMPLES

Critical to the development of an effective crisis response plan is the clinician's willingness to meet the patient at his or her current state. To this end, clinicians are encouraged to mirror the patient's language when helping them to create a crisis response plan, and to tie the intervention to their personal motives and goals for treatment. In each of our three case studies, we provide partial transcripts of treatment sessions to demonstrate how the clinicians customized the standardized set of procedures that comprise the crisis response plan to the unique needs of each individual patient.

The Case of John

Upon completing the case conceptualization, the clinician asked John what his goals for treatment were. John's immediate response was directly related to preventing suicidal behavior: "To make sure I never do this again. I don't want to put my wife or family through that ever again." The clinician therefore transitioned to the crisis response plan by tying the intervention to this goal: "Well then, how about we make a plan to reduce the likelihood of you getting that close to suicide again?" John agreed that this would be helpful. The clinician provided John with an index card and they proceeded to develop a crisis response plan together. John's crisis response plan is displayed in Figure 10.1.

The Case of Mike

As was initially described in Chapter 2, during Mike's initial consultation appointment he reported numerous symptoms of depression, heavy alcohol use, agitation, and several other risk factors. He denied suicidal thoughts or behaviors, however. Nonetheless, Mike's presentation led his clinician to assess his risk for suicide as high, which prompted the clinician to forgo the typical intake interview in order to complete a narrative assessment and a crisis response plan. Because Mike denied suicide ideation and became upset when the issue of suicide was raised, the clinician introduced the crisis response plan as a strategy for helping him to manage his emotions when feeling they were "out of control" rather than introducing the crisis response plan as a suicide prevention procedure: "Given you feel that your emotions are out of control, I'm wondering if you would be interested in talking about some strategies you could start using right away to feel a bit more in control?" By presenting the crisis response plan in this way, the clinician was able to move into the intervention while avoiding a potential power struggle. When constructing his crisis response plan, Mike was

```
┌─────────────────────────────────────────────────────┐
│  Warning Signs:  pacing                               │
│                                                       │
│                  feeling irritable                    │
│                                                       │
│                  thinking "it'll never get better"    │
├─────────────────────────────────────────────────────┤
│  • go for a walk 10 mins                              │
│  • watch Friends episodes                             │
│  • play with my dog                                   │
│  • think about my kids                                │
│     —vacation to beach in Florida                     │
│     —Christmas Day 2012                               │
│  • call/text my Mom                                   │
│    or Jennifer                                        │
│  • call Dr. Brown: 555-555-5555                       │
│     —leave msg w/name, time, phone #                  │
│  • 1-800-273-TALK                                     │
│  • go to hospital                                     │
│  • call 911                                           │
└─────────────────────────────────────────────────────┘
```

FIGURE 10.1. John's initial crisis response plan.

highly engaged in the process and quickly identified self-management strategies, reasons for living, and sources of social support. Over the course of BCBT, this plan was updated and modified several times from the version of the crisis response plan that was developed in this initial consultation session.

Mike's initial crisis response plan included four warning signs: crying, getting angry, wanting to hit things, and arguments with his wife. When asked what he has found helpful in his life for managing stress or distracting himself during difficult times, Mike quickly identified four self-management strategies: playing video games, doing woodworking in the garage, going for a walk, and practicing a breathing exercise that he had learned during martial arts many years before. With regard to sources of social support, Mike indicated he could call his friend Bill. The clinician then provided his own office phone number and the National Suicide Prevention Lifeline phone number, and reminded Mike that he could call 911 or go to the hospital. At the next session (Session 2 of BCBT), Mike reported that he had had another argument with his wife and went to go play video games, but this only angered his wife more because she felt that Mike was disengaging from the argument. Mike and his clinician therefore agreed that this option should be removed from the list; it was therefore crossed out. Over the course of subsequent sessions, Mike identified additional self-management strategies that were added to the crisis response plan: photography, writing, playing games on his phone (an option that was acceptable to his wife), and listening to music. This latter option was subsequently qualified when Mike came to session and reported that he had listened to music on one occasion but felt worse. The clinician asked Mike to describe what had happened. During this conversation, Mike explained that he had listened to some "death metal," which increased his anger. The clinician and Mike therefore clarified on his crisis response plan that he would listen to "uplifting" music. Mike's crisis response plan, including all of its modifications and changes, is displayed in Figure 10.2.

1 crying	3 wanting to hit things
2 getting angry	4 argument w/wife

~~1~~ ~~videogames~~	5 photography
2 woodwork in garage	6 writing
3 go for walk	7 games on phone
4 breathing 10 mins	8 listen to music (uplifting)

5 talk to Bill
6 Dr. Smith: 555-555-5555 (voicemail)
7 Hotline: 1-800-273-8255
8 Hospital or 911

FIGURE 10.2. Mike's crisis response plan during the final session of BCBT.

The Case of Janice

When Janice's clinician introduced the topic of the crisis response plan, Janice noted, "I think I already have one of those. I created a plan like that with my last therapist." The clinician acknowledged that this was possible, and asked Janice if she had that plan with her. Janice said she did not, but thought that it was at home. The clinician asked Janice to describe what was on her plan, to which Janice replied, "I think it has some things like playing with my dogs and calling some friends, but I don't really remember." When asked if this plan was helpful, Janice answered, "Sometimes, I guess." The clinician engaged Janice in a dialogue to further explore her thoughts and feelings about her previous crisis response plan, and discovered that she had some ambivalence about its utility and potential effectiveness. The clinician therefore offered to help Janice create a new crisis response plan that might work better for her: "It sounds like there's something about that other plan that may not work as well as you'd like. What do you think about creating a new plan now that might work better for you?" Janice agreed, and together she and her clinician created a new crisis response plan (see Figure 10.3).

In the final step of the crisis response plan, Janice expressed concern about calling 911 or going to a hospital. "I've been hospitalized before and I don't want to do that ever again," she explained. "I'm not going to go to a hospital or call the cops because that's what'll end up happening." The clinician therefore said the following: "I can understand that completely, which is why I usually include these options as the last steps rather than the first or second steps. In my experience, most people don't ever get to these steps because all the others steps work so well, but it's always good to have a safety net just in case. I'm wondering if you would be willing to add this as the final step even if you don't intend to ever use it?" Janice reasserted that she did not intend to call the police or go to a hospital but agreed to include it as the final step of her crisis response plan.

```
avoid others
"What's the point?"
not wanting to get out of bed

get a cup of coffee
listen to jazz music
spend time with my dog
text Michelle
think about kids

call my therapist
555-555-5555
call the crisis line
1-800-273-talk
    press #1 for Veterans
call 911
go to hospital
```

FIGURE 10.3. Janice's crisis response plan.

TIPS AND ADVICE FOR
THE CRISIS RESPONSE PLAN

1. **Handwrite the crisis response plan.** Asking the patient to handwrite his or her own crisis response plan personalizes the intervention and increases the patient's sense of ownership of the plan. By contrast, prefabricated crisis response plans are generally perceived as irrelevant or unhelpful. Crisis response plans that are typed and then printed also tend to receive less favorable feedback than handwritten plans and may have reduced efficacy.

2. **Use index cards instead of full sheets of paper.** Although a crisis response plan can be created using almost any type or size of paper, index cards seem to work better than full-size sheets of paper because the compact size of an index card lends itself to convenience (e.g., placement in pockets or purses). When crisis response plans are written on full sheets of paper, patients usually fold them up several times to place them in a convenient location, which seems to reduce the perceived importance of the plan.

3. **Avoid fill-in-the-blank templates.** Preprinted, fill-in-the-blank crisis response plans are generally discouraged for several reasons. First, these plans are generally perceived by patients as less personal or "customized." Second, patients who are unable to identify several (or any) items to include in each section are left with empty spaces on their crisis response plans. These empty spaces can serve to reinforce these patients' perceptions about what is lacking or missing in their lives, which can be counterproductive (e.g., "I

should have three people to call but only have one"; "I really am alone"). Third, preliminary data suggest that this approach may be less effective.

4. **When patients are unable to identify warning signs or self-management strategies, use visual cues and menus to help.** Some patients will struggle to create the crisis response plan because they lack the ability to effectively identify when they are approaching an acute emotional crisis and/or are unaware of how they can effectively manage these crises. In the former situation, patients are often unable to identify or list their warning signs. The clinician can often get around this barrier by providing a list of possible warning signs from which the patient can choose or select items that apply to him or her. A sample list of possible warning signs is provided in Appendix B.4. Likewise, when the patient is unable to identify self-management strategies for emotional crises, the clinician can provide a list of possible self-management strategies and ask the patient to identify one or two that have worked for him or her in the past. A sample list of self-management strategies is provided in Appendix B.5.

5. **Include only skills that are within the patient's ability level.** When identifying self-management strategies, the clinician should ensure the listed activities are within the patient's ability level. For instance, "relaxation" should not be listed as a self-management strategy unless the patient can effectively use this skill. The clinician can gauge the patient's skill level by asking the patient to describe (or demonstrate) how he or she uses the strategy to manage stress. The clinician should be careful not to overestimate the patient's capabilities, even with respect to relatively "simple" or basic self-management skills.

PART III

PHASE ONE

Emotion Regulation and Crisis Management

CHAPTER 11

Treatment Planning and the Commitment to Treatment Statement

The treatment plan outlines the problems to be targeted in treatment, the goals and objectives for treatment, behavioral indicators or methods for measuring progress, the interventions to be used to achieve these objectives, and the estimated number of sessions to accomplish these objectives. The treatment plan is developed based on mutual agreement among the clinician and patient and serves to guide the treatment process over time. The treatment plan typically contains several fundamental sections or components: the problem description, goals and objectives, interventions, the estimated number of sessions, and outcome. An example of a treatment plan template can be found in Appendix A.3.

Once the written treatment plan has been formalized, the clinician should introduce the commitment to treatment statement (see Appendix A.4). The commitment to treatment statement is a brief intervention designed to increase the patient's motivation and willingness to engage in treatment, and to collaboratively define the parameters for the treatment process. The primary purpose of the intervention is to facilitate an open discussion about how treatment is defined and what that definition means for both the patient and the clinician. In addition, the commitment to treatment statement provides the foundation for explaining to the patient how the clinician will respond to various forms of nonadherence or lack of engagement on the part of the patient, one of the essential elements of effective treatments for preventing suicide attempts. The commitment to treatment provides a framework for operationalizing adherence (and by extension, nonadherence) and establishes from the outset how the clinician and patient will respond to instances of nonadherence.

RATIONALE

From a clinical perspective, the treatment plan provides essential structure to the treatment process, a characteristic that is especially important when working with high-risk patients, who often have chaotic lives and struggle to regulate emotions. In many ways the treatment plan delineates the starting line, the finish line, and the boundaries of treatment, thereby enabling both the patient and the clinician to maintain a clear focus on the goals and objectives of treatment and a manner for assessing progress (or lack thereof) toward those goals. From a legal perspective, the treatment plan also serves to document the clinician's thought process specific to clinical decision making and the logic underlying the chosen interventions and the sequence in which they were introduced. The treatment plan thereby speaks to the notion of reasonable care, which relates to the legal concept of the standard of care. As discussed previously in this manual, reasonable care implies that the clinician makes treatment decisions that are consistent with the decision making of other mental health care professionals with similar training and experience (Berman, 2006). Without a documented treatment plan, it is generally assumed that no plan existed, again under the assumption that "if it isn't documented, it didn't happen," which suggests the clinician has not met generally accepted practice standards.

When complete, the treatment plan should provide an overview of the treatment process and map out the logic behind the selected interventions. The identification and prioritization of problems should lead directly to the intended goals and objectives of the treatment. Next, interventions should be selected based on their ability to achieve these goals within a designated window of time. Finally, the efficacy of these interventions should be assessed at a predetermined time to establish whether or not progress is being made and/or if any changes to the plan are warranted.

The commitment to treatment statement is intended to enhance the patient's commitment to the treatment process and the commitment to *living,* as opposed to asking the patient to give up his or her right to die by suicide. As was discussed previously, patients often feel that their personal autonomy and sense of control over their lives is restricted or impinged upon by clinicians, which can reduce their motivation to fully and openly disclose suicidal thoughts and behaviors. In reality, the patient *can* kill him- or herself or, conversely, can choose not to kill him- or herself. The commitment to treatment implicitly acknowledges this (harsh) reality, and embraces the patient's autonomy by framing BCBT as the process of learning how to live a life worth living, Committing to live sends a very different message to the patient about control and individual responsibility, both explicitly and implicitly: the focus of BCBT is not on restraining or restricting the patient's right to choose, but rather it is on recovery.

Asking the patient to voice his or her expectations for treatment also provides the clinician with the opportunity to engage in a collaborative dialogue about any unrealistic expectations the patient might hold. If, for example, the patient states the expectation that he or she should not ever be hospitalized, this reflects an unrealistic expectation for treatment. In this situation, the clinician can help the patient to revise this expectation so that it is more realistic while remaining acceptable to the patient. For instance, the clinician might use this request as an opportunity to educate the patient about the process by which the decision to hospitalize the patient is made:

SAMPLE CLINICIAN SCRIPT

Although I cannot promise to never hospitalize you, I can promise you that I will work with you to maximize outpatient safety at all times, which would reduce the likelihood that we would need to pursue hospitalization. Let's talk a little bit about how I make decisions about hospitalization. For me, hospitalization is the "last stop," so to speak, not the first. Brief cognitive-behavioral therapy is an outpatient treatment, and I'm committed to that approach. In BCBT we don't have to hospitalize patients very often, but every once in a while it's necessary to help keep them safe during especially high-risk periods. If you ever experience a time like that, you and I will have a conversation about your safety together so that you're able to be a part of the process. In our work together, we'll use this flowchart to make decisions about hospitalization. As long you and I are able to work together to develop plans that can keep us from getting to this last stop, we probably won't have to get to hospitalization, but we can't take it off the table completely. What are your thoughts about this decision-making process? Is that similar to or different from what you've experienced in treatment before?

When completed effectively, the commitment to treatment statement can be a useful tool for the clinician later on in the treatment process should the patient drop out of treatment early or become nonadherent. Premature dropout tends to occur at the end of the first phase of treatment (i.e., around Session 5 or 6). At this point in treatment, the patient has often experienced symptom relief and the presenting problem has sufficiently resolved that continuing treatment is perceived to be unnecessary. Reviewing the commitment to treatment statement can be a useful strategy for motivating the patient to reengage fully with the therapy. Because of patients' tendency to drop out of therapy early, the clinician can even raise the issue of premature termination as a point of discussion during the initial review of the commitment to treatment statement.

TROUBLESHOOTING TIPS

What if the patient becomes nonadherent during BCBT? Nonadherence can manifest in BCBT in several ways, the most common of which include no-showing for appointments, failure to complete homework assignments or to practice skills as recommended, and discontinuation of medication. If these behaviors emerge during the course of BCBT, clinicians should ask about the behaviors directly and help the patient to problem-solve any barriers to full adherence. For example:

Did something get in the way of your completing your practice assignment this week? Would it be helpful to change something about the plan so that you can practice it more? For example, should we change how many times you do it, what time of day you do it, or where you do it?

What if the patient remains nonadherent? If a patient continues to demonstrate nonadherence (e.g., persistently failing to complete practice assignments), the clinician should invite the patient to reconcile the discrepancies among these behaviors, the treatment plan, and his or her commitment to treatment. For example:

> We've talked several times about barriers to completing your practice assignments, but it seems like this continues to be an issue. It may be helpful to review the goals we established at the outset of treatment and our commitment to treatment. If we review our treatment plan and commitment to treatment, how would you say practice assignments fit with them? How do you think we're doing with respect to this plan and this commitment?

What if the Patient Drops Out of BCBT Early? If a patient discontinues BCBT earlier than planned or expected, the clinician should contact the patient and invite the patient to share his or her thoughts about continued participation in treatment. The clinician can also review the treatment plan and commitment to treatment statement and ask the patient to describe how early dropout aligns with each. For example:

> When we first started working together, we agreed that we would prioritize your risk for suicide, your depression, your sleep problems, and your sense of self-worth. How would you say we're doing on these goals? Would you say that we've achieved these goals? We also made an agreement that outlined how we would work together. Let's go through this together to see how we're doing there. The first item we agreed to was attending appointments. How would you say that's going? The second item we agreed to was setting goals. How would you say that's going?

The clinician can continue to go through the commitment to treatment statement to assess the patient's perceptions of treatment progress. In many cases, this review of the treatment plan and commitment to treatment statement will encourage the patient to reengage in treatment. In other cases, patients may express the desire to discontinue BCBT prematurely despite the use of motivational enhancement techniques. If the patient is unwilling or uninterested in continuing BCBT despite these attempts to reengage, the clinician should inform that patient that he or she can reengage treatment again in the future, and then document the content of this conversation, including a description of the specific procedures and strategies used by the clinician in an attempt to reengage the patient.

HOW TO DO IT

The problem description section of the treatment plan lists concise descriptions of the primary problems that will receive attention in treatment. In BCBT, the primary problem is always "suicide risk" because treatments that do not explicitly focus on suicide risk as the primary outcome are less effective for preventing suicide attempts. Additional problems should be identified and prioritized in collaboration with the patient (e.g., insomnia, depression, substance use, relationship problems).

The goals and objectives section outlines the intended outcome(s) associated with each problem. Specific to suicide risk, the primary goal in BCBT is to "reduce risk for suicide attempts." The clinician is cautioned against establishing "zero suicide ideation" or "no thoughts of suicide" as a treatment goal, as this may not be a realistic outcome for some patients, especially those who are chronically suicidal and experience high-frequency, low-intensity suicidal thoughts. For chronically suicidal individuals, thinking about suicide has become such an overlearned cognitive response to internal and external triggers that complete elimination is impractical or infeasible; setting this as a goal could therefore facilitate hopelessness and despair, thereby increasing risk and the likelihood of an adverse outcome. For secondary problems in treatment (e.g., depression, insomnia), treatment goals might include "reduced depression" or "increase hours of sleep per night." When setting treatment goals, the clinician should ensure that goals are specific and measurable, so they can be objectively assessed over time. For example, "feeling better" is not sufficiently specific and may be hard to measure accurately, whereas "feeling less depressed as indicated by decreased scores on a depression symptom checklist" is both specific and measurable.

In the interventions section, the treatment plan should list specific interventions and strategies designed to directly address each identified problem. In this section, the clinician selects those interventions from the BCBT protocol that appropriately address each identified problem. For the primary problem of suicide risk, the clinician lists the crisis response plan; for patients reporting sleep disturbance, the clinician can list sleep hygiene and stimulus control; for patients reporting depression, the clinician can list activity planning and cognitive restructuring; and so on. Because BCBT does not preclude the receipt of other indicated forms of treatment, the clinician should also consider the addition of treatment and intervention options external to BCBT, such as psychiatric medication, substance abuse treatment, and group therapy.

The clinician next provides an estimated time frame for accomplishing each goal. In the case of suicide risk, the clinician should list 12 sessions, which is the average number of sessions in the BCBT protocol. For secondary problems, the clinician can list the anticipated number of sessions dedicated to each problem. In the case of insomnia, for instance, the clinician might designate two sessions, one for the initial introduction and education about sleep hygiene and stimulus control, and one for a follow-up review of these issues.

The final section of the treatment plan is designed to assess progress toward the stated goal, whether fully achieved, partially achieved, or unachieved. Outcome assessment should be conducted at the mutually established time of the planned review of treatment progress, which usually occurs at or around the time of the 12th session of BCBT.

The clinician then provides the patient with a copy of the commitment to treatment and invites him or her to read each of the bullets out loud. The bulleted statements on the commitment to treatment statement outline several behavioral indicators of patient adherence including regular attendance, setting goals, honest disclosure of thoughts and feelings, completing assignments, and taking medications as prescribed. The clinician discusses each of these points individually and invites the patient to share his or her thoughts about each point, as this process can often elicit information regarding the patient's perceptions or beliefs about treatment, and his or her past experiences (both good and bad) in mental health therapy. In addition to outlining expectations for the patient, the clinician should also ask the patient to identify any expectations he or she might have for the treatment process as a whole and the clinician in particular.

Step 1: Explain the Rationale for a Treatment Plan

The clinician introduces the notion of a treatment plan and briefly explains its utility for maintaining focus in treatment for both the clinician and the patient.

SAMPLE CLINICIAN SCRIPT

An important part of treatment is making sure that you and I agree upon what we're trying to accomplish and how to get there, and whether or not we're making adequate progress. I'd therefore like for us to create a treatment plan together. The purpose of the treatment plan is to write down our plan of action. This plan will list out the most important problems we want to focus on, what we want to change about those problems, and the specific strategies we're going to use to solve those problems. We'll also talk about how we'll know if you've reached your goals. We'll write this plan down so we can refer back to it later on. Would that be OK with you?

Step 2: Prioritize Suicide Risk

The clinician explains that the primary treatment goal is to reduce the patient's risk for suicide and elicits the patient's buy-in regarding the prioritization of outpatient safety.

SAMPLE CLINICIAN SCRIPT

The first problem that we'll be working is suicide risk, which may not be much of a surprise to you. I want to prioritize this issue since we need to ensure your safety and also because we won't make much progress on any other problems if you die by suicide. What are your thoughts about prioritizing safety?

Given this is the primary problem, I would suggest our goal should be to reduce your risk for making a suicide attempt. What do you think? In order to achieve this goal, we'll primarily use your crisis response plan. We'll work on improving and refining your crisis response plan over the course of the entire treatment, so I would estimate that it'll take us about 12 sessions to achieve this goal. Does that sound acceptable to you?

TROUBLESHOOTING TIPS

What if the patient says he or she wants to prioritize other issues over safety? If patients express a strong desire to list problems other than suicide risk or safety as the primary treatment goals, clinicians should ask them how they would rank-order all of their treatment goals, including safety, and then describe their rationale for this ordering. Clinicians can also ask patients to describe how safety is relevant to their other goals. For example:

I can see how and why these other goals are so important to you. If you were to rank these goals and safety in order of importance, how would you rank them? What are your reasons for ranking things in this order? What role would you say safety plays in achieving your goals?

In many cases, this line of questioning will help patients to recognize how safety may be a precondition for their other goals, thereby increasing its relative ranking. If a patient acknowledges that safety is an important treatment goal but persists in prioritizing other goals over safety, clinicians should accept the patient's preference and list safety after his or her other goals. This avoids the potential for causing harm to the therapeutic alliance.

What if the patient says he or she doesn't want to prioritize safety at all? If a patient is unwilling to include safety as a treatment goal or precondition in any capacity, the clinician should engage the patient in a discussion about the appropriateness of outpatient treatment. Because outpatient treatment requires a reasonable level of safety for the patient, safety issues cannot be ignored. If the patient is unwilling to address and/or commit to safety-related issues, a higher level of care (e.g., partial hospitalization, inpatient hospitalization) may be more appropriate.

Step 3: Identify and Collaboratively Establish Additional Treatment Goals

The clinician invites the patient to identify his or her own personal treatment goals. These goals are collaboratively prioritized and the clinician matches BCBT interventions that directly address each goal. For example, if the patient expresses the desire to reduce depression, the clinician could select activity planning, ABC Worksheets, and Challenging Questions Worksheets to address depression-related symptoms. Examples of how to connect BCBT interventions to common patient goals are provided in Table 11.1.

SAMPLE CLINICIAN SCRIPT

Now let's talk about and prioritize a few other problems to work on. We've talked about a number of problems in your life; which of these problems would you say is most important to you to fix? What would you like to be different about this problem? If I were to see you in everyday life and just sort of walk past you on the street, how would I know if this problem is solved? What would you be doing differently that you're not doing now?

TABLE 11.1. BCBT Procedures That Match with Common Patient-Identified Goals

Patient goal	Crisis Response Plan	Sleep Stimulus Control	Relaxation Skills Training	Mindfulness Skills Training	Reasons for Living/ Survival Kit	ABC Worksheet	Challenging Questions Worksheet	Patterns of Problematic Thinking Worksheet	Activity Planning	Coping Cards
Reduce depression	X			X	X	X	X	X	X	X
Reduce anxiety/agitation	X		X	X		X	X	X	X	X
Reduce anger	X		X	X		X	X	X	X	X
Increase positive mood	X			X	X	X	X	X	X	X
Improve sleep		X	X	X						
Improve relationships					X	X	X	X	X	
Increase energy		X							X	
Reduce alcohol consumption	X			X		X	X	X	X	X
Improve self-worth						X	X	X	X	X
Improve stress management	X		X	X		X	X	X	X	X

That's a goal that we can definitely work on together. There's a specific strategy that you and I can work on together to address that. It's called [intervention name]. Let's list that as a part of our treatment plan.

The clinician repeats this process for each identified problem.

Step 4: Review the Commitment to Treatment Statement

The clinician provides a copy of the commitment to treatment statement to the patient and invites him or her to read it out loud, one section at a time, so it can be discussed collaboratively. After each bullet, the clinician asks the patient to describe his or her reactions to that particular bullet and addresses any concern the patient might have.

SAMPLE CLINICIAN SCRIPT

Now that we've developed a formal plan of action for working together, I'd like to talk just a little bit about our expectations for the treatment process and accomplishing these goals. This document is called a commitment to treatment statement, and it outlines a number of things that contribute to faster and better outcomes in treatment. I'd like us to read each of these bullets together and then talk about them one by one so we make sure we're on the same page. Why don't you go ahead and read the first sentence there and the first statement underneath it.

[Possible open-ended questions to facilitate discussion:]

What are your thoughts about that?

Does that seem reasonable to you?

Is that something you think you could commit to?

What would make it hard to commit to that item?

What has been your experience with this issue in past treatment you've received?

[When the patient reaches item #9:] In this section we will add any expectations that you have about treatment or of me as your clinician. What do you expect from me as a part of us working together?

ILLUSTRATIVE CASE EXAMPLES

Sample treatment plans for John, Mike, and Janice are provided in Figure 11.1. (See Appendix A.3 for a blank version of this treatment plan template, which the clinician can copy and use with patients.) As can be seen, suicide risk is prioritized for all three cases, and the crisis response plan is listed as the primary intervention. Means restriction, which will be discussed in detail in Chapter 12, is added as an intervention for John and Mike because of their ownership of firearms. Secondary treatment goals target risk factors that contribute directly to each patient's suicide risk; the specific order of these treatment goals are selected

				Estimated No. of	
Treatment Plan for: *John*					
Problem No.	**Problem Description**	**Goals/Objectives**	**Intervention**	**Estimated No. of Sessions**	**Outcome**
1.	Suicide risk	Reduce risk for suicide attempts	Crisis response plan, means restriction	12	
2.	Low self-esteem	Reduce self-criticism as indicated by reductions in Suicide Cognitions Scale score	ABC Worksheets, Challenging Questions Worksheets	5	
3.	Insomnia	Improve sleep quality as indicated by reductions in Insomnia Severity Scale score	Sleep stimulus control, relaxation	2	

Outcome: 0—Not accomplished, 1—Partially accomplished, 2—Accomplished

				Estimated No. of	
Treatment Plan for: *Mike*					
Problem No.	**Problem Description**	**Goals/Objectives**	**Intervention**	**Estimated No. of Sessions**	**Outcome**
1.	Suicide risk	Reduce risk for suicide attempts	Crisis response plan, means restriction	12	
2.	Alcohol use	Reduce alcohol consumption to < 5 drinks per week	Referral to substance abuse tx, relaxation, cognitive reappraisal	12	
3.	Relationship problems	Improve marriage quality as indicated by 10-point improvement on relationship satisfaction questionnaire	Crisis support plan, activity planning, cognitive reappraisal	5	

Outcome: 0—Not accomplished, 1—Partially accomplished, 2—Accomplished

(continued)

FIGURE 11.1. Sample treatment plan templates for John, Mike, and Janice.

Treatment Plan for: *Janice*					
Problem No.	Problem Description	Goals/Objectives	Intervention	Estimated No. of Sessions	Outcome
1.	*Suicide risk*	*Reduce risk for suicide attempts*	*Crisis response plan, means restriction*	*12*	
2.	*Stress management*	*Increase ability to manage stress*	*Relaxation, ABC Worksheets, Challenging Questions Worksheets*	*7*	
3.	*Improve self-worth*	*Reduce self-criticism*	*ABC Worksheets, Challenging Questions Worksheets*	*4*	

Outcome: 0—Not accomplished, 1—Partially accomplished, 2—Accomplished

FIGURE 11.1. *(continued)*

based on each patient's preferred prioritization scheme. In all cases, specific interventions from the BCBT protocol are selected for each of these goals, and the anticipated number of sessions that will be dedicated to each problem is recorded. In the case of John, referral to a substance abuse treatment program is recommended in addition to BCBT.

The Case of Mike

As noted in earlier chapters, Mike was reluctant to report suicidal thoughts and intentions despite making statements strongly implying that he was indeed experiencing such thoughts (i.e., "I should just do it"). The clinician asked some follow-up questions about this statement, but Mike continued to deny suicidal intent. Despite this, the clinician assessed his risk to be elevated and included suicide risk as a treatment priority. Below is a partial transcript of their treatment planning discussion. Note how the clinician respects Mike's autonomy while navigating the delicate issue of identifying suicide risk as a treatment priority despite Mike's discomfort with the topic:

CLINICIAN: What I'd like to do next is develop a treatment plan. A treatment plan is basically our written agreement about what we'll be trying to accomplish together and how we plan to get there. Treatment plans can also provide us with a way to determine if we're making progress or if we're off track. Does that make sense?

MIKE: Yeah, that makes sense.

CLINICIAN: OK, good. What we'll want to do here is list the most important problems or issues. Once we have that list, I can make recommendations about the specific things we should do to target those issues. What would you say are your primary goals for working together? What would you most like to work on or change?

MIKE: Definitely cutting back on my drinking. If I could stop drinking, that would solve a lot of my problems.

CLINICIAN: OK, that makes a lot of sense, given what we've talked about already. Let me ask a question to make sure I fully understand your goal here. Are you wanting to completely stop drinking alcohol altogether, or are you thinking more along the lines of cutting back on drinking?

MIKE: Stopping altogether. I gotta stop drinking, otherwise I'll keep having problems with my wife.

CLINICIAN: Yeah, OK. So no drinking at all. What about on the weekends when you guys are at a barbeque with friends, or you're watching the football game on TV? Are you wanting to avoid drinking then, too, or would it be OK to have a couple of beers in those situations?

MIKE: Well, I think it would be OK to have a few beers with friends, or even a glass of wine for dinner. I don't have any problems when I'm doing that. It's when I'm by myself and am drinking a whole lot that things are a problem.

CLINICIAN: OK, that makes sense. I just wanted to make sure we were on the same page because some people want to stop drinking completely but others have a different goal.

MIKE: Yeah, I understand. I appreciate that. It's good to be clear because if my wife and I go out for dinner or hang out with friends and I have something to drink, I would probably get really down on myself when that's really not the problem I'm having.

CLINICIAN: Right, that's what I'm thinking, too. So what should we set as our goal?

MIKE: Well, if I have only a few drinks on the weekend or have a drink at dinner, that shouldn't be more than five drinks total during a week.

CLINICIAN: OK, so we want to set as your goal to drink less than five drinks per week?

MIKE: Yeah.

CLINICIAN: Do you think five is a realistic number?

MIKE: Yeah, because we only have wine with dinner maybe once a week, and then if we go out or go visit friends, drinking only three or four drinks is a good number. I don't get out of control and it's sort of a social thing.

CLINICIAN: OK, five it is. What else would you say is a goal you're hoping to accomplish?

MIKE: I want to improve my relationship with my wife.

CLINICIAN: OK, that makes sense. We can definitely do that. If your relationship were to improve, what would be different about it?

MIKE: Well, I guess we would fight less often and I would feel better about the relationship and feel happier.

CLINICIAN: Mm-hmmm, OK. Well, maybe one thing we can do to track our progress is have you fill out a brief questionnaire that asks about marriage quality. Some of the items ask about disagreements and arguments, so that's relevant to what you're talking about, and other items ask about satisfaction and feeling close to your partner. Since the questionnaire has been used in a lot of different studies, we can use the overall score as a benchmark for improvement. An increase of 10 points, for instance, is typically used as an indicator of significant and meaningful improvement in relationship quality. What do you think about using a questionnaire like that to track your progress on this goal?

MIKE: That makes sense. I can do that.

CLINICIAN: OK, then let's include that as a treatment goal. Any other goals?

MIKE: Well, I guess I have other goals but I kind of feel like if I fix these problems the other problems will get better. Like anger is another problem, but I know that I get angry mostly when I'm arguing with my wife. If we can improve our marriage, then I wouldn't be so angry all the time, you know?

CLINICIAN: That makes sense to me. We'll keep anger in mind, but like you said, it may make more sense to focus on these goals first.

MIKE: Yeah.

CLINICIAN: OK, this sounds great. There is another goal I'd like for us to work on, if you'd be willing to entertain another possibility?

MIKE: Sure.

CLINICIAN: I'd like for us to also work on addressing suicide risk, and to lower your risk for suicide.

MIKE: Well, like I said before, that's not really an issue for me.

CLINICIAN: Right, I remember you saying that you haven't had any suicidal thoughts and haven't attempted suicide before, so I can see why it might be confusing that I'm bringing up this issue.

MIKE: Yeah.

CLINICIAN: Well, let me explain my reasoning. You've described a whole lot of stress in your life lately: anger, sleep problems, worry, self-criticism, sadness, relationship problems, and financial strain. You've also talked about how you feel out of control of your emotions, especially when drinking a lot. All of these problems increase the likelihood of suicide, even among people who haven't been thinking about suicide. My guess is that you've heard about people who die by suicide having these types of these problems?

MIKE: Yeah, I've heard of that, but I wouldn't ever do that.

CLINICIAN: Well I'm glad to hear that. The challenge is that a lot of people who think about suicide or try to kill themselves feel like they would never do it, but when things get out of control and they're having all these problems, they sort of forget about that. So what I'd like to do is keep this issue on our minds even if it's not a major problem for you right now, so that we prevent it becoming an issue in the future. It's sort of like how we plan ahead to prevent bad outcomes even if we're not in a bad situation now.

MIKE: Like how?

CLINICIAN: Let's use alcohol as an example. Most people don't plan to get into car accidents when they've been drinking. I can't think of anyone who says to themselves, "I'm going to drink and then drive and then get into an accident." Because most of us don't want this to happen, we plan ahead and take steps to avoid it, even if we're not drinking at that moment. Before we go out to the bars, for instance, we identify a designated driver or we plan to take a taxi home. We put this plan into place before we start drinking in order to avoid drinking-related issues later on, right?

MIKE: Yeah, I guess so.

CLINICIAN: We can do the same with suicide. Maybe you're not struggling with suicidal thoughts right now, but like you said, the problems you're having are common among people who do struggle with these thoughts. So what I'm proposing is that we monitor this and make sure we have a plan in place as a safety precaution, just like we plan ahead when we're going out drinking with friends. Does that make sense?

MIKE: Yeah, it does. I just don't know . . .

CLINICIAN: It sounds like you're uncomfortable with this topic.

MIKE: I'm not uncomfortable with the topic, I'm just not sure if we need to write this down on my paperwork.

CLINICIAN: Oh, I see. Well, let me ask this: What do you think would happen if we were to include suicide risk as a treatment goal?

MIKE: Well, that means there's something really screwed up with me and people will want to lock me up. I can't afford to get locked up in a hospital. That would ruin my job, put me in debt, and all sorts of issues.

CLINICIAN: So if we include suicide risk as a treatment goal, you're worried that you'll be hospitalized, which has a whole lot of negative consequences?

MIKE: Yeah, definitely.

CLINICIAN: OK, that makes sense to me. Maybe it would helpful then to talk about how I make decisions about hospitalizing patients for suicide risk?

MIKE: Yeah, that would be really good. I've been wondering about that.

CLINICIAN: OK, no problem. Well, the simple answer is that it all comes down to safety. As we've discussed already, we'll track your progress every time we meet, typically with symptom scales and other questionnaires designed to see how well you're doing. We'll also talk every time we meet about how things are going, if the strategies we're learning and practicing are helpful, and so on. Based on this combination of information, I'll make a decision about the safety of treatment. If it seems as though our work provides sufficient safety, then we'll continue meeting on an outpatient basis. If it seems as though your risk has increased so much that safety no longer seems likely, that's when I would recommend hospitalization. Now, it's important to keep in mind, first, that there's a lot of room between meeting once a week and being hospitalized. You and I might decide, for example, that we should meet twice a week or maybe three times a week to help get you through a bad patch, or maybe we'll have phone calls in between our meetings to check in and provide you support. I generally prefer to do this before jumping to hospitalization. No matter what, we'll always talk about these decisions together; I wouldn't make the decision without your input and thoughts. The reason I

PHASE ONE: EMOTION REGULATION AND CRISIS MANAGEMENT

do this is because I know that you'll get better faster if you're fully on board with treatment and we're working together as a team. Does that make sense?

MIKE: So you don't just decide to hospitalize people against their will?

CLINICIAN: I've actually never had to do that. I have recommended hospitalization before, but when I did, it was only after the patient and I talked about it and we agreed that it was the best course of action at that time. I've never had to recommend hospitalization against someone's will, and it's something I hope to continue. This is why I raised this issue with you. I've found that when my patients and I are working together to track and monitor suicide risk, even if they're not feeling suicidal at the beginning of treatment, we tend to be on the same page and rarely disagree about treatment decisions.

MIKE: That's interesting.

CLINICIAN: Yeah, it's worked out pretty well. I'll add that I don't see any reason why it would be any different for you.

MIKE: Really?

CLINICIAN: Yeah, really. Does that help explain how I go about making decisions about hospitalization?

MIKE: Yeah, that's really helpful.

CLINICIAN: OK, good. I'm glad we hashed that out.

MIKE: Me too.

CLINICIAN: So now that we've talked about that in detail, I'm wondering what your thoughts are about us including suicide risk as one of our treatment goals?

MIKE: It makes sense. Even though it's not an issue now, it could be in the future, so it's probably best for us to have a plan in place.

CLINICIAN: I agree. We've already done a few things to address this issue, but let's talk about some other things we could also do.

In this exchange, the clinician opened the topic of treatment planning by inviting Mike to articulate his personal treatment goals rather than immediately pushing for suicide risk as a treatment goal, a move that would have likely been met with reluctance and defensiveness. Once Mike's priorities were identified, the clinician raised the issue of suicide risk by asking for Mike's permission to introduce a new goal. When Mike expressed concern about this issue, the clinician did not show defensiveness in return, but rather responded with openness and transparency. This led to the identification of Mike's concern regarding hospitalization. Once this was identified, the clinician invited Mike to describe his specific concerns about hospitalization and then engaged him in a frank discussion about clinical decision making, again demonstrating a high level of transparency. Such transparency conveys respect for the patient, as it communicates that he or she is seen as an autonomous individual with legitimate concerns that are treated with respect. The clinician further communicated respect for Mike's autonomy by clearly explaining that Mike will be involved in treatment decisions rather than being the passive recipient of the clinician's decision making. This reduced Mike's anxiety and enabled him and the clinician to include suicide risk as a treatment goal despite his lack of endorsement of suicidal thoughts or behaviors. By respecting Mike's position and his experience, the clinician has enlisted Mike as an ally in the shared goal of suicide prevention without coercion.

TIPS AND ADVICE FOR TREATMENT PLANNING AND COMMITMENT TO TREATMENT STATEMENTS

1. **Prioritize suicide risk, but not at the expense of patient autonomy.** BCBT prioritizes suicide risk as its primary treatment, and clinicians are encouraged to explicitly document this on the treatment plan. However, BCBT does not require that suicide risk be listed at the top of the treatment plan in all cases. If a patient insists on prioritizing another goal above suicide risk, the clinician should follow his or her lead. Preserving the therapeutic alliance and keeping the patient engaged is more important than writing the words "suicide risk" at the top of a form.

2. **Remember to preserve and respect patient autonomy.** Although the commitment to treatment statement is designed to enhance patient motivation and engagement in treatment, clinicians should not use it as a tool to coerce a patient. Because the commitment to treatment helps frame treatment as a process for developing a meaningful life as opposed to a process for avoiding death, it can be useful to stimulate talk about change and orient the patient toward growth. When used as a tool that restricts autonomy, however, it can actually undermine motivation and engagement.

CHAPTER 12

Means Safety Counseling and the Crisis Support Plan

Means safety counseling, also referred to as means restriction counseling, entails two distinct but interrelated actions (Harvard University School of Public Health, n.d.): (1) assessing whether an individual at risk for suicide has access to a firearm or other lethal means for suicide, and (2) working with the individual and his or her support system to limit access to these means until the individual is no longer feeling suicidal. Of the many interventions and strategies developed to prevent suicide, restriction of access to lethal means has garnered the most empirical support and is arguably the only intervention that has consistently led to reductions in suicide across diverse samples and populations (Bryan, Stone, & Rudd, 2011; Mann et al., 2005). At the population level, means safety is most effective when the means we want to restrict access to is common and is highly lethal (Mann et al., 2005). Although means safety has long been considered an important component of clinical work with suicidal patients, clear guidance and recommendations for discussing means safety with patients have only recently emerged (Britton et al., 2016; Bryan et al., 2011).

Means safety counseling can be complemented by the crisis support plan, an intervention that explicitly incorporates the involvement and support of a significant other in the suicidal patient's life. As a complement to means safety counseling, the crisis support plan is designed to increase the likelihood of patient adherence to risk management strategies and treatment recommendations and to enhance social connectedness between the suicidal patient and a significant other. To complete the crisis support plan, the clinician invites the patient to bring a significant other to attend a session with him or her. Ideally, this significant other is the person the patient identified to help with means safety counseling.

Complete removal of access to lethal means is often desired, but this is not always practical or feasible. Means safety therefore also includes the placement of barriers between suicidal individuals and their preferred or chosen method. For example, use of trigger locks, cable locks, and/or gun safes have been suggested for suicidal individuals who own firearms but are unwilling to remove them from their home (Bryan et al., 2011). In some cases, these barriers can effectively render a method unusable (a trigger lock or cable lock prevents the gun from being fired) or sufficiently inconvenient (storing a gun unloaded in a gun safe with the ammunition stored in a separate location) to allow enough the individual enough time to calm down from his or her crisis.

RATIONALE

Means safety counseling is based on three primary assumptions: (1) periods of acute suicidal distress are brief, (2) additional suicide attempts are unlikely if someone survives a suicidal crisis, and (3) easy access to lethal means is the strongest determinant of suicide attempt outcome (i.e., fatal versus nonfatal). This first assumption aligns with the fluid vulnerability theory, which posits that suicide risk is inherently dynamic over time, with periods of acute risk being relatively brief and time limited, and it is supported by research indicating that the majority of individuals who make a suicide attempt made the final decision to act within 1 hour of the suicide attempt (Simon et al., 2001). More recent data provide even more nuanced information: the final decision regarding the suicide attempt method typically occurs approximately 2 hours prior to the attempt, the final decision regarding the location of the attempt typically occurs approximately 30 minutes prior to the attempt, and the final decision to act typically occurs approximately 5 minutes prior to the attempt (Millner, Lee, & Nock, 2016). Because this narrow window of time makes it impractical for the clinician and supportive others to intervene, means safety procedures can prevent a fatal outcome during a period of intense emotional distress. The second assumption is supported by findings that only 10% of individuals who survive a medically severe suicide attempt later die by suicide (Owens, Horrocks, & House, 2002). This suggests that individuals who survive a suicidal crisis, even a crisis that entails a suicide attempt, are unlikely to make another suicide attempt at all, let alone a fatal attempt.

The third assumption is often surprising to clinicians. Among clinicians, the medical seriousness of a suicide attempt is often presumed to be a function of the severity of the individual's suicidal intent, which is based on the assumption that individuals who possess a very strong desire for suicide will choose more lethal methods. Research does not support this assumption, however: suicidal intent is actually a relatively weak correlate of attempt lethality (Brown, Henriques, Sosdjan, & Beck, 2004; Pirkola, Isometsä, & Lönnqvist, 2003; Swahn & Potter, 2001). A much stronger correlate is ease or convenience of access to the method (Eddleston, Buckley, Gunnell, Dawson, & Konradsen, 2006; Peterson, Peterson, O'Shanick, & Swann, 1985). These findings indicate that suicidal individuals tend to select methods that are readily available to them in their moment of acute distress. From a practical perspective, what this means is that even individuals with relatively mild suicidal intent can nonetheless make a highly lethal attempt if they have access to highly lethal methods (e.g., firearms). Conversely, individuals with relatively severe suicidal intent can make a low-lethality attempt if they only have access to methods with low lethality profiles (e.g., cutting). In short, a suicidal patient cannot die by suicide if he or she does not have the means for doing so, despite the presence of a strong desire or intent for death.

These three assumptions are keenly important when considering firearms, which have an especially high lethality profile. In the United States, firearms are the most commonly used method for suicide, accounting for over half of all suicide deaths. Because easy access to a highly lethal method like firearms can be so dangerous for suicidal individuals, clinicians should screen or ask every patient about the presence of firearms in the home, even if the patient states he or she is considering an alternate method for suicide. This can be accomplished via screening items on intake paperwork or assessment scales, or via direct inquiry by the clinician. Suicidal patients may also report access to firearms during the course of the narrative assessment.

The crisis support plan is designed to build social support and to increase the likelihood of success for other interventions including the crisis response plan and means safety. Relationship problems are among the most common activating events associated with suicide attempts (Bryan & Rudd, 2012; Frey & Cerel, 2015; Smith, Mercy, & Conn, 1988), whereas social support is among one of the most robust factors that reduce risk for suicide attempts (Bryan & Hernandez, 2013; Joiner, 2005). Chronic relationship problems, in particular, are associated with more severe suicidal crises and greater frequency of suicide attempts (Bryan, Clemans, Leeson, & Rudd, 2015). The crisis support plan can be especially helpful for patients who are experiencing strained relationships because it can align the patient and significant other together against the problem of suicide. In some cases it can also function as a method for reducing the negative influence of relationship problems on the patient's emotional state.

HOW TO DO IT: MEANS SAFETY COUNSELING

The general approach to means safety counseling should take into account the strong likelihood of *ambivalence,* a psychological state characterized by mixed, even contradictory, feelings. Specifically, patients may recognize the increased risk from having easy access to potentially lethal methods of suicide but may also feel a strong desire to maintain or preserve their ability to access these methods. That desire may be influenced by a number of factors including sociopolitical views (e.g., belief in the right to bear arms), safety-related assumptions and worldviews (e.g., the desire to protect oneself and one's family), and autonomy (e.g., preserving the option to kill oneself). If the clinician argues too strongly in favor of means safety, the patient is much more likely to take the opposing side by arguing against safety procedures. This tendency is known as "reactance" and is a well-understood principle of ambivalence and behavior change (Britton et al., 2016). The clinician should therefore approach means safety counseling by guiding the patient to argue in favor of safety procedures. This can be accomplished via several relatively simple and straightforward strategies following four core processes of motivational interviewing (Miller & Rollnick, 2012): engaging, focusing, evoking, and planning.

Engaging

At the start of the conversation, the clinician introduces the notion of means safety and invites the patient to openly express his or her initial thoughts about the topic. The clinician should listen carefully to the patient's thoughts and perceptions to obtain critical information about how to best proceed with the discussion and how to best align with the patient against the problem of suicide and access to lethal means. For example, the clinician might engage the patient by asking about firearms in general: "I understand that you are a gun owner. What types of guns do you own?" By opening with a nonthreatening question that invites the patient to share his or her thoughts and perceptions about guns, the clinician can gain useful clues for how to approach the conversation. A patient who describes owning long guns (e.g., rifles, shotguns) for the purposes of hunting and sporting, for instance, may benefit from a different approach than a patient who describes small arms (e.g., handguns, pistols) for the purposes of self-defense and protection. In the former case, safe storage procedures may be seen as more acceptable than the in the latter case.

Focusing

The clinician must ensure that the topic of means safety is directly addressed but should do so in a guiding way that keeps patients engaged in the conversation while maintaining their autonomy. A guiding approach falls between a directive approach (i.e., taking charge of the conversation), which can reduce the patient's willingness to engage in the conversation, and a following approach (i.e., allowing the patient to take charge of the conversation), which can result in the conversation moving completely off of the topic of means safety. For example, a clinician can focus the conversation on the topic of means safety by raising the issue of safety in particular and then asking the patient if he or she would be willing to discuss the topic: "That reminds me of something I wanted to talk about: safety. Would you be willing to talk a bit about the safety procedures you follow as a gun owner?" By raising the issue in this way, the clinician balances taking charge of the conversation without completely relinquishing control. In addition, the clinician invites the patient to discuss what safety procedures he or she has already taken rather than assuming that none have been taken, which could imply that the patient does not value safety.

Evoking

After the patient agrees to discuss means safety, the clinician invites the patient to talk about his or her personal reasons for restricting access. In essence, the clinician sets up a situation in which it is possible for the patient to talk him- or herself into restricting potential means for suicide. For example, the clinician might ask the patient to discuss his or her opinions or thoughts about safe storage procedures: "What are your thoughts about securing or locking up firearms at home?" As a part of this process, it is common for the patient to also want to talk about arguments *against* means safety. The clinician should allow the patient to voice these arguments and then reflect them in a respectful and nonjudgmental way. Sometimes the patient will not be ready to restrict his or her access to potential methods for suicide; in these cases, the clinician should keep in mind that the process of change can take longer for some patients than others, and that change can also occur in between sessions. Simply raising the issue may be an important first step to eventual change. Revisiting the topic during future sessions can ensure the topic remains "on the table," with incremental changes toward means safety being supported over time.

Planning

When the patient starts talking about change, the clinician should introduce the possibility of establishing a written plan to restrict access to means: "A lot of people find it's helpful to write down their safety plan; can I help you to create one for you and your home?" The clinician can introduce the means safety plan and receipt (see Figure 12.1) as a mechanism for developing and documenting a written plan. Similar to any other plan of action that is developed in treatment, the clinician should help the patient set specific goals and identify specific individuals to help enact the plan. In the means safety plan and receipt, the clinician and patient identify someone in the patient's life who will help to enact the safety plan and then verify that the plan was put into place. The clinician and patient write down the mutually agreed-upon plan (e.g., "give firearms to my friend"; "put trigger lock on my gun"; "lock up extra meds in safe and give key to wife") and the conditions under which the safety plan would no longer be needed and/or the patient can regain access to the method. Once the safety plan is enacted, the patient can have the supportive other confirm this by signing the plan.

When conducting means safety counseling, the clinician should aim to provide a menu of options for the patient to choose from. This respects the patient's autonomy and preserves a sense of control over the decision, and also preserves the patient's responsibility for his or her own safety. The clinician should also approach this topic from the perspective of safety promotion as opposed to suicide prevention, as the latter can sometimes be experienced by the patient as a constraint on his or her autonomy. For example, the clinician might talk about "gun safety" as opposed to "restriction of access to guns." Finally, the clinician should consider asking the patient to involve a family member, friend, or another significant other to assist with securing access to lethal means or enhancing their safety. Once a means safety plan is agreed upon, the clinician and patient formalize the plan in writing. The means the safety plan should detail the specific steps to be taken to reduce easy access to potentially lethal means, the person who will assist with the plan, and the conditions under which access to the potential method will be returned. A sample template for the means safety plan can be found in Appendix A.5.

A list of talking points for the clinician to refer to when conducting means safety counseling is provided in Figure 12.1, and is presented as an aid to help clinicians guide their discussion with the patient. As noted above, the efficacy of this approach will increase if the clinician uses evoking strategies that encourage patients to identify and elicit these points themselves rather than their being introduced by the clinician.

1. Suicide desire can increase very rapidly.

2. Having easy access to lethal methods of suicide can be dangerous during crises.

3. Increasing safety by temporarily reducing access to lethal methods can reduce the chance of bad outcomes.

4. If complete removal of a method is not possible, other options can still increase safety:

   a. Giving the method to a trusted friend or family member.

   b. Locking up the method in a way that is difficult to access.

   c. **For firearms:**
      - Dismantle the firearm and give critical piece to a significant other
      - Store the firearm in tamper-proof safe secured by a significant other
      - Store the firearm unloaded, and store the ammunition in a separate location
      - Use a trigger lock or cable lock

5. Hiding unlocked means (especially firearms) is not sufficient since hidden items can be found with minimal difficulty.

6. In the case of joint custody situations for children or adolescents who are suicidal, ensure that lethal means are secured in all homes regularly visited by the patient.

7. Involving a family member or friend to help enact the safety plan can increase the likelihood of success.

FIGURE 12.1. Recommended talking points for means safety counseling.

Step 1: Raise the Issue of Outpatient Safety and Screen for Access to Firearms

The clinician initiates means safety counseling from the perspective of maximizing outpatient safety.

SAMPLE CLINICIAN SCRIPT

We've talked quite a bit about what's been going on your life lately and the problems you've been facing. I appreciate you being willing to share all of that with me, even though it hasn't been easy. Given all that's been going on lately, I wonder if you'd be willing to talk a bit more about how we can maximize your safety while you're in this treatment.

TROUBLESHOOTING TIP

What if the patient says that he or she doesn't want to talk about safety? If the patient responds negatively to this focusing question, the clinician can respond by inviting the patient to share his or her reasons for this perspective. For example:

If we were to talk about safety issues in treatment, how do you think that would go or what do you think would happen?

In many cases, a patient's reluctance to talk about safety issues relates to concerns about restriction of autonomy (e.g., removal of firearms, hospitalization). If the patient addresses these concerns, the patient will often be more likely to discuss safety-related issues.

Step 2: Educate the Patient about Gun Safety

The clinician provides a brief explanation for focusing on gun safety and guides the patient to discuss the points outlined in Figure 12.1. The clinician asks the patient to identify and discuss reasons for temporarily securing any firearms that he or she might have access to.

SAMPLE CLINICIAN SCRIPT

One big issue regarding safety involves firearm safety. The reason I'd like to talk about gun safety is because having easy access to guns when you're upset could lead to bad outcomes. Research has shown, for instance, that households that do not follow safe storage procedures like locking up or securing a firearm are much more likely to have gun-related fatalities. What are your thoughts about securing or locking up firearms at home?
[Possible open-ended questions to facilitate discussion:]

What do you think about someone having access to guns when they're really upset and are suicidal?

What might be some benefits of temporarily limiting your access to firearms?

If complete removal of the guns is not possible, what are some other options for practicing good gun safety while you're going through this treatment?

What do you think about putting together a plan for this?

Step 3: Develop a Written Plan for Means Safety

The clinician and patient collaboratively develop a written plan for means safety and identify someone in the patient's life who can assist with the implementation of the plan.

SAMPLE CLINICIAN SCRIPT

Now that we've identified some specific steps we can take to increase your safety, what might you want to do about this? A lot of people find that it's helpful to write down their safety plan. Can I help you to create one for you and your home? Involving a family member or friend to help us enact our plan can increase the likelihood of success. Is there anyone in your life who could help us put this plan into action? Do you think it would be helpful to have that person come in with you next time to talk some more about this plan and gun safety in general?

TROUBLESHOOTING TIPS

What if the patient says he or she doesn't want to write down the plan? If patients say they do not want to create a written plan, the clinician should suggest writing down the plan for their own benefit. For example:

> OK, that's fine. I'll just jot down the plan here for myself so I don't forget it. I'll keep a copy in my notes so we can reference it in the future. Let's go over the plan together again to make sure I got it right.

The clinician and patient can then review each component of the means safety plan. Afterwards, the clinician can provide a copy of the written plan to the patient, thereby accomplishing the task in a subtle, indirect way:

> OK, I think I've got it. Does this seem correct to you? I'll just go ahead and make a copy for you real quick, that way you can keep it in your treatment log or somewhere else in case you need to refer back to it again like I probably will.

What if the patient says it wouldn't be helpful to bring in a significant other to discuss the safety plan? If patients do not want to bring in a significant other, the clinician should respect this decision but reinforce the importance of involving them nonetheless. For example:

> That's OK. Even if they aren't able to come in with you to meet together, we can still ask them to help. Would you be willing to talk about this plan with them and ask them to confirm that the plan has been put in place by signing our plan? That way we know for sure if they're on board and willing to help.

[After finishing the plan:] On a scale of 0 to 10, with 0 being "not at all" and 10 being "definitely," what would you say is the likelihood that you will implement this plan for increasing your safety during treatment?

[If the rating is lower than 7 out of 10:] Is there any part of this plan that reduces your likelihood for using it? What could we change about this plan to make it more likely that you would use it?

HOW TO DO IT: THE CRISIS SUPPORT PLAN

In a joint session conducted with the patient's identified source of support (usually a spouse, friend, or family member), the clinician begins by asking the patient to describe his or her suicidal mode to the significant other. Asking the patient to educate the significant other in his or her own words provides a mechanism for gauging whether or not the patient understands the case conceptualization and can clearly articulate his or her unique factors and circumstances related to suicide risk. Placing the patient in the role of the "teacher" also implicitly supports the notion that the patient has mastery over his or her problems. The clinician next invites the patient to describe the crisis response plan and to share the specific steps that the plan entails. Here again, asking the patient to be the teacher provides a mechanism for the clinician to assess the patient's knowledge base and also reinforces the philosophy of self-management, since the patient is explicitly stating in his or her own words what "my" customized plan is for managing "my" crises.

The clinician then provides a written copy of the crisis support plan to both the patient and the significant other, and they review the plan as a group. In the first section of the crisis support plan, the patient and the significant other identify several ways the significant other can support the patient. For example, the patient and significant other might go for a walk together, practice breathing exercises together, give each other a hug, watch a movie together, or play video games together. Because many suicidal patients struggle to articulate their needs effectively to others, this step can serve as basic interpersonal communication skills training and can even derail or undermine negative relational patterns that contribute to the patient's emotional distress. The clinician then reviews the basic principles of means safety counseling and invites the significant other to assist with safety precautions. Finally, the clinician reviews crisis management procedures with the significant other. This final step is critical so that the supportive other does not mistakenly assume that he or she is solely responsible for managing crises and realizes that calling for help in an emergency is not just acceptable, but is also encouraged.

As a final step, the clinician asks the patient and the significant other if they have any questions or concerns about the plan and concludes by asking the significant other to rate the likelihood that he or she will be able to implement the plan on a scale ranging from 0 (not at all likely) to 10 (very likely). If the significant other provides a low likelihood rating, the clinician should ask him or her what about the plan would need to be changed or revised to increase its likelihood for use. A crisis support plan template is available in Appendix A.6.

Step 1: Review the Suicidal Mode

The clinician invites the patient to explain the concept of the suicidal mode to the significant other and also explain how the suicidal mode applies to him or her.

SAMPLE CLINICIAN SCRIPT

[Patient], I'd like to start off by asking you to share with [significant other] your suicidal mode. Would you be willing to explain to him/her what the suicidal mode is, and also show him/her the personalized suicidal mode that we have been working on so far in treatment?

[Significant other], if at any time you have any questions or need any clarifications, please let us know.

[When the patient has finished:] [Significant other], what questions do you have about the suicidal mode and how we have used this to understand what has been going on with [patient]?

Step 2: Review the Crisis Response Plan

The clinician invites the patient to explain the purpose and rationale for the crisis response plan and then review the steps involved in his or her crisis response plan.

SAMPLE CLINICIAN SCRIPT

We've used this notion of the suicidal mode to help guide what changes to make and what steps to take, especially in a crisis. The first step we took was to develop what's called a crisis response plan. [Patient], could you explain what the crisis response plan is and share your plan with [significant other]?

[When the patient has finished:] [Patient], how has this plan been helpful for you so far?

Step 3: Introduce the Crisis Support Plan

The clinician next introduces the crisis support plan and explains the rationale for the intervention. The clinician emphasizes that the crisis support plan is designed to improve patient safety and to enhance treatment outcomes.

SAMPLE CLINICIAN SCRIPT

What I'd like to do next to go over what we call a crisis support plan. The crisis support plan is similar in many ways to the crisis response plan that was just described, but this support plan has a much more explicit role for including supportive others. The purpose of the crisis support plan is to identify concrete strategies for supporting [patient] and for increasing overall safety, both of which will lead to better outcomes in treatment. Here's a copy of the plan; let's go over this together.

Step 4: Identify Helpful Supportive Actions

The clinician facilitates a discussion between the patient and the significant other to identify simple behavioral strategies that the significant other can enact to support the patient during a crisis.

SAMPLE CLINICIAN SCRIPT

In this first section is a place where we can list some simple strategies that you can take to help support [patient] on a day-to-day basis.

[Patient], what are some things that [significant other] could do or say to encourage you and support you? How often and when would you like for [significant other] to do this?

[When a strategy is suggested:] [Significant other], is that reasonable for you to do? Do you think you could do that?

Step 5: Provide Means Safety Counseling

The clinician and patient collaboratively conduct means safety counseling for the significant other and review the means safety plan. The significant other is invited to assist with means safety. The means safety plan is revised or edited as needed based on the input of the significant other.

SAMPLE CLINICIAN SCRIPT

The next thing I'd like to do is talk about making the home as safe as possible for [patient], especially with respect to firearms [or other suicide method]. [Patient] and I have talked about gun safety and developed an initial safety plan that we'd like to share with you so we can get your thoughts about it and also see if you might be able to help us to put it into action. Let's go over some of the main points together.

[The clinician reads bullets under item 3 of the crisis support plan, displayed in Appendix A.6. After each item:]

What are your thoughts about that?

Do you think this step is doable?

Are there any challenges to doing this?

Step 6: Review Emergency Procedures and Obtain Buy-In

The clinician reviews emergency procedures to be taken in the event of a crisis or imminent suicide risk, which includes transporting the patient to the hospital and/or calling 911. Upon completion of the crisis support plan, the clinician should gauge buy-in by asking the patient and the supportive other to rate the likelihood that they will enact the plan on a scale ranging from 0 to 10, with 0 indicating "not at all likely" and 10 indicating "very likely."

SAMPLE CLINICIAN SCRIPT

Now one thing I would like to make clear is that you shouldn't ever feel like you have to manage an emergency on your own. If [patient] is ever in a severe crisis, you should call for professional help. Here's my phone number, so you can call me if you have questions or need assistance. Because I won't always be immediately available, let me give you the National Lifeline number as well in case you need to talk with someone right away and I'm not available. The National Lifeline is a network of suicide crisis counselors who will answer the phone 24/7. Their toll-free number is already written down here on this plan. If you're in an emergency situation, take [patient] to the closest hospital or call 911 for support.

Do you have any questions about these emergency steps? How about any questions about the plan as a whole?

[After finishing the plan:] On a scale of 0 to 10, with 0 being "not at all" and 10 being "definitely," what would you say is the likelihood that you will put this plan into action?

[If rating is lower than 7 out of 10:] Is there any part of this plan that reduces your likelihood of using it? What could we change about this plan to make it more likely that you would use it?

ILLUSTRATIVE CASE EXAMPLES

The Case of Mike

The clinic's intake paperwork included screening items for firearm ownership, but Mike had skipped these items. After completing a crisis response plan, Mike's clinician therefore asked about firearm ownership. Note how the clinician uses guiding:

CLINICIAN: As I was looking over your paperwork before we met today, I noticed that you missed the item that asks about firearm ownership. It was the only one you missed.

MIKE: Yeah, I don't really want to answer that question. Are you even allowed to ask me about that?

CLINICIAN: Yes, I'm allowed to ask. In fact, mental health clinicians are encouraged to ask their patients about firearms in the same way that some doctors ask about wearing seat belts or using safe sex practices: it's about safety and prevention of injury or other health problems.

MIKE: Oh, OK. I just don't want anyone thinking I'm crazy and trying to take my guns away from me when I haven't done anything wrong.

CLINICIAN: Yeah, I understand. I know that can be a common concern, but I'll admit I've not actually heard of anyone actually having their guns taken away after talking to a psychologist. Well, I guess I should say it's not ever happened to any of my patients before, and I'm thinking they would've told me if it had. Do you know of anyone that's happened to before?

MIKE: No, not personally.

CLINICIAN: Have you heard of that happening to someone outside of your personal circle?

MIKE: No. I mean, you hear stories but I can't give you a name.

CLINICIAN: Yeah, same for me. I've heard lots of stories, too, but never any names. It does raise an interesting question, though: Why do you think someone like me would ask this question?

MIKE: Well, probably because of people shooting themselves, but I'm not going to do that.

CLINICIAN: You're right, it's because of suicide.

MIKE: I'm not having those thoughts, though.

CLINICIAN: Yes, I saw here on your paperwork that you said you weren't, and you said before that you weren't having those kinds of thoughts. You have, however, said that you've been feeling really down and haven't been sleeping well and have been drinking more than usual, right?

MIKE: Yeah.

CLINICIAN: And we spent some time talking about all the stress in your life.

MIKE: Yeah, but that doesn't mean I'm going to blow my brains out.

CLINICIAN: Yes, that's correct. Having problems and feeling bad doesn't mean you're always suicidal. However, those things can make it hard to concentrate and make decisions, right?

MIKE: Yeah.

CLINICIAN: That was something we had talked about today as well: how you feel like you're not able to make good decisions anymore and you feel like you can't take it. Because of this, you've been drinking more and getting angrier.

MIKE: Yeah.

CLINICIAN: So tell me what your thoughts are about someone having easy access to firearms when they're having lots of problems in their lives, feeling down and overwhelmed, drinking more than usual, and having trouble making decisions, even if they're not suicidal.

MIKE: Well, drinking and guns aren't a good idea.

CLINICIAN: Why not?

MIKE: Well, you're impaired and can't think straight, so you could end up doing something stupid. It's like drinking and driving. You may not mean to do something stupid but you could end up in a bad place anyway if you drive.

CLINICIAN: And the consequences can be pretty steep.

MIKE: Yeah, definitely.

CLINICIAN: So heavy alcohol use and guns can be a dangerous combination?

MIKE: Yeah.

CLINICIAN: What about the other issues we talked about? Things like getting angry easily and not sleeping much? How does that go along with easy access to firearms?

MIKE: Well, those aren't good combinations either. Angry people who have guns are scary, and if you aren't sleeping then you probably aren't going to be as safe.

CLINICIAN: So those are safety issues, too?

MIKE: Yeah.

CLINICIAN: So if I'm understanding you correctly, the issues you're currently dealing with increase risk for bad outcomes when combined with firearms.

MIKE: Yeah, I guess so.

CLINICIAN: What are your thoughts about how this might apply to you?

MIKE: Well, it's probably not too safe for me to be sleeping with a gun under my bed.

CLINICIAN: Yeah, I think you're probably right. How about we spend some time talking about some different options for addressing this safety concern?

MIKE: OK.

In this exchange, the clinician uses all four processes of motivational interviewing: engaging, focusing, evoking, and planning. First, the clinician engages Mike by inviting him to share his thoughts about screening for firearm safety. Next, the clinician maintains a focus on means safety in a way that does not take charge of the conversation while also ensuring that Mike does not take charge of the conversation. The clinician also uses evoking strategies by asking Mike to share his thoughts about combining firearm access with the various problems he has reported. In this way, the clinician has guided Mike to argue in favor of means safety. Finally, the clinician transitions Mike into an active planning stage by suggesting a conversation about various options for means safety.

The Case of John

After John was released by the psychiatric unit and brought in for his initial walk-in consultation appointment for BCBT, the clinician conducted means safety counseling with him and his friend. John and his friend agreed to temporarily store John's rifle at the friend's home until the end of treatment. The issue of means safety was raised again during the third session of BCBT, when John was accompanied by his wife, Alice. The clinician completed the crisis support plan with both John and Alice, during which means safety was addressed again. During the course of this discussion, John and Alice expressed different opinions and thoughts about ongoing means safety procedures, specifically with respect to the purchase of a gun safe. Although John was in favor of this option, Alice expressed concern about its cost. As is seen in this partial transcript of their discussion, careful questioning by the clinician using all four principles of motivational interviewing enabled John and Alice to resolve this issue and come to a mutual agreement about gun safety:

CLINICIAN: So if I understand you correctly, the two of you have talked about getting a gun safe before in order to increase safety in general, but you haven't actually done this yet because of its cost, although it sounds like the roles have reversed here in terms of who's in favor and who's not.

JOHN: Yeah, there always seemed to be more important things to spend our money on, but now I'm thinking this should maybe take priority. Now she's saying we can't afford it even though she was the one who was constantly wanting to buy one before.

CLINICIAN: Hmm, that's interesting. Alice, what's your take?

ALICE: He's right that I've been harping on him for about a year to buy a gun safe. I just think it's safer to have one and to keep the gun in there, and now that we're talking about having a baby, I don't want them playing with a gun.

CLINICIAN: So it sounds like safety is pretty important to you.

ALICE: Oh, yes. I'd just as soon not have the gun in the house at all, but it's important to John to have it.

JOHN: I just feel safer with a gun so I can protect my family if someone tries to break in. Before I just didn't think it was that big of a priority, but now I'm seeing that safety is pretty important.

CLINICIAN: So we're all in agreement that safety is important?

JOHN AND ALICE: Yes.

CLINICIAN: OK, good. So that doesn't really seem to be a topic of debate there. Where are you two not seeing eye to eye?

JOHN: Well, I think I should get the gun safe now, but she thinks we should wait because we can't afford it, which totally confuses me because before all this happened she was the one wanting to get the gun safe so badly.

CLINICIAN: Alice, is that accurate?

ALICE: Technically, yes. It's not that I don't want to get a gun safe or whatever. I know that's important and I don't want John to hurt himself.

CLINICIAN: So you do want a gun safe and you want John to be safe as well, but something is getting in the way of your supporting the purchase of a gun safe right now.

ALICE: I guess so.

CLINICIAN: I wonder what you think would happen if you were to get a gun safe?

ALICE: Well, then he'd want his gun back from his friend, and I just don't know if that's a good idea right now.

CLINICIAN: Tell me more about that.

ALICE: Well, just a few weeks ago he had taken that thing out to shoot himself while I was talking with him on the phone. That was the scariest moment of my life, and he wouldn't listen to me or respond to me. I thought I was about to hear my husband kill himself on the phone with that gun. It was horrible. I just don't want that gun back around, at least not yet. I don't know if he's ready to have that gun back.

JOHN: Babe, if we get the gun safe, it'll be OK.

ALICE: But it'll still be in our home. It's too soon.

CLINICIAN: If I'm understanding you right, what you're saying, Alice, is that you're still scared about what happened and worry that it may not be safe enough to have the gun back in the house, even if it's in a gun safe. Is that right?

ALICE: Yeah, pretty much.

CLINICIAN: So it's not that you're opposed to a gun safe; you're concerned about your husband's safety.

ALICE: Yes, and I worry that maybe he's trying to just do this so he gets his gun back while our guard is down.

CLINICIAN: I see. That's a very valid concern. What do you think, John?

JOHN: That's not what I'm doing. I'm not trying to trick anyone.

CLINICIAN: I don't think you're trying to trick us either. At the same time, Alice is worried about your safety and—correct me if I'm wrong, Alice—isn't ready for the gun to be back in your home just yet.

ALICE: That's right.

CLINICIAN: John, what do you think about Alice saying she's not ready for the gun to be back in the home just yet.

JOHN: I can understand that.

CLINICIAN: OK, good. Does this mean that the primary concern here is more about when we bring the gun back home than whether or not we have a gun safe?

JOHN: What do you mean?

CLINICIAN: Well, it sounds like we're all in agreement about safety, and we're all in agreement that a gun safe is a good idea. Am I right about that?

JOHN AND ALICE: Yes.

CLINICIAN: Where we're not yet in agreement is when the gun comes home and gets put into that safe.

ALICE: Yeah, I think that's right.

CLINICIAN: How about you, John?

JOHN: That makes sense. What if we just bought the gun safe now so we at least have it, then later on when more time has passed we can get my rifle and store it in the safe. It doesn't have to be right now, though.

CLINICIAN: Oh, that's an interesting idea. What do you think about that, Alice?

ALICE: That sounds find to me. I'm OK with getting the safe, but I just don't want that gun back right now.

JOHN: That's fine, babe. I don't have to have it back right away. We can wait a while.

CLINICIAN: So did we just come to an agreement here?

ALICE: Yeah, I think so.

JOHN: Yeah.

CLINICIAN: OK, well I guess you guys will do some shopping for a safe and then we'll revisit the issue of returning the rifle later on. I usually recommend we have that conversation during the last session of treatment. That would be around 2 to 3 months from now. How's that sound?

JOHN: That's fine with me.

ALICE: Yeah, that's good.

CLINICIAN: OK, well that gives you a little bit of time to find a safe and make sure you have the money for it.

TIPS AND ADVICE FOR
MEANS SAFETY COUNSELING AND CRISIS SUPPORT PLANS

1. **Be mindful of language.** We have found that using the language "means restriction" (especially "firearm restriction") often increases the patient's defensiveness. Using the language "means safety" elicits less intense negative reactions.

2. **Let the patient argue in favor of means safety.** Clinicians should encourage patients to provide the rationale for means safety. This can often be accomplished by asking them what their thoughts are about suicidal individuals having access to firearms (e.g., "On the topic of safety, I wonder what your thoughts are about suicidal individuals having easy access to firearms? I wonder what you would think about a family member or friend having access to their firearms if they were suicidal?"). If the patient can provide reasons in support of means safety, the clinician can subsequently refer back to his or her own words and arguments (e.g., "How does that fit with you said before about the dangerousness of firearms when suicidal?").

3. **Keep trigger locks and cable locks available for patients.** Clinicians can facilitate firearm safety by keeping a supply of trigger locks and/or cable locks in their office. These can often be obtained from local law enforcement for reduced (or even no) cost.

4. **Become familiar with state and local laws dictating firearm possession and storage.** Gun laws can vary considerably across different jurisdictions. Knowing these laws can help clinicians and patients generate options for firearm safety plans. Some states, for example, allow for law enforcement agencies to temporarily store citizens' firearms to facilitate their safety.

CHAPTER 13

Targeting Sleep Disturbance

Stimulus control and sleep hygiene are two cognitive-behavioral approaches for reducing sleep disturbance and insomnia. Stimulus control is based on the principles of learning theory and classical conditioning, with the primary goal being to strengthen the associations among the bed and sleep-related behaviors (e.g., relaxing, laying down, falling asleep) while simultaneously weakening the associations among the bed and behaviors that are unrelated to sleep (e.g., reading, watching television). Stimulus control is the most effective stand-alone cognitive-behavioral intervention for insomnia, and typically contributes to 50–60% improvements in insomnia (Taylor, McCrae, Gehrman, Dautovich, & Lichstein, 2007). Sleep hygiene entails psychoeducation focused on reducing behaviors that could possibly interfere with sleep (e.g., excessive caffeine use, nicotine use at night, exercising too soon before bedtime) and adjusting environmental conditions that might contribute to sleep problems (e.g., temperature or climate control, excessive light or noise). Because it is often used in conjunction with other medical and cognitive-behavioral treatments, the efficacy of sleep hygiene as a stand-alone intervention is unknown. Nonetheless, it is frequently used in combination with stimulus control.

Stimulus control entails several primary and interrelated principles:

- **Bed is for sleep and sex only.** When the patient engages in activities other than sleep and sex in bed (e.g., watching television, eating, reading, studying), the bed becomes associated with nonsleeping activities. When the patient restricts the bed to only sleep and sex, however, the bed becomes associated with sleep, which increases the likelihood that the patient will quickly fall asleep when he or she gets into bed.

- **Get out of bed if you have not fallen asleep within 15 minutes of getting into bed.** This guideline functions as an extension of the previous one: lying in bed for an

159

extended period of time, during which time the patient is typically becoming increasingly frustrated or stressed, contributes to the development of an association of the bed with sleeplessness. By getting out of bed, one disrupts this learned process. When getting out of bed, the patient should engage in activities that are relaxing and/or unstimulating. Activities such as cleaning, watching television, playing video games, or surfing the Internet may not be ideal since they can be mentally activating. The latter three options can also be unhelpful because they entail looking at a bright light source, which can also trick the brain into thinking that it is daytime.

- **Return to bed only when sleepy.** The patient should be educated about the difference between feeling "tired" and feeling "sleepy." Being tired entails being physically or mentally exhausted but does not necessarily include the sensation of sleepiness. The patient should therefore be instructed to get into bed only when feeling *sleepy* (e.g., dozing off).

RATIONALE

The exact mechanisms by which sleep disturbance is associated with increased risk for suicidal thoughts and behaviors are not fully understood, although a few general models have been proposed. The first of these models relates to emotional overarousal. Arguably the predominant model within the suicide prevention literature, there is strong reason to believe that sleeplessness is an indicator of physiological overarousal or agitation, each of which are independent risk factors for suicide (Busch et al., 2003; Hall et al., 1999), especially among men (Bryan, Hitschfeld, et al., 2014). According to this model, sleep disturbance contributes to negative emotion states via increased autonomic arousal. A second possible model relates to neurocognitive disruption resulting from sleep disturbance. According to this perspective, sleep disturbance contributes to declines in problem solving (Harrison & Horne, 2000) and emotional reactivity (Gujar, Yoo, Hu, & Walker, 2011).

Similarly unknown are the specific dimensions of sleep disturbance that are most relevant to the emergence of suicidal thoughts and behaviors. Hall (2010) has described four discrete but interrelated dimensions of sleep disturbance: sleep duration, sleep continuity, sleep architecture, and sleep quality. *Sleep duration* refers to the total amount of sleep that a person achieves, and is typically operationalized as the total time in bed minus the amount of time needed to fall asleep and the amount of time spent awake during the night. This is most often assessed by asking patients to report how many hours of sleep they usually get at night (or during a 24-hour period), although greater accuracy can be achieved using sleep diaries or objective measures of sleep duration (e.g., actigraphs, electroencephalogram [EEG]). *Sleep continuity* focuses on the individual's ability to initiate and maintain sleep. Similar to sleep duration, sleep continuity is often assessed via self-report and/or objective measures like actigraphs. *Sleep architecture* refers to the pattern of electrical activity in the brain that corresponds with various sleep stages, notably rapid-eye-movement (REM) versus non-rapid-eye-movement (NREM) sleep. This dimension of sleep disturbance requires objective measurement schemes that measure electrical activity in the brain during periods of sleep. Finally, *sleep quality* refers to the individual's subjective appraisal of his or her sleep, and is usually assessed via self-report methods, of which many different scales and strategies exist.

Of these four dimensions, sleep quality has received the greatest amount of attention in suicide research, and has consistently been shown to be correlated with suicidal thoughts and behaviors above and beyond the effects of other risk factors like sociodemographics and depression (Woznica, Carney, Kuo, & Moss, 2015). A growing body of evidence suggests that sleep disturbance is an important risk factor for suicide and in many cases incrementally predicts suicide ideation, attempts, and death even when controlling for other risk factors such as depression (Barraclough & Pallis, 1975; Bernert, Joiner, Cukrowicz, Schmidt, & Krakow, 2005). Additional research indicates that patients who report sleep disturbance die by suicide significantly sooner after their last medical appointment as compared to patients who do not report insomnia (Pigeon, Britton, Ilgen, Chapman, & Conner, 2012). Interestingly, different patterns have been observed in military personnel and veterans. In this population, the association of sleep disturbance with suicidal thoughts and behaviors is mediated by co-occurring depression (Bryan, Gonzalez, et al., 2015), which suggests that mood disturbance has a closer association with suicide risk than sleep disturbance in military personnel and veterans.

Despite our knowledge gaps, the accumulation of evidence suggests that individuals who are dissatisfied with their sleep and/or perceive that they have poor sleep are more likely to experience suicidal thoughts and behaviors. It remains unclear, however, the degree to which these appraisals reflect actual deficits in sleep versus exaggerated or distorted perceptions of sleep parameters. Given the well-established link between subjective sleep quality and suicide risk, procedures and interventions that target subjective sleep quality could reduce suicidal thoughts and behaviors. Emerging evidence supports this perspective. In a recent observational cohort study of patients treated with cognitive-behavioral therapy for insomnia (CBT-I), suicide ideation was found to significantly decline over the course of treatment (Trockel, Karlin, Taylor, Brown, & Manber, 2015). In this study, change in severity of suicide ideation was significantly predicted by change in self-reported sleep quality, such that improvements in sleep quality were correlated with reductions in suicide ideation. Targeting sleep disturbance therefore appears to have a positive impact on suicide risk reduction.

HOW TO DO IT

A simple and straightforward strategy for conducting stimulus control and sleep hygiene is to list the primary guidelines and recommendations for each on a patient handout (see Appendix A.7, Improving Your Sleep) and then review the handout with the patient. As each item is reviewed, the clinician asks the patient if the guideline applies to him or her and, if it does, invites the patient to discuss the reasonableness of implementing each strategy. After reviewing the entire handout, the clinician and patient review those areas that were identified for possible change. The clinician then asks which changes the patient is willing and able to make right away. The clinician may need to use motivational enhancement strategies to increase the patient's willingness to make changes to his or her sleep behaviors, especially for stimulus control procedures, of which some can be difficult or unpleasant to implement (e.g., getting out of bed if the patient does not fall asleep within 15 minutes). Because it can take several weeks for insomnia to improve noticeably after initiating stimulus control and sleep hygiene, these interventions are best implemented early in BCBT.

To complete stimulus control and sleep hygiene, the clinician provides the insomnia handout to the patient and invites him or her to review each section. The clinician asks the patient to identify areas that could be changed to improve his or her sleep, and then helps the patient plan to develop a plan for making these changes.

Step 1: Introduce Stimulus Control and Sleep Hygiene

The clinician introduces stimulus control and sleep hygiene, explains the rationale for the intervention, and provides a patient handout to facilitate the discussion.

SAMPLE CLINICIAN SCRIPT

We've talked about how sleep has been a problem for you and how that's something that you'd like to work on. Insomnia falls under the physical domain of the suicidal mode, so if we can make some improvements in this area, we'll be addressing a physical aspect of what's been going on. Is insomnia an issue that you'd be willing to talk about today? What I'd like to do is go over some sleep guidelines that are called "stimulus control" and "sleep hygiene." These guidelines have been shown to be the most effective methods for improving sleep. Here's a handout that lists all of the guidelines for you.

Step 2: Review Stimulus Control and Sleep Hygiene Principles

The clinician provides the insomnia handout (see Appendix A.7) to the patient and invites the patient to read each of the guidelines one at a time. The clinician then asks the patient if the guideline is relevant to his or her life, and if so, how it is relevant. If the guideline is relevant, the clinician asks the patient to mark it for later reference.

SAMPLE CLINICIAN SCRIPT

What I'd like to do is read through these together, and then talk about how each item might apply to you. Let's start here with the first item. Could you read that out loud for us? What are your thoughts about that item? Is that something that applies to your own sleep habits?

   [If yes:] Tell me a bit more about how that is relevant to you. Since that one applies to you, let's go ahead and just mark that one with a check mark and we'll come back to that later. Let's move on to the next one. Could you read the next item out loud for us?

   [If no:] OK, let's move on to the next one then. Could you read the next item out loud for us?

Step 3: Formalize a Plan and Elicit Patient Buy-In

In the final step of stimulus control and sleep hygiene, the clinician asks the patient to consider all of the relevant items and to select those behaviors that can be changed immediately. The agreed-upon changes should be formalized into a change plan and assigned by the clinician. If the patient verbalizes reluctance or concerns about changing his or her sleep behaviors, the clinician should use motivational enhancement strategies appropriately. Once a change plan is in place, the clinician should gauge buy-in by asking the patient to rate the likelihood that he or she will enact the plan on a scale ranging from 0 to 10, with 0 indicating "not at all likely" and 10 indicating "very likely."

> **SAMPLE CLINICIAN SCRIPT**
>
> So now that we've gotten through all of these, it seems as though you've identified a number of changes that you could make to improve your sleep. As we look at all of the changes that you say apply to you, I wonder which of these you could change today? What would you need to do to make that change? Let's write that down.
>
> [After finishing the plan:] On a scale of 0 to 10, with 0 being "not at all" and 10 being "definitely," what would you say is the likelihood that you will make these changes to your sleep habits?
>
> [If rating is lower than 7 out of 10:] Is there any part of this plan that reduces your likelihood for using it? What could we change about this plan to make it more likely that you would use it?

ILLUSTRATIVE CASE EXAMPLE

Mike reported significant problems with falling asleep and staying asleep. These problems had been ongoing for several years but had worsened in the months immediately preceding his self-referral for BCBT. Because improved sleep was one of Mike's primary treatment goals and it seemed to be closely tied to his agitation and emotional distress, the clinician decided to introduce stimulus control and sleep hygiene during their third session. As they reviewed the Improving Your Sleep Handout, Mike identified the following possible areas for change: getting out of bed when he is unable to fall asleep within 15 minutes, using his bed for sleep and sex only, avoiding alcohol, engaging in regular exercise, unwinding before bed, and establishing a regular sleep schedule. Mike indicated that he could make changes to all of these behaviors starting immediately. Upon follow-up, however, he had not made any of the changes. Mike and his clinician subsequently engaged in the following dialogue:

CLINICIAN: What got in the way of making these changes?

MIKE: I'm not really sure. They're all easy enough. I mean, I didn't drink any alcohol, but I had already been doing that.

CLINICIAN: So you were able to keep that change in place?

MIKE: Yeah, but that was the easiest one because I was already doing it.

CLINICIAN: Oh, I see. So some of these are harder than others?

MIKE: Yeah, I guess so.

CLINICIAN: Which one would you say is the hardest change to make?

MIKE: Probably getting out of bed after 15 minutes. I realize that's a pretty simple thing to do in many ways, but that one just seems really hard when I'm lying there in bed and just want to go to sleep.

CLINICIAN: Yeah, that's the one that most people find hardest. You're right, though: it's a pretty simple thing to do that ends up being really hard in practice. So which one of these would be the easiest change to make?

MIKE: Probably setting a bedtime routine and unwind period.

CLINICIAN: What about that one is the easiest?

MIKE: Well, I kind of already have a routine, but I don't necessarily do it at a consistent time. So if I just set a consistent time for going to bed, I could set a consistent time for unwinding.

CLINICIAN: If you were to set a consistent time for going to bed, what would that be?

MIKE: Probably 11:00 P.M. I'm usually in bed by then.

CLINICIAN: How long do you typically stay awake after getting into bed?

MIKE: Maybe an hour or so.

CLINICIAN: So you're usually asleep by midnight?

MIKE: Yeah, on most nights.

CLINICIAN: Well, since we want to maximize the amount of time that you're asleep in bed and minimize the amount of time that you're lying awake in bed, what if we set your bedtime to midnight? That way you'd fall asleep pretty soon after getting into bed.

MIKE: That makes sense.

CLINICIAN: Then what time should we start the unwinding process?

MIKE: That should be at 11:00 P.M. That gives me an hour to get settled and stuff.

CLINICIAN: That sounds like a good plan. When do you think you could start doing that?

MIKE: Probably tonight.

CLINICIAN: What if we were to start that tonight and see how it goes, then if it goes well we can come back to this list and pick the next easiest thing to do on the list? How does that sound?

MIKE: I like that.

CLINICIAN: OK, then let's start with unwinding at 11:00 P.M. and bedtime at midnight, and then we'll start working on these other changes. That way we start with the easy stuff and work our way up.

At the next appointment, Mike reported that he had followed this plan and had taken several other steps on his own: bringing a chair into his bedroom so he could watch TV and read without lying in bed. When asked about this additional change, Mike replied, "Well, once I got started on the unwinding thing, I realized that reading helps me do that. So I moved a chair into my room to do that while following the other guidelines." Over subsequent sessions, Mike continued to make additional changes to his sleep behaviors. The clinician was able to motivate Mike to make these changes by troubleshooting his barriers and devising a simple method to sidestep these barriers: rank-ordering all of the proposed changes and starting with the most attainable change. Once Mike had experienced some initial momentum, it was easier for him to continue with additional changes.

TIPS AND ADVICE FOR
TARGETING SLEEP DISTURBANCE

1. **Familiarize yourself with CBT-I.** The stimulus control principles used in BCBT are based on the principles of CBT-I. In addition to addressing these behavioral aspects of sleep disturbance, CBT-I also targets distorted thoughts and beliefs about sleep (e.g., "I must get 8 hours of sleep every night or I can't function"; "Tomorrow will be horrible if I don't get to sleep"). Clinicians who are familiar with CBT-I principles will be able to more effectively target sleep disturbance during BCBT.

2. **Be alert for possible breathing-related sleep disorders.** Breathing-related sleep disorders such as sleep apnea will not respond to stimulus control. Possible signs of a breathing-related sleep disorder include snoring and gasping for air while asleep (usually reported by sleep partners) and daytime fatigue despite a sufficient duration of sleep. Patients with possible breathing-related sleep disorders should be referred to their physicians for further evaluation, include a possible sleep study.

CHAPTER 14

Relaxation and Mindfulness Skills Training

Relaxation training is a very common cognitive-behavioral intervention used to teach patients how to manage their physiological arousal. Mindfulness training is an increasingly popular cognitive-behavioral intervention that can appear similar, on its surface, to relaxation training. Although similar in many ways, the two interventions differ from each other with respect to the specific domains they target: relaxation skills target the physiological domain, whereas mindfulness skills target the cognitive domain. By activating the parasympathetic nervous system, relaxation training has the effect of reducing negative emotional states associated with physiological arousal such as anxiety, fear, generalized distress, and anger. Many different versions of relaxation training have been described, of which the two most common are arguably diaphragmatic breathing and progressive muscle relaxation:

• **Diaphragmatic breathing.** Diaphragmatic breathing consists of very slow, deep inhales that completely fill the lungs, followed by very slow exhales. Diaphragmatic breathing is sometimes referred to as "belly breathing" because of the abdominal distension that occurs as a result of the downward expansion of the diaphragm during the inhale. When initially teaching and demonstrating diaphragmatic breathing, the clinician often provides verbal suggestions to heighten the relaxation effect (e.g., "As you breathe out, let your shoulders slump").

• **Progressive muscle relaxation.** Progressive muscle relaxation consists of alternately tensing a muscle group and then relaxing the muscle group by releasing the tension. In progressive muscle relaxation, the patient tenses or tightens a muscle group (e.g., the feet) and holds the tension for several seconds, then releases the tension. The patient then moves to the next muscle group (e.g., the calves) and holds these muscles in a state of tension for

166

several seconds, then releases the tension. The patient progresses through the body, repeating this process of tensing the muscles, holding the tension, and then releasing the tension. The side-by-side placement of sustained tension followed by the release of this tension provides a heightened awareness of relaxation, thereby augmenting its perceived effect.

Other relaxation strategies (e.g., imagery and autogenic relaxation) also exist and, although not described here, are viable alternatives to diaphragmatic breathing and progressive muscle relaxation.

In contrast to relaxation, which focuses on autonomic arousal, mindfulness is a method for teaching patients how to become more aware of their thoughts, internal psychological experiences, and behaviors, and how to better regulate the attention that is directed toward these different internal experiences. Many of the maladaptive thoughts and behaviors that are experienced by the suicidal patient occur automatically because they have been reinforced and consequentially overlearned. Suicidal individuals also tend to have elevated cognitive reactivity, which is the process by which changes in mood trigger cognitive reactions that are otherwise dormant (Ingram, Miranda, & Segal, 2006). Individuals with core suicidal beliefs are therefore more likely to experience frequent episodes of acute distress and maladaptive behaviors when they experience a negative shift in mood (e.g., depression, anger, anxiety). Such individuals often feel unable to control or manage their behavior and might be perceived by others as "overreacting" to triggering events. In short, the suicidal patient responds to life situations based on habitual patterns rather than intentional decision making.

Mindfulness training is intended to offset this vulnerability by strengthening the patient's awareness of his or her internal states and the context within which these states are experienced, thereby enabling him or her to respond to life situations in a more intentional way. For example, a suicidal patient with the core belief "I am a failure" may interpret an undesirable or unfortunate life event as evidence of failure, even if his or her actions or decisions had little to do with the actual outcome. This automatic assumption may contribute to feelings of guilt or shame. The suicidal patient might then dwell upon his or her perceived failure in an attempt to "undo" or "fix" the problem, which ultimately leads to even greater emotional distress. Rumination of this kind can consume a great deal of the patient's attention and cognitive resources, thereby causing him or her to lose awareness of the present moment. The suicidal patient therefore becomes "trapped" in misery, rendering him or her unable to redirect attention toward more pleasant and reinforcing life experiences that would otherwise be able to counteract or undermine the misery. In many cases, this automatic responding occurs with little, if any, awareness or insight on the part of the suicidal patient. Suicidal individuals therefore engage in maladaptive cognitive and behavioral patterns because they are unable to redirect their attention toward experiences that could undermine these patterns.

Mindfulness is neither distraction nor detachment from uncomfortable internal experiences. The purpose of mindfulness is actually the opposite of distraction: to enable the individual to experience internal states without judgment, thereby enabling deliberate and adaptive responding. Mindfulness accomplishes this not by reducing the negative internal state (e.g., depression), but rather by broadening the individual's awareness such that the negative internal state no longer consumes all or most of his or her attention. Mindfulness therefore does not *eliminate* the problem, but it enables the patient to place the problem within a larger context, thereby making it more subjectively (and perhaps objectively) manageable. A number of mindfulness exercises have been developed and described. To date, there are no data suggesting any one exercise is more effective than others.

RATIONALE

Relaxation training has well-established empirical support as an intervention for reducing emotional distress, depression, agitation, and anxiety (Jain et al., 2007; Luebbert, Dahme, & Hasenbring, 2001; Stetter & Kupper, 2002). It is therefore a core emotion regulation skill for the full range of psychological and behavioral disorders. Of the many different relaxation strategies that exist, progressive muscle relaxation has additionally proven to be effective for the treatment of insomnia (Taylor et al., 2007). In addition to its utility as an emotion regulation skill, relaxation training may therefore also be a useful intervention for suicidal patients who report sleep disturbance.

Mindfulness exercises are a common ingredient of treatments that effectively reduce suicide ideation and suicide attempts (Katz, Cox, Gunasekara, & Miller, 2004; Linehan, 1993; Miklowitz et al., 2009; Rudd et al., 2015) and are useful with suicidal patients due to the method's ability to reduce cognitive reactivity (Lynch et al., 2006). Although mindfulness exercises appear on the surface to be very similar to relaxation exercises, and both mindfulness and relaxation effectively reduce general distress (Jain et al., 2007; Kabat-Zinn et al., 1992; Speca, Carlson, Goodey, & Angen, 2000; Stetter & Kupper, 2002), research indicates that relaxation and mindfulness operate via different mechanisms. Specifically, whereas relaxation exercises act upon the physiological domain, mindfulness exercises act upon the cognitive domain. This is supported by research finding that mindfulness reduces cognitive rumination whereas relaxation does not (Jain et al., 2007). Furthermore, mindfulness also appears to boost *positive* emotions much more than relaxation (Jain et al., 2007). Because relaxation and mindfulness skills target separate domains of the suicidal mode and are associated with different outcomes, both are included in BCBT.

HOW TO DO IT

Relaxation training begins with psychoeducation focused on autonomic arousal and the stress response. Most patients have at least a basic knowledge of autonomic nervous system functioning, typically with respect to the concept of the "fight-or-flight" response. After explaining how relaxation can be beneficial for reducing physiological and emotional arousal, the clinician invites the patient to practice relaxation together in session. The clinician then proceeds to verbally walk the patient through the relaxation exercise. A sample relaxation script is provided in Appendix B.6. Upon completion of the exercise, the clinician helps the patient to gain greater awareness of the intervention's effect through Socratic questioning.

Mindfulness training begins with psychoeducation focused on how attentional bias can influence the subjective experience of stress. For many patients, the notion that emotional distress can be mitigated by allowing oneself to experience the distress, as opposed to suppressing or avoiding the distress, will be new. After explaining how mindfulness can be beneficial for reducing rumination and putting things into perspective, the clinician should invite the patient to practice mindfulness together in session. The clinician then proceeds to verbally walk the patient through the mindfulness exercise. A sample mindfulness script is provided in Appendix B.7. Upon completion of the exercise, the clinician helps the patient to gain greater awareness of the intervention's effect through Socratic questioning.

Step 1a (Relaxation): Introduce Relaxation Training and the Autonomic Nervous System

The clinician begins by introducing the concept of relaxation and educating the patient about autonomic nervous system activation and deactivation.

SAMPLE CLINICIAN SCRIPT

Let's talk a little bit about the physical aspects of getting emotionally upset. When you get emotionally upset, how do you know that you're upset? What changes in you physically to tell you that you're angry, for instance, instead of happy? What other physical changes have you noticed when you're stressed or upset?

These changes are a result of your stress response. All of us have a stress response that's designed to keep us safe when we're in a dangerous or threatening situation. Perhaps you've heard of the "fight-or-flight" response? Explain to me what the fight-or-flight response is.

When we're stressed out, our body prepares to either fight for our lives or to run away as quickly as possible. In order to do this, our heart starts beating faster, we start to sweat, we get a dry mouth, our breathing gets rapid and shallow, our muscles get tense, and all sorts of other changes occur. When you're stressed out or upset, your body is responding in this way. Being in a constant state of stress can be exhausting, though; it wears down the body and the mind. Based on what we've been talking about thus far, I think this may apply to you: you're getting worn out from all the stress. Would you say that's accurate or would you disagree with that?

The good news is that we can actually manage our stress response by doing some very simple strategies such as slowing down our breathing and focusing on the tension in our muscles. Have you ever learned any sort of relaxation or breathing techniques before?

[If yes:] Would you mind explaining to me what you've learned and show me how to do it?

[If no:] I'd like to show you a really simple technique. Would you be interested in learning one?

Step 1b (Mindfulness): Introduce Mindfulness Training and Attentional Bias

The clinician introduces the concept of relaxation and educates the patient about attentional bias.

SAMPLE CLINICIAN SCRIPT

Let's talk about how what you pay attention to when stressed out can keep you emotionally upset. You've said that when you get upset, you often feel completely overwhelmed, and you can't think about anything other than whatever problem you're facing and the stress that you're feeling. Some people say it's sort of like having "tunnel vision." Is that sort of what it's like for you?

I could definitely see how that would make it hard for you to make decisions and keep the bigger picture in mind. When we're stressed out, it definitely becomes harder to see the bigger picture and keep things in perspective. Our attention narrows in on the problem itself, and it becomes hard to see anything else. Our perceptions of that problem can then become colored by the assumptions and beliefs we have about ourselves, others, and the world. So if we generally think that we are bad people, then when we are stressed out we will focus on those aspects of the situation that line up with the notion of being a bad person and will ignore those aspects of the situation that contradict this assumption. Likewise, if we believe we're incapable of managing stress then we will tend to focus on those aspects of the situation that match that assumption.

When you get upset, do you try not to think about the problem or think about being upset? Does trying not to think about it work? Does it make things worse? The interesting thing is that the more we try not to think about something, the bigger of an issue it seems to become. It's sort of a paradox: trying not to think about something makes you think about it more. One possible way to respond to stress is to try not to think about it. Another possible way to respond to stress is to allow yourself to think about it, but to take a step back from the problem and look at it more objectively, without trying to interfere with it or judging it. Have you ever tried to just notice problems and thoughts and feelings, but without trying to change them?

If you'd be willing to try, I'd like to teach you how to do this. Learning how to just notice thoughts and feelings, as opposed to trying to avoid them or get rid of them, can help us to take a step back and see the bigger picture. It doesn't necessarily make the problem go away, but it can make the problem seem less overwhelming. Would you like to learn this technique?

Step 2: Invite the Patient to Practice an Exercise

The clinician invites the patient to practice a brief relaxation or mindfulness exercise together in session and guides him or her through the procedure.

SAMPLE CLINICIAN SCRIPT

What I'd like for you to do is make sure you're sitting comfortably straight in your seat. What that means is I want you to sit up straight without slouching, but I don't want you to sit up so straight that you're stiff and rigid. If you'd like you can close your eyes while we do this, but you don't have to. Some people find it's easier to do at first if they close their eyes, but if you don't want to you can find a point on the wall or the floor and just fix your gaze on that point instead so your eyes don't wander around.

The clinician reads the relaxation script detailed in Appendix B.6 or the mindfulness script detailed in Appendix B.7.

Step 3: Process the Experience

After completing the exercise, the clinician uses guiding questions to help the patient to recognize its effectiveness and value. Although open-ended questions are ideal, in some cases the patient will have limited insight and/or ability to fully recognize the effects that relaxation had on him or her.

SAMPLE CLINICIAN SCRIPT (RELAXATION)

[Possible open-ended questions to facilitate processing and integration:]

> What was that like for you?
>
> What did you notice changing inside of you when you were doing that?
>
> What changed about the tension in your muscles/your heart rate/your breathing?
>
> Describe what you noticed.
>
> How did you know that you were getting more relaxed?
>
> Where in your body did you feel more relaxed?
>
> Was any part of that difficult or hard to do?
>
> What was the easiest part of that?
>
> What did you like best about that activity?

SAMPLE CLINICIAN SCRIPT (MINDFULNESS)

[Possible open-ended questions to facilitate processing and integration:]

> What was that like for you?
>
> Describe what you noticed.
>
> Were you able to shift your focus and attention?
>
> What was hard about shifting your attention?
>
> What was easy about shifting your attention?
>
> What was different about your stressful thoughts this time as compared to all the other times you have had them?
>
> What was it like to remain calm while thinking about stressful things?

Step 4: Formalize a Plan and Elicit Patient Buy-In

In the final step of skills training, the clinician asks the patient if he or she would be willing to practice the relaxation or mindfulness skill on a regular basis and then develops a plan that specifies the frequency, timing, and duration of practice. Once a plan is in place, the clinician should gauge buy-in by asking the patient to rate the likelihood that he or she will practice relaxation as planned on a scale ranging from 0 to 10, with 0 indicating "not at all likely" and 10 indicating "very likely."

SAMPLE CLINICIAN SCRIPT

So as you can see, this is something that is pretty easy to do and doesn't take much time. Most people find that if they practice this daily, or even a few times per day, they can see improvements in their stress level. How often do you think you would be able to reasonably practice this technique? How many minutes do you think you could reasonably practice this for each time? Is there any particular place or situation where you would be especially likely to practice? Are there any times where it might be good to practice because it might help you out?

[After finishing the plan:] On a scale of 0 to 10, with 0 being "not at all" and 10 being "definitely," what would you say is the likelihood that you will practice relaxation on a daily basis?

[If rating is lower than 7 out of 10:] Is there any part of this plan that reduces your likelihood for using it? What could we change about this plan to make it more likely that you would use it?

ILLUSTRATIVE CASE EXAMPLE

Janice's clinician introduced relaxation training during the fifth session as a skill designed to directly target deficits in stress management. This decision was made in response to Janice's disclosure during the previous session that she had made another suicide attempt. Although Janice used her crisis response plan and several coping skills, she reported feeling on edge, adding that she "felt like I needed something to help calm me down." The following exchange occurred:

CLINICIAN: Could you describe in more detail what feeling on edge is like?

JANICE: Well, like feeling restless, like I can't sit still and my muscles are all tense.

CLINICIAN: So when you say you need something to calm you down . . .

JANICE: I mean something to help me relax, like so I could lie down to take a nap or whatever.

CLINICIAN: OK, that makes sense. Have you ever learned any sort of relaxation exercises before?

JANICE: Just the breathing stuff you taught me.

CLINICIAN: OK, then let's teach you how to do another breathing exercise that will help your muscles to be less tense and calm down more than the other exercise you've been using.

Upon completing the relaxation exercise, Janice and her clinician discussed the exercise together:

CLINICIAN: What was that like for you?

JANICE: I liked it.

CLINICIAN: Good! What did you like in particular?

JANICE: Well, I liked that my body doesn't feel so tight anymore, and my heart slowed down and wasn't beating so hard.

CLINICIAN: Yeah, that's a pretty common thing people notice. What else changed inside you while you were doing this?

JANICE: Well, I felt as though I was falling asleep there for a second.

CLINICIAN: Yeah, I noticed that your head started to droop forward toward your chest.

JANICE: Yeah. It was kind of peaceful, like I could just chill out.

CLINICIAN: So you felt calm?

JANICE: Yes, definitely.

CLINICIAN: Is this something you think you could do on a regular basis then?

JANICE: Yes, I'm going to do this every night when I'm going to bed. I can also do it in the morning when I get to work because I usually start getting tense then.

CLINICIAN: That sounds like a great plan. Let's write that down.

TIPS AND ADVICE FOR RELAXATION AND MINDFULNESS SKILLS TRAINING

1. **Practice voice modulation.** Clinicians who have not used relaxation or mindfulness exercises with their patients should be sure to practice how to guide a patient through the script effectively. Especially key to maximizing the effect of the exercises is voice modulation, which includes softening one's voice and speaking in a rhythmic pattern.

2. **Mindfulness does not entail avoidance or suppression.** A common misunderstanding of mindfulness is that it is designed to stop one's thinking or to otherwise "blank out" or erase one's thoughts. The purpose of mindfulness, however, is not to stop one's thinking; rather, the purpose is to observe one's thinking without judgment or interference. If a patient reports that mindfulness is not helping (or has "stopped working"), the clinician should seek to determine if the patient holds this misconception. If so, the clinician should reeducate the patient and practice with him or her again.

CHAPTER 15

The Reasons for Living List and the Survival Kit

Suicidal individuals who seek out treatment are often ambivalent about suicide: they both want to die and to live at the same time. During emotional crises, however, suicidal individuals often focus on their reasons for dying more so than their reasons for living. Reminding suicidal patients of their reasons for living during crises can counteract this effect. The reasons for living list and survival kit are two interventions that accomplish this objective by explicitly identifying the reasons why the patient does *not* want to die, which reinforces his or her desire to live. The survival kit is referred to as a "hope box" in cognitive therapy for suicide prevention (Wenzel et al., 2009). Although these two terms refer to the same intervention, they may have different levels of appeal and acceptability to different subgroups of patients. For example, the term "survival kit" may be more acceptable to male patients, whereas the term "hope box" may be more acceptable to female patients (especially adolescents).

The two interventions are very similar in purpose and design, but the survival kit differs from the reasons for living list by using tangible objects to serve as physical reminders of the patient's positive life experiences. These interventions may not directly reduce the patient's desire to die, but by enhancing his or her desire to live, they can create enough ambivalence about suicide in the short term that the patient may delay his or her decision to act upon the suicidal urge. Outside the boundaries of an acute crisis, as the patient recalls and reflects upon his or her reasons for living, the orientation toward life is strengthened and the orientation toward death is weakened.

RATIONALE

The primary purpose of the reasons for living list is to increase cognitive flexibility by undermining the patient's tendency to focus on death- and suicide-related information. Cognitive bias toward suicide is associated with risk for future suicide attempts (Cha et al., 2010; Nock et al., 2010) and causes the suicidal patient to focus attention on beliefs and memories that trigger and/or sustain suicidal crises. Because of this bias, suicidal individuals report fewer reasons for living than nonsuicidal individuals (Strosahl, Chiles, & Linehan, 1992) and also underestimate the likelihood that positive events will happen to them in the future (MacLeod et al., 1993). Suicidal individuals are able to consider just as many potential *negative* future events as nonsuicidal individuals, however, indicating that impairments in future orientation among suicidal individuals are restricted to the ability to consider *desirable* outcomes as opposed to more generalized or global impairments. The reasons for living list therefore helps patients consider potential positive outcomes in life in addition to possible negative outcomes, which reduces hopelessness in the short term (MacLeod & Tarbuck, 1994).

Similar to the reasons for living list, the primary purposes of the survival kit are to reduce cognitive rigidity, to enhance cognitive flexibility, and to induce positive emotional states, each of which contributes to the desire for life. The ability to maintain and increase one's positive emotional experience is referred to as *savoring* (Bryant, 2003). The survival kit facilitates savoring skills through two specific strategies: enabling the patient to maintain his or her focus on the positive emotional state, referred to as *being present* skills, and enabling the patient to share this experience with another person, referred to as *capitalizing* skills (Quoidbach, Berry, Hansenne, & Mikolajczak, 2010). Being present skills are associated with increased frequency and intensity of experiencing positive emotions (Bryant, 2003; Erisman & Roemer, 2010; Quoidbach et al., 2010), whereas capitalizing skills heighten the effect of positive emotional experiences beyond the experience of the emotional state itself (Gable, Reis, Impett, & Asher, 2004). The sharing of positive events with others (e.g., the clinician) is also associated with greater life satisfaction (Quoidbach et al., 2010).

Reasons for living also serve to reduce risk for suicide even among patients with a strong desire to die by generating ambivalence. Research indicates that a very strong desire to die is associated with increased risk for death by suicide only among patients who also report no desire to live (Brown, Steer, Henriques, & Beck, 2005). Of note, even a small to moderate desire to live is sufficient to offset the risk associated with the strong desire to die. Helping the patient to remember what is worth living for, even if these reasons are relatively underdeveloped, can therefore be a powerful counterbalance to the desire to die.

As was discussed in Chapter 10, the crisis response plan includes an explicit discussion of the patient's reasons to live. This component of the crisis response plan overlaps with these interventions. In the original BCBT protocol, reasons for living were not included as a part of the crisis response plan; they were integrated into the treatment as the two separate procedures described here. However, the reasons for living list and survival kit interventions proved to be especially popular components among BCBT patients and were among the most frequently recalled interventions from the treatment. Our subsequent research indicated that the desire to live played an especially powerful role in reducing suicide attempts among patients who received BCBT and seemed to be a primary mechanism of change (Bryan, Rudd, et al., 2016). We therefore integrated a reasons for living task into the crisis response plan in an attempt to enhance its potency. Although the addition of a reasons for living discussion did not increase the crisis response plan's effects on suicidal thoughts and behaviors, it contributed to a significant increase in positive mood states like hope and calmness and led to significantly larger reductions in perceived burdensomeness. Targeting a patient's reasons for living therefore seems to have an especially potent effect on suicide risk.

HOW TO DO IT: THE REASONS FOR LIVING LIST

To create a reasons for living list, the clinician simply asks what the patient's reasons are for *not* killing him- or herself. It is reasonably common for suicidal patients to state that they have no reasons for living. In this case, the clinician can follow up by asking the patient what prevents him or her from making a (or another) suicide attempt. To heighten the emotional salience of this intervention, the clinician should invite the patient to discuss his or her reasons for living in as much detail as possible. The patient's reasons for living should then be handwritten by the patient on the back side of the crisis response plan or on an index card that can be laminated. Reviewing reasons for living should also be added as a self-management strategy to the crisis response plan (e.g., adding "Review my reasons for living" to the second section of the crisis response plan). Adding the patient's reasons for living to the back side of the crisis response plan helps to connect this intervention to other foundational crisis management and emotion regulation strategies.

Step 1: Introduce the Concept of Reasons for Living

The clinician introduces the concept of reasons for living and explains the rationale for the intervention.

SAMPLE CLINICIAN SCRIPT

I'd like to spend some time today talking about what keeps you alive despite the stress that you've experienced and the problems you've faced. Have you noticed that when you're the most upset or in crisis, it's hard to remember good memories and to think about positive things in life? That's because we have this mental filter that causes us to focus on things that match what we're feeling in the moment. So if we're feeling depressed it's easier to remember depressing things. If we're feeling afraid it's easier to remember other anxiety-provoking or fearful things. If we're suicidal it's easier to remember reasons why we want to die, but it's hard to remember our reasons for wanting to live. This doesn't mean that when we're suicidal we don't have any reasons for living, just that it's hard to remember them. If we can take a moment to remember those reasons for wanting to live, however, it can help us to get unstuck and to maintain a bigger perspective on what's happening to us.

Step 2: Identify the Patient's Reasons for Living

The clinician asks the patient to list his or her reasons for living. If the patient does not understand the question, the clinician can reword the question by asking the patient to identify reasons for not making a suicide attempt.

SAMPLE CLINICIAN SCRIPT

What are your reasons for living, or for not killing yourself? With all that has been going on in your life, what helps to keep you alive and going on a day-to-day basis?

Step 3: Increase the Emotional Salience of the Patient's Reasons for Living

The clinician engages the patient in a discussion about his or her reasons for living and asks the patient to describe specific details about the identified reasons for living in order to increase the vividness of the patient's memory. The clinician should then ask the patient to vividly imagine one or more reason for living in session as practice.

SAMPLE CLINICIAN SCRIPT

[Possible open-ended questions to facilitate discussion:]

> Tell me more about that.
>
> Describe to me what happened.
>
> What about that makes you want to stay alive?
>
> Why would you consider that to be a reason for living?
>
> What do you find so enjoyable about that?
>
> Why is that person so important to you?
>
> As you think about these reasons for living, how does your mood change?

[After a sufficient number of reasons for living have been identified:] Of these many reasons for living, what would you say is the strongest or most important reason to you? Why is that reason so much more important than the other reasons for living?

What I'd like for you to do now is close your eyes and think about that reason for living in great detail. When you think about [reason for living], imagine what it sounds like, looks like, and feels like. Remember a positive story about this reason for living, and describe it to me out loud with as much detail as you can, so that I can understand exactly what you're thinking about. As you're thinking about [reason for living], take a moment to notice how that changes your mood and your thoughts. What specific changes occur to your thoughts and feelings when you think about [reason for living]?

Step 4: Write Down the Reasons for Living

The clinician invites the patient to handwrite his or her reasons for living on the back side of the crisis response plan card or on an index card that can be laminated.

> **SAMPLE CLINICIAN SCRIPT**
>
> Let's write these reasons for living down in a place where you'll be able to easily remember them. Because thinking about your reasons for living is so helpful when you're in crisis, many people find it's helpful to write down their reasons for living on the back of their crisis response plan. That way it's easily accessible when you're trying to solve a problem. What do you think about updating your crisis response plan by writing your reasons for living on the back side of the card?

Step 5: Develop a Plan for Reviewing the Reasons for Living and Elicit Patient Buy-In

In the final step of the reasons for living list, the clinician asks the patient if he or she would be willing to read the list on a regular basis and then develop a plan that specifies the frequency, timing, and duration of practice. Of note, the clinician should make sure that the practice plan includes reviewing the list even when the patient is feeling OK and/or is not in crisis, as this repeated rehearsal will facilitate learning and cognitive flexibility. Once a plan is in place, the clinician should gauge buy-in by asking the patient to rate the likelihood that he or she will review the reasons for living list as planned on a scale ranging from 0 to 10, with 0 indicating "not at all likely" and 10 indicating "very likely."

> **SAMPLE CLINICIAN SCRIPT**
>
> What I'd like for you to do is to review your reasons for living several times a day so you can practice remembering them. This will make it easier for you to remember your reasons for living when you're stressed out. Do you think you would be able to take this card out a few times each day, read the list, and take a minute or two to imagine the things on this list? How many times per day do you think you could take out this card and read this list? How many minutes at a time do you think you could reasonably imagine or mentally picture each of these items? Is there any particular place or situation where you would be especially likely to practice? Are there any times where it might be good to practice because it might help you out?
>
> [After finishing the plan:] So it sounds like we have a plan in place. Using a scale from 0 to 10, with 0 indicating "not at all likely" and 10 indicating "very likely," how likely is it that you'll follow this plan to practice this skill?
>
> [If the rating is lower than 7 out of 10:] Is there any part of this plan that reduces your likelihood for using it? What could we change about this plan to make it more likely that you would use it?

HOW TO DO IT: THE SURVIVAL KIT

To construct a survival kit, the clinician asks the patient to identify objects that elicit positive emotions because they serve as physical reminders of positive life experiences, enjoyable or meaningful activities, or supportive relationships. For example, photos of family members, inspirational quotes or passages, trinkets or mementos from trips and vacations, or small gifts received from friends or loved ones are common objects that are included in a survival kit. The patient gathers these objects and then places them in a container (e.g., a shoebox, an envelope, a tackle box) so they can be easily accessed at a later date. Upon building the survival kit, the patient brings it to session to review with the clinician. As the clinician reviews the contents of the survival kit, he or she asks the patient to explain why each object or item was included in the survival kit. Reviewing each individual item in session serves as skills practice since it typically induces positive emotions in the moment, which is the primary purpose of the activity. Reviewing each item also affords the clinician the opportunity to determine if any of the included objects are potentially iatrogenic (e.g., photos of a family member who sexually abused the patient). If an iatrogenic object is identified, the clinician uses Socratic questioning to help the patient recognize the object as such, thereby guiding the patient to choose to exclude the object.

Once the survival kit is constructed, the patient is encouraged to review its contents on a daily basis to induce positive emotions and to practice remembering positive life experiences. The patient is also encouraged to review the contents of the survival kit during crises or periods of emotional distress. The survival kit should therefore be added to the crisis response plan as a self-management strategy.

Step 1: Introduce the Survival Kit and Invite the Patient to Construct One

The clinician introduces the concept of the survival kit, describes its purpose, and then invites the patient to construct one for him- or herself.

SAMPLE CLINICIAN SCRIPT

We've talked a little bit about how even though you have experienced a lot of challenges in life, there have nonetheless been some positive times and bright spots along the way. Being able to remember happier times and events in our lives can help us to face other challenges, cope with stress, and live a life that's worth living. As you know, thinking about positive life experiences doesn't necessarily solve the problems you're currently facing or make them disappear, but it can make those problems seem less overwhelming and in some cases it can help you think of solutions or alternatives to addressing the problem. Thinking about positive memories can therefore serve as a sort of "survival kit" when we're facing problems.

What I'd like to do today is talk about how you can create a survival kit for yourself.

In this survival kit we're going to place objects and items that remind you of positive experiences from your life. For example, some people put pictures of friends and family in their survival kit; others put inspirational passages or readings in their survival kit; others will put mementos from vacations, trips, or life accomplishments in their survival kit. Once we have the survival kit built, what you can do is go through the contents of the kit when you're experiencing problems. This will help you to keep perspective on the problem, reduce the likelihood of getting overwhelmed, and maybe even help you to generate some solutions. Would you like to hear more about how we can create a survival kit for you?

Since the purpose of the survival kit is to store objects that remind you of positive life experiences, the first step in building one is to find a container of some kind to keep your items in. Most people just use a shoebox or something like that, but others have used a large envelope or a tackle box or a backpack instead. What sort of container would you like to use for your survival kit?

The next step in building a survival kit is figuring out what we want to put inside of it. Again, we're looking for physical objects or items that remind you of positive life experiences or good things in life. What might be some objects you could place in your survival kit? Let's write some of these items down so that when you go home you'll be able to remember what we talked about.

Step 2: Develop a Plan for Creating the Survival Kit and Elicit Patient Buy-In

The clinician asks the patient if he or she would be willing to create a survival kit for the next appointment. The clinician should gauge buy-in by asking the patient to rate the likelihood that he or she create the survival kit on a scale ranging from 0 to 10, with 0 indicating "not at all likely" and 10 indicating "very likely."

SAMPLE CLINICIAN SCRIPT

It sounds like we have a plan, then. Do you think you would be able to build your survival kit before our next appointment and then bring it with you so we can look through it together? On a scale from 0 to 10, with 0 indicating "not at all likely" and 10 indicating "very likely," how likely is it that you'll build a survival kit before our next appointment?

[If the rating is lower than 7 out of 10:] Is there any part of this plan that reduces your likelihood for using it? What could we change about this plan to make it more likely that you would use it?

Step 3: Review the Contents of the Survival Kit (Follow-Up Session)

During the follow-up session, the clinician and the patient review the contents of the survival kit together. The clinician facilitates this process by inviting the patient to "tell the story" of each item and/or explain the rationale for including each item. The clinician assesses whether or not the item might be iatrogenic, and when a potentially iatrogenic item is identified, discusses with the patient whether or not the item should be maintained in the survival kit.

SAMPLE CLINICIAN SCRIPT

So I see you brought in your survival kit with you. Did you have any questions about building it, or any challenges or difficulties in building it?

Why don't we go through the kit together? What's the first item you have? Tell me the story about this item, and why you decided to include it in your survival kit.

[For potentially iatrogenic items:] This item is sort of interesting. I'd like to talk some more about it. As you were telling me about this item, I couldn't help but wonder if it also has some less good aspects in addition to its positive aspects. In particular, I'm wondering if it might cause you to feel more stressed or upset when you're facing a problem? We've spent some time talking about how [the person, place, or situation associated with the item] has caused you problems and stress in the past, and/or hasn't been especially helpful for you. In light of that, I wonder if this object might cause you to remember those negative experiences instead of the positive experiences? What are your thoughts about that? Would you say that this object activates your suicidal mode or deactivates your suicidal mode?

[If the patient is reluctant to remove an iatrogenic object:] Since there are both positive and less positive parts about this object, how about we create a "maybe" pile over here and place this object there temporarily while we go through all the other items? We can come back to this one later and see what we think about it once we've talked about all the other items you have.

[If all objects are potentially iatrogenic and need to be removed:] As you can see, this can be a bit harder than it might seem at first, but that's exactly why we are doing this activity. It sounds like one lesson learned from this is that it can be challenging to differentiate between those aspects of our life that are helpful and those that are unhelpful. Now that we know a little bit more about what might be unhelpful, we'll be able to more easily identify things that are helpful. Let's take some time to do that.

What are some things you used to enjoy doing that you don't do anymore? Let's see if we can find some pictures of those things online, and then we can print them up and place them in your survival kit.

Who are some people that have supported you in the past without making you feel guilty, ashamed, or bad about yourself? Do you have any pictures of them on your phone or on your social media page? Let's print some pictures of them and add them to your survival kit.

Have you ever read anything that made you feel good about yourself or inspired you in some way? Let's see if we can find a passage online and print that up to include in your survival kit.

Good. Now that we've added a few new items for your survival kit, do you want to add additional items or objects that represent these same people, places, or events? For instance, do you have any small mementos or gifts that represent these positive experiences? Would you be willing to add those objects to your survival kit before the next session?

Step 4: Develop a Plan for Reviewing the Contents of the Survival Kit and Elicit Patient Buy-In

In the final step of the survival kit, the clinician invites the patient to review the contents of the survival kit on a regular basis and then develops a plan to specify the frequency, timing, and duration of doing so. Initially, the clinician should encourage the patient to practice accessing and reviewing the contents of his or her survival kit even when feeling OK and/ or relatively calm, as this will facilitate learning and the acquisition of savoring skills. Once a plan is in place, the clinician should gauge buy-in by asking the patient to rate the likelihood that he or she will review the contents of the survival kit on a scale ranging from 0 to 10, with 0 indicating "not at all likely" and 10 indicating "very likely."

SAMPLE CLINICIAN SCRIPT

What I'd like for you to do is to review your survival kit at least once a day so you can practice remembering positive experiences in life. This will make it easier for you to face problems that arise in your life, especially when you're stressed out. Do you think you would be able to take a few minutes each day to go through your survival kit and remember why you placed each of these objects in it? Where do you think you'll keep your survival kit? Are there any times of the day that work better for you for going through the survival kit for a few minutes?

[After finishing the plan:] So it sounds like we have a plan in place. Using a scale from 0 to 10, with 0 indicating "not at all likely" and 10 indicating "very likely," how likely is it that you'll go through your survival kit at least once a day between now and the next time we meet?

[If the rating is lower than 7 out of 10:] Is there any part of this plan that reduces your likelihood for using it? What could we change about this plan to make it more likely that you would use it?

ILLUSTRATIVE CASE EXAMPLES

The Case of Mike

When the reasons for living task was first introduced to Mike, he initially expressed some confusion because this implied that he was suicidal. As seen below, the clinician responded to this by noting that it is possible to have reasons for living even if one is not suicidal. Also note how the clinician increased the emotional salience of Mike's reasons for living by asking him to tell stories about each reason for living.

CLINICIAN: What I'd like to do next is spend some talking about your reasons for living.

MIKE: What do you mean?

CLINICIAN: Reasons for living are things that keep us going on a day-to-day basis despite stress and adversity. Reasons for living often give us a sense of purpose or meaning in life.

MIKE: But wouldn't that just be helpful for people who want to kill themselves?

CLINICIAN: It's definitely helpful for people thinking about suicide, but it's also helpful to know our reasons for living even when we're not suicidal. All of us have reasons for living, even if we aren't thinking about suicide. For most of us, these reasons for living help us to feel good about ourselves even when things aren't going our way. They're sort of like our reasons to get up in the morning and do the things we do, and to keep going when things are tough. You certainly don't have to be suicidal to experience tough times in life, and you certainly don't have to be suicidal to know what's worth living for.

MIKE: Yeah, that makes sense.

CLINICIAN: OK, good. So then what would you say are your reasons for living?

MIKE: Well, definitely my wife.

CLINICIAN: Mm-hmm. What is it about her that makes life worth living?

MIKE: Well, she's a really great person, very supportive, very kind. We have our problems, for sure, and we seem to fight a lot, but she's really important to me.

CLINICIAN: Can you describe a favorite memory you have with your wife?

MIKE: Yeah, I guess it would be the first Christmas we spent together. It was just the two of us that year because we weren't able to go visit family. We celebrated at my apartment and spent most of the day together. We cooked dinner, which was really fun, and then it started snowing really hard, so that night we went out and built a snowman together, which was so completely silly. I hadn't done that since I was a kid. And of course we ended up having a snowball fight with each other. Well, the kids that live underneath me heard us and came out and joined in, so it was me and her against these kids. It was really funny because we were just killing them. They were so uncoordinated. Once that was done we went back inside and changed and just spent the night watching movies and eating leftovers. I don't know why that Christmas stands out to me; we've had so many since. I guess it's just because it was our first and we were young, and we didn't have all the stress we do now.

CLINICIAN: That's a great memory. It definitely sounds like that was a great Christmas. I noticed that as you were telling that story, you started to smile.

MIKE: Yeah. How could I not? It was a really great day.

CLINICIAN: So thinking about positive memories helps you to feel better, even when things aren't going well in life?

MIKE: Yeah, I guess so. It's like there are still good things in life even though things get bad sometimes. It also helps remind me that me and my wife have had some really good times, so it's not all bad.

CLINICIAN: Yeah, interesting. It sounds like you're saying it puts things in perspective?

MIKE: Yeah, definitely. It's not all bad.

CLINICIAN: Well, we certainly haven't fixed all of your marriage issues, but it's helpful to take a step back and remember the good times.

MIKE: Yeah.

CLINICIAN: It sounds like it's sometimes hard for you to remember these fun memories.

MIKE: Oh yeah, definitely. I certainly don't think about any of this when we're arguing with each other.

CLINICIAN: Maybe we should jot this down on an index card to help kick-start your memory in the future. That may help you remember to keep things into perspective.

MIKE: OK, we can do that. That would probably help.

The Case of Janice

Janice was instructed to complete a survival kit during the second session and to bring it with her to the third session. She returned to the third session with a shoebox that was decorated on the outside with scrapbooking supplies. "I wanted to make it look nice so that it would stand out a bit on my shelf, so that whenever I see the box I remember what's inside." The clinician commended her for this decision. He then asked Janice to show him what she had included in her survival kit and to explain the story of each item. Janice's survival kit contained the following:

- A photo of her daughter at a young age playing in the backyard with their dog at that time. "This is my favorite picture of her daughter; it always puts a smile on my face."
- A pocket-sized book of inspirational quotes with several dog-eared pages. "These are the pages with my favorite quotes. I like them because they help remind me about what's important in life."
- A birthday card from a member of her church that she had received for her birthday several months before. "I didn't expect it from her at all and couldn't believe that someone remembered my birthday. It was very sweet of her to do."
- A military medal that she had been awarded while serving in the military. "This medal isn't an especially important one, but I put it in here because it reminds me of serving my country, and that's something I'm proud of."
- An empty bottle of cologne from her ex-husband. "It reminds me of how lucky I am to be away from him. He ended up being very abusive, so choosing to leave him was one of the more important decisions of my life."

Because this last item was related to an especially challenging time in Janice's life, the clinician decided to ask her more about it. Note how the clinician helps Janice to critically evaluate her reasons for including this item in her survival kit and guides her to discover how it actually facilitates negative mood, thoughts, and memories that sustain the suicidal mode, rather than fostering positive mood and thoughts.

CLINICIAN: Tell me more about this cologne bottle.

JANICE: Well, when we first got married, things were fine. But over the years my ex became increasingly controlling and abusive, both emotionally and physically. He would yell at me all the time and criticize me, and tell me how I was ugly and stupid. Eventually he started hitting me as well. I put up with that for about 3 years before I finally left him and got divorced. He was just an awful person and, in many ways, is the source of all my problems and mental health issues.

CLINICIAN: I see. I guess that would explain why you seemed to be getting tense while you were telling me about him. I can see that tears have come to your eyes.

JANICE: Yeah, it's not easy to talk about him.

CLINICIAN: I bet. Which leads me to wonder about something: if thinking about him gets you tense and emotionally upset, should we keep this reminder of him in your survival kit?

JANICE: Well, I put it in there to remind me of how my life is better without him.

CLINICIAN: That makes sense. It sounds like things are much better now.

JANICE: Oh yeah, way better, although I'm still sort of dealing with him and what he did to me.

CLINICIAN: He's had quite a lasting impression on your life . . .

JANICE: Uh-huh.

CLINICIAN: . . . and that impression isn't particularly positive.

JANICE: Definitely not.

CLINICIAN: So when you think about your ex-husband, it brings up all of these negative feelings and thoughts and memories, even though it's also a good thing that he's gone.

JANICE: Yes.

CLINICIAN: Well, given the purpose of this survival kit is to help you feel positive emotions and remember good times for life, it seems in many ways like this cologne bottle does the opposite. What do you think?

JANICE: Yeah, I agree. I see what you're saying. I should take this out.

CLINICIAN: Yeah, that makes sense. I think that's a good idea.

JANICE: I should probably just get rid of it, period.

CLINICIAN: There's another idea. What are your thoughts about that?

JANICE: Well, now that I think about it, I've held on to this because I thought it was my way of reminding myself about my good decisions, but now I realize that all it does is make me think about the bad times we had. I just need to throw it away

CLINICIAN: That makes a lot of sense to me.

TIPS AND ADVICE FOR
THE REASONS FOR LIVING LIST AND THE SURVIVAL KIT

1. **Use both the reasons for living list and the survival kit.** The reasons for living list may be most effective when combined with the survival kit. Because the reasons for living list and the survival kit have a similar purpose but differ in terms of physical structure, they can serve as complementary interventions that can facilitate use across a wider range of contexts and situations than either intervention alone. For example, the reasons for living list is the more transportable of the two interventions; it can therefore serve as an "extension" of the survival kit in situations where access to the survival kit is impractical or inconvenient, or where discretion is preferable. The clinician should therefore seek to link the reasons for living list with the survival kit to enhance the effectiveness of each individual intervention.

2. **Patients cannot leave a session with an empty survival kit.** An important guideline for using the survival kit is that the patient cannot leave the session with an empty survival kit. Very rarely will the patient construct a survival kit in which *all* of the included objects are potentially iatrogenic, but in some cases the clinician and patient may find that a new survival kit is needed to replace the one originally constructed. When this occurs, the clinician should help the patient to identify new, non-iatrogenic objects to place in the survival kit prior to concluding the session. For instance, if the patient enjoys mountain biking or hiking at a particular location, the clinician might search online for images of a mountain bike or a map of hiking trails at the patient's preferred location and then print these images during the session to add to the survival kit. Similarly, the clinician and patient might search online together for favorite quotes or inspirational passages, then print these for inclusion in the survival kit.

3. **Augment interventions with appropriate smartphone apps.** An electronic version of the survival kit, referred to as the "virtual hope box," has recently been developed as a smartphone app and is now available for download. The virtual hope box app enables the patient to construct a survival kit on his or her smartphone from the photos, songs, websites, and phone numbers stored on the patient's phone. The patient can then access the app at any time with a higher level of discretion than can be achieved with the traditional survival kit. Suicidal patients find the virtual hope box app beneficial, useful, and easy to use and tend to use it more than the conventional survival kit (Bush et al., 2014). Patients generally prefer to use *both* the virtual hope box app and the conventional survival kit together because each has unique strengths or qualities that are desirable and complementary. The clinician should therefore consider using both a conventional survival kit and the virtual hope box app with suicidal patients who have smartphones and are willing to download the app.

PART IV

PHASE TWO

Undermining the Suicidal Belief System

CHAPTER 16

ABC Worksheets

The ABC Worksheet is one of several cognitive appraisal techniques for teaching the patient how to identify automatic negative thoughts, assumptions, and core suicidal beliefs that increase vulnerability to suicidal mode activation. The ABC Worksheet is a foundational skill for cognitive reappraisal, specifically by helping patients to identify their cognitive biases. The ABC Worksheet teaches the patient to recognize several interrelated and automatic processes: how automatic thoughts emerge in response to triggering events, how automatic thoughts reflect underlying core beliefs, and how emotional states and behaviors are influenced by the thoughts one has in response to life events. Although many different types of ABC Worksheets have been developed and used in various treatment manuals, in BCBT we selected to incorporate the ABC Worksheets developed by Resick and colleagues (2007) for cognitive processing therapy for PTSD. We selected this particular version of the worksheet for two primary reasons. First, trauma is commong among suicidal patients, and many suicidal beliefs are often related to or influenced by traumatic experiences. Second, many of our BCBT patients had previously completed cognitive processing therapy and were therefore familiar with using the worksheet. Given these circumstances, we have found the ABC Worksheet developed for cognitive processing therapy to be simple and easy for patients to understand, and highly useful for targeting many of the suicidal beliefs that are frequently encountered in BCBT. The ABC Worksheet can be found in Appendix A.8. The suicidal patient is often unaware of how he or she is negatively interpreting triggering events (whether internal or external) and how these interpretations are driving maladaptive behaviors and negative emotional reactions. The ABC Worksheets therefore serve to teach basic self-monitoring skills, which effectively "slow down" the negative chain of events that leads from triggering event to automatic thought to emotional or behavioral consequence. This in turn reduces the likelihood that the patient will respond to an external or internal trigger in an overlearned manner. The ABC Worksheet is an especially useful first intervention to implement during the second phase of treatment.

RATIONALE

Cognitive reappraisal is a common skill set among treatments that reduce suicide attempts (Brown, Ten Have, et al., 2005; Linehan, Comtois, Murray, et al., 2006; Rudd et al., 2015). Consistent with the fluid vulnerability theory of suicide, core suicidal beliefs lend long-term, persisting vulnerability to suicide attempts. Among psychiatric outpatients, suicidal beliefs such as hopelessness, perceived burdensomeness, self-hatred, perceived defectiveness, and shame differentiate those who have made a suicide attempt from those who have thought about suicide but not made an attempt and those who have never been suicidal (Bryan, Rudd, Wertenberger, Etienne, et al., 2014). Core suicidal beliefs also predict future suicide attempts better than suicide ideation, a history of suicide attempts, and emotional distress (Brown, Beck, Steer, & Grisham, 2000; Bryan, Clemans, & Hernandez, 2012; Bryan, Morrow, Anestis, & Joiner, 2010; Bryan, Rudd, Wertenberger, Etienne, et al., 2014; Joiner, Van Orden, Witte, Selby et al., 2009; Kanzler, Bryan, McGeary, & Morrow, 2012). Taken together, these findings support the fluid vulnerability theory's contention that core suicidal beliefs serve as chronic vulnerabilities to suicide regardless of acute emotional distress. The specific targeting of core suicidal beliefs is a key mechanism of action that distinguishes those treatments that effectively reduce the risk for suicide attempts following treatment. In order to effectively target these cognitive vulnerabilities, suicidal patients must first learn how to recognize the automaticity with which these underlying beliefs contribute to their emotions and actions.

HOW TO DO IT

ABC Worksheets should be completed as a collaborative writing project as opposed to merely a verbal exercise. Practically speaking, this means that when the patient is working on ABC Worksheets, he or she should handwrite responses directly onto the worksheet because this will increase emotional engagement with the task. Likewise, the clinician should be aware that completing the ABC Worksheet (and all other worksheets described in subsequent chapters) as a written task works better than simply reviewing its content verbally. This aligns with the skills training philosophy of effective treatments: translating cognitive reappraisal into a behavior skill set increases its effectiveness.

The main section of the ABC Worksheet contains three boxes: the A box represents the activating event (i.e., "What happened to me?"), the B box represents the belief (i.e., "What do I think about it or say to myself?"), and the C box represents the emotional consequences (i.e., "What do I feel?"). Underneath the ABC boxes are two questions that serve to facilitate the process of cognitive reappraisal. The first question, *Are the thoughts in "B" helpful?*, is designed to help the patient to distinguish between automatic thoughts and beliefs that are adaptive and those that are maladaptive. Underneath this question, the ABC Worksheet includes a final question designed to facilitate cognitive reappraisal: *What is a more helpful thing I can say to myself in the future when in a similar situation?* Note that these questions do not ask patients to determine if their beliefs are "realistic" or "reasonable" and do not ask them to produce a "more realistic" or "more reasonable" thought. This is because, to the suicidal patient, certain negative beliefs truly are perceived as realistic and reasonable; asking the patient to determine if his or her perceptions are realistic or reasonable therefore often results in an affirmative response. Using functionally based language (e.g., *helpful* and *unhelpful*) also avoids the judgmental and self-critical aspects of cognitive reappraisal that can be implied by words such as *realistic* and *reasonable* (e.g., "I'm an unreasonable person with unrealistic thinking").

When teaching the ABC Worksheet, the clinician should first review how life events, thoughts, and emotions are interconnected. The clinician has the patient learn how to do the ABC Worksheet using his or her index suicidal episode or suicide attempt as an example. The clinician asks the patient to identify the triggering event that led to the suicidal episode or suicide attempt and to write this event in the A box. Because most patients can easily identify the emotions they felt during a given incident but are more likely to struggle to identify their automatic thoughts and core beliefs, a practical strategy for the ABC Worksheet is to temporarily skip the B box and proceed to the C box next. The clinician then asks the patient to identify the emotions that he or she felt in response to this trigger and to write these emotions in the C box. Finally, the clinician asks to the patient to identify what thoughts were going through his or her mind in response to the triggering event and to write this down in the B box. Most patients will identify an automatic thought for the B box. Once the automatic thought is identified, the clinician should use Socratic questioning to identify the core belief that underlies the automatic thought.

A common strategy for uncovering core beliefs is the *downward arrow technique*. In the downward arrow technique, the clinician asks the patient to determine the implications of the automatic thought using an "if . . . then" assumption formula: "If [automatic thought] is true, then what does that say about you as a person?" In some cases, the patient will not initially respond to the downward arrow with a core belief, but will instead respond with another automatic thought or an assumption. In this case, the clinician responds with another downward arrow: "And if that's true, what does that say about you as a person?" The downward arrow technique is highlighted in John's case study, which is described below

After the ABC boxes have been completed, the clinician asks the patient to answer the two cognitive reappraisal questions. Once a new, more helpful thought or belief has been identified, the clinician asks the patient to consider how the new belief affects his or her emotions as compared to the original belief. To ensure skill mastery, patients should complete several ABC Worksheets per session as well as several between sessions. In addition to focusing on the index suicidal episode, the clinician also asks the patient to complete worksheets that are focused on other triggering events and situations in his or her life so that skill generalization can occur.

Step 1: Introduce the Concept of the ABC Worksheet

The clinician introduces the concept of the ABC Worksheet and then briefly reviews the general cognitive-behavioral model for conceptualizing and targeting emotional distress.

Today I'd like for us to start focusing on the thoughts you have during stressful situations and the beliefs or "rules" you have acquired during your life that influence your decisions. As a reminder, we've talked about how what you say to yourself mentally in various situations can determine how you feel and what you do in response to situations in life. For example, if a person generally thinks that they're a failure in life, when they make a relatively small mistake they might think to themselves, "I screwed up again, like I always do," and they're likely to feel guilty or sad. Because this person feels so bad, they might withdraw from others or drink alcohol to feel better. In contrast, someone who generally thinks that they are a smart and competent person would probably respond to that same mistake in a different way, perhaps by thinking to themselves, "Oops, that's a bummer; we all make mistakes sometimes." This person recognizes that mistakes happen sometimes, fixes the mistake, and then moves on with what they were doing. Although this second person might be frustrated or annoyed about making a mistake, they don't necessarily feel sad or guilty because they realize that sometimes mistakes just happen. So the assumptions and beliefs we have about ourselves can influence how we interpret life events, how we feel, and how we act. Does that make sense?

Today I want to spend some time focusing on how your thoughts and beliefs contributed to your suicidal crisis, and how they continue to contribute to the negative emotions and distress you feel on a regular basis. To do this we're going to use what's called an ABC Worksheet. The ABC Worksheet is designed to help us identify the thoughts, beliefs, and assumptions that underlie the decisions we make and the actions we take in life.

Step 2: Complete an ABC Worksheet
Focused on the Index Suicidal Episode or Suicide Attempt

The clinician assists the patient in completing an ABC Worksheet focused on the index suicidal episode or crisis. The clinician explains each component of the ABC Worksheet and guides the patient with Socratic dialogue to identify automatic thoughts and beliefs and to recognize how cognition, emotion, and behavior are interconnected. When the patient identifies an automatic thought, the clinician uses the downward arrow technique or other Socratic questioning to identify the underlying core belief. The clinician hands the patient a copy of the ABC Worksheet and asks the patient to fill in each section of the worksheet in his or her own writing.

This worksheet has several sections that I'll explain as we work through this together. These three boxes here are the main section of the worksheet, and are where the name "ABC Worksheet" comes from. This first box is the A box. "A" stands for "activating event." In this box we want to answer the question that's right above the box: "What is going on?" Also, "What happened?" So let's think back to the suicidal crisis that occurred right before we started working together. What was the event or the situation that activated or triggered your crisis? Go ahead and write that down in the A box.

Now what we're going to do next is actually skip this middle box and go over to this box on the right. This is the C box. "C" stands for "consequences." When we talk about the consequences of a situation, we're most interested in the emotion you felt afterwards. So this question here for the C box asks, "What do I feel as a result?" Also, "What emotion do I feel?" So if we go back to your suicidal crisis again, when that stressful situation occurred, what were you feeling afterwards? Go ahead and write that down in the C box.

Now let's look at this middle box. The reason I skipped the middle box is that sometimes knowing how we felt in a situation can help us figure out what we were thinking at the time. This middle box is the B box, and the "B" stands for "belief." This is where we want to note what your thoughts were at the time. An easy way to figure out what you were thinking is to ask yourself the questions written on the worksheet: "What do I tell myself?" Also, "What goes through my mind?" So in your suicidal crisis, when that stressful situation occurred and you were feeling [emotion], what were you telling yourself and was going through your mind at that time? Write down that thought here in the B box.

[If the patient identifies an automatic thought but not a core belief:] Let's talk about that thought a little bit more. Let's assume that your thought at that time is completely true and accurate. If this thought is true, what does that say about you as a person?

So as a recap, during your suicidal crisis, this activating event sort of set things in motion. In response to this event, you started to think very negative things about the situation and yourself, which caused you to feel upset. Now let's look at this next question here: "Are the thoughts in B helpful?" So in that situation, was it helpful to you to say these things about yourself? In general, do you find it's helpful to think these negative things about yourself? What makes these thoughts and beliefs so unhelpful? Go ahead and write that down on the line here.

If these thoughts and beliefs are so unhelpful, what is something else that you can tell yourself in the future when you're in a similar situation? Go ahead and write that down as well.

Now that you see how this process works, do you have any questions? Does this make sense? Good; let's practice with another worksheet.

Step 3: Complete Several ABC Worksheets Focused on Other Stressful Situations

In order to facilitate skill acquisition and generalization, the clinician has the patient complete several more ABC Worksheets that are focused on other stressful situations in the patient's life. The clinician provides additional copies of the ABC Worksheet and guides the patient through the completion of each.

SAMPLE CLINICIAN SCRIPT

For this worksheet, let's focus on a different time when you felt stressed out or upset. Tell me about a recent situation when you felt stressed or upset. Just like the last worksheet, let's go through each of these sections one at a time so we can identify your thoughts and beliefs and then figure out whether or not they were helpful.

Let's start with A, the activating event. What happened or what was going on? Write that down in the A box.

Next is C, the consequence. What did you feel as a result or what emotion did you feel? Write that down in the C box.

Last is B, the belief. What did you say to yourself or what was going through your mind at that time? And if that's true, what does that say about you as a person? Write that down in the B box.

So in this situation, when the activating event occurred, you started to tell yourself these things in the B box, and that caused you to feel these negative emotions.

Were these thoughts in B helpful for you in that situation? Why not? Write that down here.

If these thoughts are so unhelpful, what is something else you can say to yourself in the future if you find yourself in a similar situation? Write that down here.

Great job. I think you're getting the hang of this. What questions do you have about how to do this worksheet? How might this be helpful to practice?

Step 4: Develop a Plan for Practicing ABC Worksheets in between Sessions

In the final step of the ABC Worksheet, the clinician invites the patient to complete at least one worksheet per day before the next appointment. At least one of these worksheets should be focused on the index suicide attempt or suicidal episode. The clinician then gauges buy-in by asking the patient to rate the likelihood that he or she will complete the worksheets as prescribed on a scale ranging from 0 to 10, with 0 indicating "not at all likely" and 10 indicating "very likely." The clinician then provides the patient with a sufficient number of blank ABC Worksheets to complete the assignment.

SAMPLE CLINICIAN SCRIPT

Like all the other skills we've talked about thus far, practice makes perfect. Now that you've done a few of these, you can see that they don't take much time at all to complete. Do you think you would be able to complete at least one ABC Worksheet a day between now and the next time we meet? You can focus on any situation you want, but at least one of these worksheets should be focused on the original suicidal crisis that brought you in to treatment. Does that make sense? Here is a stack of ABC Worksheets for you to take with you.

[After finishing the plan:] So it sounds like we have a plan in place. Using a scale from 0 to 10, with 0 indicating "not at all likely" and 10 indicating "very likely," how likely is it that you'll complete at least one ABC Worksheet per day between now and the next time we meet?

[If rating is lower than 7 out of 10:] Is there any part of this plan that reduces your likelihood for practicing these worksheets? What could we change about this plan to make it more likely that you will complete them?

ILLUSTRATIVE CASE EXAMPLE

For his first ABC Worksheet, John and his clinician decided to focus on the argument with his spouse that activated his suicidal crisis. This event was selected first because it was most proximally related to his suicidal crisis. As can be seen in Figure 16.1, John wrote "argument with my wife" in the A box, which designated the activating event. John wasn't able to identify his thoughts and beliefs, however, so the clinician directed him to the C box next, which identified his emotional response. John indicated that he felt guilt, anger, and sadness during the argument with his wife. To help identify his suicidal beliefs, John and the clinician engaged in the following exchange:

CLINICIAN: If you think back to that argument, what would you say was running through your head at that time? What sorts of things were you saying to yourself?

JOHN: I don't really remember.

CLINICIAN: I know it can be hard to remember the details of that day. When it's hard to remember what we were thinking, we can sometimes look at our emotions for some clues. This is because certain types of thoughts go with certain types of emotions.

JOHN: What do you mean?

CLINICIAN: Let's take the thought "I'm a failure" as an example. If you were to tell yourself, "I'm a failure," would you expect to feel happy afterward?

A Activating Event (What happened?)	B Beliefs (What do I tell myself?)	C Consequences (What emotion do I feel?)
Argument with my wife	She's right, it's all my fault. I'm a failure and always will be.	Guilt Anger Sadness
Is the belief above in box "B" helpful? No, because it just makes me want to give up and drink more.		
What is something else I can tell myself in the future when in a similar situation? I'm not perfect, but I do some things right.		

FIGURE 16.1. ABC Worksheet from John.

JOHN: No.

CLINICIAN: Why not?

JOHN: Well, telling yourself a failure probably means you're upset or feeling down or something like that.

CLINICIAN: That's right! Thinking about being a failure fits with feeling down or sad but doesn't fit with feeling happy. Let's do another one. If you were to tell yourself, "I'm not safe," would you expect to feel relaxed and calm?

JOHN: Probably not.

CLINICIAN: Why not?

JOHN: If you're not safe then probably you aren't relaxed.

CLINICIAN: What would be feeling instead of relaxed?

JOHN: I don't know. Fear, I guess.

CLINICIAN: You're right again! Thinking that you're not safe fits with feeling afraid or anxious, but it doesn't fit with feeling relaxed or calm. Some thoughts fit with some emotions but not others. If you know the emotions that you're feeling, then, you can often help figure out what you're telling yourself.

JOHN: That makes sense.

CLINICIAN: OK, great. So then if you were feeling guilty, angry, and sad, what types of thoughts do you think you were having?

JOHN: (*After a long pause*) I think I was telling myself how she's always right and it's my fault that we have problems.

CLINICIAN: Yeah, that would seem to fit here.

JOHN: Yeah, I think I get this now.

CLINICIAN: OK, go ahead and write that down. Here's my next question: if it's true that she's right and it's all your fault, what does that say about what kind of person you are?

JOHN: It means I'm a bad husband and a failure. I was thinking I always will be.

CLINICIAN: That's a pretty strong thought. Let's write that down, too.

Once his core belief was identified, John and the clinician completed the worksheet together. John indicated that blaming himself and calling himself a failure was not helpful because it only made him "want to drink more and give up." When asked what he could say in the future when having arguments with his wife, John replied, "I'm definitely not perfect but I do some things right." The clinician directed John to record this alternative thought as well.

TIPS AND ADVICE FOR
ABC WORKSHEETS

1. **Continue to reinforce skills learned in the first phase of BCBT.** Although the focus of BCBT shifts to the cognitive domain, clinicians should nonetheless continue to ask the patient about his or her use of crisis response planning and other emotion regulation skills.

2. **Target core beliefs, not automatic thoughts.** Automatic thoughts entail the individual's immediate reactions to activating events. Automatic thoughts therefore depend on the context and, as a result, are highly variable. Core beliefs lie underneath automatic thoughts and tend to be stable across different contexts. Because automatic thoughts are influenced by core beliefs, the former can be used to uncover the latter. For example, a patient may have the automatic thoughts "I screwed up again" and "I always make mistakes" when he or she makes an error. Both of these automatic thoughts may reflect the underlying core belief "I'm a failure," which exists across all settings and situations. By targeting the core belief, clinicians can address a more central vulnerability that cuts across situations and contexts.

3. **Encourage patients to write their responses on the worksheets.** Although a good deal of cognitive work is conducted verbally through the use of Socratic dialogue, patients can translate these concepts into tangible skills by writing their responses on the worksheet. By writing out their responses, patients can "see" their beliefs in a new way that can facilitate more rapid change. Use of the worksheets also provides a concrete method for clinicians to track patient skills practice and treatment adherence.

4. **Cognitive rigidity does not necessarily reflect clinical regression.** As patients transition from the first to the second phase of BCBT, clinicians often report feeling as though their patients have "regressed." In most cases, this is because patients had been progressing well during the first sessions of BCBT, but then they suddenly seem to stall once they start working on the ABC Worksheets. This apparent slowdown does not necessarily reflect clinical regression, however; rather, it may instead reflect the shift in focus to the cognitive domain, which has not been directly targeted in treatment until now. Because the cognitive domain takes center stage at this point in BCBT, the patient's cognitive rigidity comes to the forefront. Clinicians may need to "take it slow" during this transition period, but they should not delay or prematurely abandon cognition-oriented work.

CHAPTER 17

Challenging Questions Worksheets

The Challenging Questions Worksheet is a second cognitive appraisal technique designed to teach the patient how to critically evaluate the core beliefs that make him or her more vulnerable to suicidal mode activation. The Challenging Questions Worksheet builds on the foundational cognitive reappraisal skills learned from the ABC Worksheets. From a sequencing perspective, the clinician should therefore introduce the Challenging Questions Worksheet only after the patient has demonstrated mastery of the basic self-monitoring skills that underlie the ABC Worksheets (i.e., recognition of how situational variables, cognition, and emotion are interrelated). Challenging Questions Worksheets facilitate patients' ability to recognize the maladaptive or unhelpful nature of their overlearned core suicidal beliefs, thereby enabling them to consider more adaptive alternative beliefs that are inconsistent with suicidal mode activation and reducing vulnerability for later suicide attempts. Similar to the ABC Worksheets, the Challenging Questions Worksheets used in BCBT were adapted from those developed for cognitive processing therapy (Resick et al., 2017). These worksheets should be completed as a collaborative written activity as opposed to being limited to a verbal exercise. The Challenging Questions Worksheet can be found in Appendix A.9.

RATIONALE

As noted in the previous chapter, cognitive reappraisal is a common element of treatments that reduce suicide attempts (Brown, Ten Have, et al., 2005; Linehan, Comtois, Murray, et al., 2006; Rudd et al., 2015). The primary purpose of cognitive appraisal is to replace core suicidal beliefs with more adaptive beliefs and positive cognitive styles that reduce risk for suicide, such as optimism (Bryan, Ray-Sannerud, Morrow, & Etienne, 2013b; Hirsch & Conner, 2006; Hirsch, Conner, & Duberstein, 2007; Hirsch, Wolford, Lalonde, Brunk, &

Parker-Morris, 2009), meaning in life (Bryan, Elder, et al., 2013; Dogra, Basu, & Das, 2011; Heisel & Flett, 2008), hope (Dogra et al., 2011), pride (Bryan, Ray-Sannerud, et al., 2013c), and self-efficacy (Bryan, Andreski, et al., 2014). Guilt and shame may be particularly important targets for cognitive appraisal given their strong relationships with suicidal thoughts and behaviors (Bryan, Morrow, Etienne, & Ray-Sannerud, 2013; Bryan, Ray-Sannerud, Morrow, & Etienne, 2013a; Bryan, Roberge, Bryan, & Ray-Sannerud, 2015; Hendin & Haas, 1991). Further supporting this possibility is newer evidence suggesting that the capacity to forgive oneself for perceived transgressions and wrongdoing is associated with decreased risk for making a suicide attempt (Bryan, Theriault, & Bryan, 2014). The Challenging Questions Worksheet helps to undermine guilt, shame, self-blame, and other maladaptive beliefs through the development of cognitive flexibility. As patients' cognitive flexibility increases and their cognitive rigidity declines, they become better equipped to evaluate themselves, others, and the world in a more balanced manner. This, in turn, reduces the risk for making suicide attempts in the future.

HOW TO DO IT

At the top of the Challenging Questions Worksheet is an area for the patient to write down a maladaptive suicidal (or other) core belief. Underneath this section is a list of several questions that direct the patient to critically evaluate the core belief identified at the top of sheet. Because the patient should work on only one core belief per worksheet, writing the specific core belief in the top section provides a visual reference point (and reminder) about which core belief is specifically being evaluated. When teaching the Challenging Questions Worksheet, the clinician reviews the ABC Worksheets with specific reference to the cognitive reappraisal questions at the bottom of the ABC Worksheet (i.e., "Are the thoughts in 'B' helpful? What is something else I can tell myself in the future when in a similar situation?"). The clinician notes that the Challenging Questions Worksheet is the next step in learning how to think about life events in a different way and explains that the worksheet serves to strengthen the patient's ability to determine if his or her thoughts and beliefs are helpful. The clinician has the patient learn how to do the Challenging Questions Worksheet using a core suicidal belief as an example and asks him or her to write this belief in the section at the top of the worksheet. The clinician then asks the patient to read the first question and consider how it applies to the identified belief at the top of the worksheet. The clinician uses Socratic questioning to help the patient to identify alternative and more adaptive perspectives about his or her belief. Once the patient identifies a more functional or adaptive perspective, the clinician invites the patient to write this new perspective down on the worksheet. The clinician and patient repeat this process until all of the questions have been answered.

When working on the Challenging Questions Worksheet for the first time, many patients have difficulty challenging their core beliefs and considering alternative perspectives. This is common even for those patients who are responding very well to treatment and have made considerable progress. The clinician should keep in mind that difficulties with this task are not necessarily an indication of a lack of progress in treatment; rather, they are a reflection of the automaticity of the suicidal belief system. In short, the patient's maladaptive beliefs are so overlearned that they continue to persist even when a patient's symptoms have started to remit and his or her emotional distress has been reduced. Early in the process of teaching cognitive reappraisal skills, the clinician should keep in mind that the clinical goal is not to help the patient to completely abandon overlearned beliefs, but rather to help the patient acknowledge the *possibility* of an alternative perspective, even if he or she does not believe in or fully accept the alternative.

To ensure skill mastery, patients should complete several Challenging Questions Worksheets per session as well as several Challenging Questions Worksheets between each session. The clinician asks the patient to complete at least one worksheet focused on a suicidal belief that was present during the index suicidal episode.

Step 1: Introduce the Concept of the Challenging Questions Worksheet

The clinician introduces the concept of the Challenging Questions Worksheet and then briefly reviews the general concept of cognitive appraisal.

SAMPLE CLINICIAN SCRIPT

Over the past week or so we've been focusing a lot on the ABC Worksheets to learn how our thoughts and beliefs in certain situations contribute to emotional distress. When completing the ABC Worksheets, you were asked to determine if your thoughts and beliefs were helpful for you and, if not, to think of something else you could say to yourself in the future to reduce the likelihood that you'll experience these negative emotions. As you're starting to learn, what we say to ourselves and the "rules" we follow in life have a major impact on how we feel and how we choose to act in response to stressful situations. By evaluating our thoughts and beliefs, we can better identify those thoughts and beliefs that are unhelpful and then identify more helpful or balanced ways to think about things.

Today I'd like for us to take the next step by teaching you a more advanced skill for doing this. To learn this skill, we'll use a new worksheet called the Challenging Questions Worksheet. The Challenging Questions Worksheet will provide you with a series of questions that you can ask to determine if a belief is helpful or not. If you determine that a belief is not helpful as a result of asking these questions, you'll also be better positioned to figure out how to think about what's happening to you in a more helpful way.

Step 2: Complete a Challenging Questions Worksheet Focused on a Suicidal Belief

The clinician assists the patient in completing a Challenging Questions Worksheet focused on a suicidal belief that was present during the index suicidal episode. The clinician explains each component of the Challenging Questions Worksheet and guides the patient with Socratic dialogue to evaluate the suicidal belief. When the patient provides a response that supports the suicidal belief (i.e., no evidence of change), the clinician uses Socratic questioning to uncover information that would counter the core belief and then asks the patient if the alternative perspective is possible, even if he or she does not fully believe or accept it. The clinician hands a copy of the Challenging Questions Worksheet to the patient and asks him or her to fill in each section of the worksheet in his or her own writing.

SAMPLE CLINICIAN SCRIPT

This worksheet has two main sections. Up here at the top is where we can write down a particular thought or belief that we want to focus on when completing the worksheet. When doing these worksheets, we'll always focus on just one belief at a time. Underneath this section is a series of questions that we'll be asking with respect to the belief and then writing down our answers. As we'll see shortly, these questions are designed to put your belief on trial, so to speak. We'll use the questions to help us determine if the belief is helpful or if it is unhelpful.

Let's start by choosing a belief to focus on. If we think back to the suicidal episode that brought you in for treatment, what are some of the things you were thinking in the time leading up to your suicide attempt [or crisis]? Let's go ahead and write that belief down here on this blank line. Now what we'll do is ask each of these questions down here as it relates to this belief. In other words, we're going to be figuring out how helpful this belief is by asking all of these questions.

Go ahead and read the first question there out loud. How would you answer that as it relates to this belief? Write down your answer underneath that question.

[The clinician repeats for all subsequent questions on the worksheet:] Let's go to the next one. How would you answer that question? Write down your answer underneath the question here.

Very good. Now that you've done the whole worksheet, what are your thoughts about this? What questions do you have about doing this worksheet? Let's practice another one.

Step 3: Complete Several Challenging Questions Worksheets Focused on Other Maladaptive Beliefs

In order to facilitate skill acquisition and generalization, the clinician completes several more Challenging Questions Worksheets focused on other suicidal or maladaptive beliefs. The clinician provides additional copies of the Challenging Questions Worksheet and guides the patient through the completion of each.

SAMPLE CLINICIAN SCRIPT

For this worksheet, let's focus on a different belief that we've talked about being unhelpful. Just like the last worksheet, let's go through each of the questions together so we can better figure out if the belief is helpful or not. What belief should we focus on for this worksheet? Go ahead and write that down at the top.

Let's start with the first question. Go ahead and read that out loud and then let me know how you would answer that. Write down your answer underneath.

[The clinician repeats for all subsequent questions on the worksheet:] Go ahead to the next one. What is that question and how would you answer it? Go ahead and write down your answer underneath.

Great job. I think you're getting the hang of this. What questions do you have about this worksheet? How might this worksheet be helpful to practice on a regular basis?

Step 4: Develop a Plan for Practicing Challenging Questions Worksheets in between Sessions

In the final step of the Challenging Questions Worksheet, the clinician invites the patient to complete at least one worksheet per day before the next appointment. At least one of these worksheets should be focused on a suicidal belief that was present during the index suicide attempt or suicidal episode. The clinician gauges buy-in by asking the patient to rate the likelihood that he or she will complete the worksheets as prescribed on a scale ranging from 0 to 10, with 0 indicating "not at all likely" and 10 indicating "very likely." The clinician then provides the patient with a sufficient number of blank Challenging Questions Worksheets to complete the assignment.

SAMPLE CLINICIAN SCRIPT

Now that you've done a few of these, you see how they should be done. Do you think you would be able to complete at least one Challenging Questions Worksheet a day between now and the next time we meet? You can focus on any belief you want, but at least one of these worksheets should be focused on a belief you had during your last suicide attempt or suicidal crisis. Does that make sense? Here is a stack of Challenging Questions Worksheets for you to take with you.

[After finishing the plan:] So it sounds like we have a plan in place. Using a scale from 0 to 10, with 0 indicating "not at all likely" and 10 indicating "very likely," how likely is it that you'll complete at least one Challenging Questions Worksheet per day between now and the next time we meet?

[If rating is lower than 7 out of 10:] Is there any part of this plan that reduces your likelihood for completing these worksheets? What could we change about this plan to make it more likely that you will complete the worksheets?

ILLUSTRATIVE CASE EXAMPLE

Building on his initial work with the ABC Worksheets, John chose to work on the core belief "I'm a failure" for his first Challenging Questions Worksheet. John's responses can be found in Figure 17.1. For the second question on the worksheet (i.e., "Is this belief based on facts or is it something you've just gotten used to saying?"), John initially responded that his belief was based on facts. When questioned about this response, John described a number of mistakes and errors he had made as evidence to support the contention that the belief was based on facts. Instead of disagreeing outright with John's conclusion, however, the clinician engaged him in a series of questions to introduce the possibility that the belief might also be something that John had gotten used to saying:

CLINICIAN: It sounds like there are lots of instances in which you've told yourself that you're a failure. Do you find yourself having the thought "I'm a failure" very often?

JOHN: Yeah, I guess so.

CLINICIAN: How many times per day would you say you think about being a failure?

JOHN: I don't know. I guess at least once a day, but some days it's more.

CLINICIAN: It sounds like you have that thought quite a bit. Given how often you have that thought, would you say it's pretty easy for you to think about how you're a failure?

JOHN: Yeah, it's pretty easy to think about that.

CLINICIAN: Would you say it's become so easy to think about that the thought comes to you quickly, without having to give it much thought? Sort of like it just pops into your mind automatically?

JOHN: Yeah, I guess so. Yeah. It's like it's just always there when I screw up.

CLINICIAN: Got it. So if I understand you right, this thought about being a failure comes to mind quickly, without much effort, and seems to occur over and over again, almost as though it's an automatic response. Is that right?

JOHN: Yeah, I'd say so.

CLINICIAN: Hmmm . . . Well, I don't know, but that sounds a lot like a habit.

JOHN: What do you mean?

CLINICIAN: Well, a habit is something we do over and over again without much thought, and usually we aren't even aware that we're doing it. At least that's how I think of a habit. How would you describe a habit?

JOHN: I'd probably describe it the same way.

CLINICIAN: OK, so we're on the same page there. Based on how you just explained this thought about being a failure, it really sounds a lot like it's become a habit for you.

JOHN: Well, but it's based on facts.

CLINICIAN: Right, you told me about all of the mistakes and errors you had made.

JOHN: Yes.

CLINICIAN: So maybe it's both a fact and a habit?

JOHN: Yeah, maybe.

CLINICIAN: Maybe that's it. Because you say it's based on facts, but you also talked about how it's sort of like a habit, too. What do you think?

JOHN: Yeah, I agree. That makes sense.

CLINICIAN: OK, so what do you think we should put on the worksheet?

JOHN: I guess I'll put that it's both.

CLINICIAN: OK, that sounds good. Do you think it would be helpful to also jot a few words down to explain how it's a habit? It seems like that's the part of this belief that wasn't as obvious.

JOHN: Yeah, that would be good.

In this interaction, John understandably argued that his belief about being a failure was based on facts. John's clinician was able to introduce the alternate possibility that the belief was based on habit not by disagreeing with John's perspective, which could have prompted John to defend his position, but rather by using Socratic dialogue. John started by leading John to describe the nature of his belief in a way that would align with the concept of a habit. The clinician then asked John to reconcile this description with the more general concept or definition of a habit. When John continued to maintain the perspective that his belief was factual, the clinician rolled with this and did not disagree, but rather proposed the possibility that the belief was based on both facts *and* habit, rather than one or the other. In essence, the clinician accepted a "middle ground," thereby making it possible for John to accept the possibility that his belief was habitual to some degree. This, in turn, weakened the possibility that it was based entirely on facts. Although John may not yet be ready to fully abandon the maladaptive belief, with additional practice, the strength of the belief will decline. John's full Challenging Questions Worksheet is displayed in Figure 17.1.

TIPS AND ADVICE FOR
CHALLENGING QUESTIONS WORKSHEETS

1. **Take an inch to get a mile.** A common mistake for many clinicians is to hold unrealistic expectations about patient progress when using the Challenging Questions Worksheets. Because suicidal patients have such constricted thought processes and problem-solving abilities, however, change can be sometimes be slow. When working with suicidal patients, be willing to accept small changes early on, as this will often motivate and/or reinforce bigger change later on down the road. As was demonstrated in the case of John, a clinician who merely accepts the patient's willingness to concede the possible existence of an alternative perspective can sow the seed for subsequent change. Accepting a relatively small change can therefore be an important first step in the change process.

2. **Emphasize the importance of context.** A key component of cognitive flexibility is the ability to contextualize one's beliefs, decisions, and actions. In many cases, suicidal beliefs result from the patient's tendency to disregard or ignore this context. Of the 10 questions listed on the Challenging Questions Worksheets, three are specifically designed to contextualize the patient's beliefs: question 3 ("If someone else had this belief in this same situation, would you consider it accurate?"), question 6 ("Are you only focusing on one aspect of the event and ignoring other important facts about the situation that explains things?"), and question 10 ("Are you focused on unrelated details of the situation?"). Although all 10 questions are critical for helping patients develop the capacity to critically evaluate their beliefs, these three questions are especially important for helping them to "see the bigger picture." Clinicians should therefore make sure to pay particular attention to the patient's responses to these questions.

Belief: *I'm a failure.*

1. **What is the evidence for and against this idea?** *For: I feel overwhelmed, I drink all the time, I've been divorced a lot.* *Against: I've been able to get by OK so far, I do a good job at work.*
2. **Is your belief a habit or based on facts?** *Both Fact and Habit—I'm so used to saying this that I think it's true*
3. **If someone else had this belief in this same situation, would you consider it accurate?** *Not very accurate because they've done some things right in life, too*
4. **Are you thinking in all-or-none terms?** *Yes, I think I'm a total failure even if I've just made mistakes that everyone makes*
5. **Are you using words or phrases that are extreme or exaggerated (i.e., always, forever, never, need, should, must, can't, and every time)?** *No, but I do think I'm always a failure.*
6. **Are you only focusing on one aspect of the event and ignoring other important facts about the situation that explains things?** *Yes, just focusing on my worry and anger and overreacting*
7. **What is the source of this belief? Is that source reliable?** *I'm the source. I'm not a reliable source because I only say it when I'm upset and drunk, which is not when I'm not the best judge*
8. **Are you blowing things out of proportion? Or the opposite: minimizing things?** *Yes—chances are that she won't leave me if I talk with her and work it out. It's only likely to happen if I don't take steps to control my drinking, which I can do.*
9. **Is your belief based on feelings rather than facts?** *Based mostly on stress*
10. **Are you focused on unrelated details of the situation?** *Yes, I'm focusing on how I'm afraid my wife will leave me instead of focusing on what's actually going on.*

FIGURE 17.1. Sample Challenging Questions Worksheet from John.

CHAPTER 18

Patterns of Problematic Thinking Worksheets

The Patterns of Problematic Thinking Worksheet is a third cognitive reappraisal technique used to teach patients how to identify and label different types of cognitive distortions that increase a patient's vulnerability to suicidal mode activation. Cognitive distortions are exaggerated or dysfunctional thought patterns that cause the patient to perceive life events in a biased way, thereby reinforcing negative emotions and beliefs and interfering with daily functioning (Beck, 1972; Burns, 1989). The Patterns of Problematic Thinking Worksheet is a useful tool to help patients recognize maladaptive automatic thoughts and core beliefs, especially those patients who are struggling to master the skills that underlie the Challenging Questions Worksheets (see Chapter 17). Recognizing general patterns or "categories" of maladaptive cognitions can help with these other worksheets because it can teach the patient how to more effectively evaluate his or her beliefs. Similar to the ABC Worksheets and Challenging Questions Worksheets, the Patterns of Problematic Thinking Worksheets are based on the worksheets developed for cognitive processing therapy (Resick et al., 2017) and should be completed as a collaborative written activity. The Patterns of Problematic Thinking Worksheet can be found in Appendix A.10.

RATIONALE

The explicit labeling or "naming" of maladaptive core beliefs facilitates the process of cognitive reappraisal by helping the patient to consider *how* the identified belief is maladaptive as opposed to considering *if* the identified belief is maladaptive. By presenting the patient with a list of categories and definitions that are unequivocally maladaptive and then asking him or her to consider how specific beliefs fit into one of more of these categories, the Patterns of Problematic Thinking Worksheet implicitly assumes that the core belief is maladaptive. By considering their beliefs from this implicit perspective, the worksheet helps the patient to view and consider the belief as maladaptive.

TROUBLESHOOTING TIP

What if the patient is unable (or unwilling) to see his or her beliefs as maladaptive? The inability or unwillingness to view maladaptive beliefs as such reflects underlying cognitive rigidity. If patients insist that their maladaptive beliefs are reasonable, clinicians should direct them to consider and/or evaluate their beliefs with respect to their *helpfulness.* For example:

> I can see how you might view this belief as true. I'm wondering, however, how it's helpful for you. In other words, how is it beneficial for you to repeatedly tell yourself this?

Although patients may find their beliefs to be believable or true, they rarely find these beliefs helpful. By pointing out that a belief can be unhelpful even though it may be true, clinicians can often sidestep the patient's cognitive rigidity.

HOW TO DO IT

On the Patterns of Problematic Thinking Worksheet is a list of cognitive distortions with brief definitions designed to help the patient determine which category (or categories) best describe the belief. Patients are encouraged to work on multiple core beliefs per worksheet so they can begin to identify specific patterns in their thinking. An especially helpful approach is to review maladaptive beliefs identified during earlier assignments (i.e., the ABC Worksheet and the Challenging Questions Worksheet) and categorizing them on the Patterns of Problematic Thinking Worksheet. In this way, the patient can link multiple cognitive reappraisal strategies together to more effectively undermine suicidogenic beliefs. When introducing the Patterns of Problematic Thinking Worksheet, the clinician can note that some individuals tend to have certain patterns or "styles" of thinking that contribute to their distress, and that another useful strategy for determining the helpfulness of these thoughts and beliefs is by classifying them into different categories. The clinician has the patient complete the Patterns of Problematic Thinking Worksheet using a core suicidal belief as an example, and to write this belief in the appropriate category on the worksheet. The clinician uses Socratic questioning to help the patient evaluate the belief within the context of each cognitive distortion. If the patient determines that the belief fits within a category, the clinician invites the patient to write an explanation regarding how or why it does so. The clinician and patient repeat this process until all of the cognitive distortions have been considered.

To ensure skill mastery, patients should categorize several maladaptive beliefs on Patterns of Problematic Thinking Worksheets per session, and be asked to complete Patterns of Problematic Thinking Worksheets between sessions. The clinician should be sure to direct the patient to categorize suicidal beliefs that were present during the index suicidal episode.

Step 1: Introduce the Concept of the Patterns of Problematic Thinking Worksheet

The clinician introduces the concept of the Patterns of Problematic Thinking Worksheet and then briefly reviews the general concept of cognitive appraisal.

SAMPLE CLINICIAN SCRIPT

Now that you have used the ABC Worksheets to recognize how life events, thoughts, and emotions influence each other and have started learning how to evaluate whether your thoughts and reactions to different situations are helpful by using the Challenging Questions Worksheets, I'd like for us to work on one more skill designed to help you evaluate your thoughts and beliefs.

Many of us have certain problematic patterns or "styles" of thinking that shape how we view ourselves and the world. For example, some people tend to oversimplify things by viewing life in all-or-nothing terms. These individuals see things as either black or white and have trouble seeing the gray areas of life. To them, everything has to be either one thing or its opposite; there can be no in-between. Do you know anyone who tends to oversimplify by looking at things from a black-or-white perspective? Would you say that you tend to oversimplify?

Another pattern of problematic thinking is jumping to conclusions. Individuals who jump to conclusions tend to assume that bad things are going to happen in the future based on very little information. For example, they have an argument with their partner and assume that this means their partner doesn't love them and is going to break up with them. These individuals tend to predict negative future events even if there isn't much evidence or information to support that. Do you know anyone who has a tendency to jump to conclusions? How about you? Do you tend to jump to conclusions in stressful situations?

Let's go over a few more of these patterns of problematic thinking and talk about whether or not you might have some patterns that are unhelpful. To do this we'll use the Patterns of Problematic Thinking Worksheet. This worksheet lists seven unhelpful styles of thinking. We've already talked about two: oversimplifying and jumping to conclusions. Let's review the rest together.

Exaggerating is when we blow things out of proportion or overreact to a situation, whereas minimizing is when we dismiss or overly discount the importance of something. For example, if I avoid going to a social event because I'm afraid that I will say something stupid and embarrass myself, I would be exaggerating because I'm blowing out of proportion the likelihood of a negative experience. On the other hand, if I was the leader of a team project at work, but I say that I didn't have anything to do with the project's success, then I would be minimizing because I'm discounting the important role I played in the project.

Ignoring is when we focus on the negative aspects of a situation but do not focus on the positive aspects of the situation. For example, if I get a 95% on an exam but focus only on the few items I got wrong, I would be ignoring because I'm not focusing on the fact that I got an A.

Overgeneralizing is when we assume that a single life event or situation will always happen or will never stop. For example, if I make a small mistake on a home improvement project but then tell myself, "I always screw everything up and will always be a failure," then I'm overgeneralizing because I'm assuming a single mistake will always happen or never end.

Mind reading is when we assume that we know what other people are thinking when we have no evidence to support this, especially when we assume that others are thinking negatively about us. For example, if I'm interested in meeting someone but say to myself, "They'll just think I'm an idiot," then I'm mind-reading because I'm assuming I know what someone else is thinking without any evidence.

Emotional reasoning is when we assume that something is true because we had a certain feeling. For example, I might being feeling guilty or sad in a situation so I assume that I must have done something wrong or must be a failure. This is emotional reasoning because I'm assuming it's true that I did something wrong simply because I'm feeling a particular emotion.

Step 2: Complete a Patterns of Problematic Thinking Worksheet Focused on a Suicidal Belief

The clinician assists the patient in completing a Patterns of Problematic Thinking Worksheet focused on a suicidal belief that was present during the index suicidal episode. The clinician ensures the patient understands each of the cognitive distortions listed on the Patterns of Problematic Worksheet and guides the patient with Socratic dialogue to determine if the suicidal belief serves as an example of the cognitive distortion. When the patient determines that the suicidal belief fits with a particular category, the clinician uses Socratic questioning to explain why or how the belief fits and then asks the patient to handwrite this explanation underneath the appropriate category.

SAMPLE CLINICIAN SCRIPT

When doing these worksheets, we'll focus on just one belief at a time to make things more straightforward. Here is a list of the problematic thinking patterns with a brief definition of each. Let's go through these patterns one at a time to determine if your unhelpful belief fits within each category. It's possible for the belief to fit into only one category, but it's also possible for the belief to fit into multiple categories.

Let's start by choosing a belief to focus on. If we think back to the suicidal episode that brought you in for treatment, what are some of the things you were thinking in the time leading up to your suicide attempt [or crisis]? Now let's figure out which patterns this belief fits into.

Go ahead and read that first definition there. Would you say that your belief is an example of jumping to conclusions?

[If yes:] In what way is your belief an example of jumping to conclusions? Go ahead and write that down here.

[The clinician repeats for all subsequent questions on the worksheet:] Let's go to the next one. Would you say that your belief is an example of [cognitive distortion]? In what way is your belief of example of this? Go ahead and write that down.

Very good. Now that you've done the whole worksheet, what are your thoughts about this? What questions do you have about doing this worksheet? Let's choose another belief and practice again.

Step 3: Complete Several Patterns of Problematic Thinking Worksheets Focused on Other Maladaptive Beliefs

In order to facilitate skill acquisition and generalization, the clinician helps the patient identify other suicidal or maladaptive beliefs and repeats the process. The clinician provides additional copies of the Patterns of Problematic Thinking Worksheet when needed.

SAMPLE CLINICIAN SCRIPT

Now let's focus on a different belief that we've talked about being unhelpful. Just like the last time, let's go through each of the categories together so we can better figure out what pattern it fits with. What belief should we focus on for this worksheet?

Let's start with the first pattern. Go ahead and read that out loud and then let me know if you think your belief fits there. Write down your answer underneath.

[The clinician repeats for all subsequent questions on the worksheet:] Go ahead to the next one. What is pattern and do you think your belief fits there? Go ahead and write down your why underneath.

Great job. I think you're getting the hang of this. What questions do you have about this worksheet? How might this worksheet be helpful to practice on a regular basis?

Step 4: Develop a Plan for Practicing Patterns of Problematic Thinking Worksheets in between Sessions

In the final step of the Patterns of Problematic Thinking Worksheet, the clinician invites the patient to complete at least one worksheet per day before the next appointment. At least one of these worksheets should be focused on suicidal beliefs that were present during the index suicide attempt or suicidal episode. The clinician then gauges buy-in by asking the patient to rate the likelihood that he or she will complete the worksheets as prescribed on a scale ranging from 0 to 10, with 0 indicating "not at all likely" and 10 indicating "very likely." The clinician then provides the patient with a sufficient number of blank Patterns of Problematic Thinking Worksheets to complete the assignment.

SAMPLE CLINICIAN SCRIPT

Now that you've done a few of these, you see how they should be done. Do you think you would be able to complete at least one Patterns of Problematic Thinking Worksheet a day between now and the next time we meet? You can focus on any beliefs you want, but at least one of these worksheets should be focused on the beliefs you had during your last suicide attempt or suicidal crisis. Does that make sense? Here is a stack of Patterns of Problematic Thinking Worksheets for you to take with you.

[After finishing the plan:] So it sounds like we have a plan in place. Using a scale from 0 to 10, with 0 indicating "not at all likely" and 10 indicating "very likely," how likely is it that you'll complete at least one Patterns of Problematic Thinking Worksheet per day between now and the next time we meet?

[If the rating is lower than 7 out of 10:] Is there any part of this plan that reduces your likelihood for completing these worksheets? What could we change about this plan to make it more likely that you will complete the worksheets?

ILLUSTRATIVE CASE EXAMPLE

The Patterns of Problematic Thinking Worksheet was introduced to John in the 10th session of BCBT. By this point in treatment, John and his clinician had identified a number of suicidal beliefs and had already started to challenge them using the ABC Worksheets and Challenging Questions Worksheets. Over the course of several sessions, John's clinician noticed that John often seemed to struggle to understand why his maladaptive beliefs were unhelpful. Of note, John often commented that he "knows, logically, that these beliefs don't make sense, but they just feel so true to me anyway." The clinician therefore introduced the Patterns of Problematic Thinking Worksheet with the intent to help John understand this seeming paradox. John and his clinician first reviewed the content of his previously completed ABC Worksheets and Challenging Questions Worksheets, after which the clinician asked John to categorize all of the beliefs from these earlier worksheets into the various patterns of problematic thinking, and to provide an explanation for each. John's responses are displayed in Figure 18.1.

Upon completing the worksheet, John and his clinician engaged in the following dialogue:

CLINICIAN: Anything stand out to you from this worksheet?

JOHN: Well, it seems like some of my thoughts fit under different patterns.

CLINICIAN: Yeah, that's pretty common. A lot of our unhelpful beliefs are problematic in multiple ways.

JOHN: Yeah. Another thing is that I seem to jump to conclusions and do emotional reasoning more than the others.

CLINICIAN: What do you make of that?

JOHN: I think they're probably related to each other.

CLINICIAN: How so?

JOHN: Well, I think that when I feel bad or upset, I assume there's a reason for it, so I'll think something about myself that matches the feeling even if there's no evidence for it. So emotional reasoning ends up leading me to jump to conclusions.

CLINICIAN: That's a pretty interesting observation.

JOHN: Yeah. As I look at this worksheet and we talk about it, I think that may be why I feel like things are true even though I know they aren't: the beliefs are based on my emotions.

CLINICIAN: So it's kind of like the thoughts and beliefs are coming from your emotions?

JOHN: Yeah, that has to be it. I never thought of it that way before, but whenever I feel bad

Jumping to conclusions when the evidence is lacking or even contradictory

"I shouldn't even try because I screw everything up"—assuming things won't go well even though I haven't even tried yet.

"My family would be better off without me"—assuming that I make things worse for everyone even though they would disagree

---

Exaggerating or minimizing a situation (blowing things way out of proportion or shrinking their importance inappropriately)

"It can't get any worse"—making things seem worse than they actually are

"I always screw everything up"—blowing things out of proportion when I make a mistake

---

Disregarding important aspects of a situation

"It's my fault"—Blaming myself for my friend's death even though no one injured that badly would be able to survive

---

Oversimplifying things as good/bad or right/wrong

"I'm a failure"—Saying I'm completely bad based on one mistake even though I also doing things right.

"I always screw everything up"—I ignore the things that I do right

---

Overgeneralizing from a single incident (a negative event is seen as a never-ending pattern)

"I always screw everything up"—Blowing things out of proportion based on a single mistake, even though I also do things right

---

Mind reading (you assume people are thinking negatively of you when there is no definite evidence for this)

"My family would be better off without me"—Assuming this is true when they actually love me and would miss me

---

Emotional reasoning (you have a feeling and assume there must be a reason)

"I can't take this anymore"—Assuming I can't handle things just because I feel bad

"I'm a failure"—I feel embarrassed or angry at myself, so I assume I messed up

"My family would be better off without me"—I feel ashamed and angry, so I think I make things worse for my family.

FIGURE 18.1. John's Patterns of Problematic Thinking Worksheet.

or something is when I really start to think all these things. Even if these thoughts don't make sense for the situation, I end up believing them anyway simply because I'm feeling bad.

CLINICIAN: So what do you think we should do with this new knowledge?

JOHN: Well, one thing is I can tell myself that just because I'm feeling bad doesn't mean I've done something wrong. I think that would really help.

TIPS AND ADVICE FOR
PATTERNS OF PROBLEMATIC THINKING WORKSHEETS

1. **Suicidal beliefs can fall under more than one category.** Clinicians should remember and help patients to recognize that some suicidal beliefs can fit within multiple categories. This reflects the multiple sources of bias that can influence an individual's thinking, and points to various potential approaches to evaluating and restructuring their thoughts.

2. **Identify "styles" of thinking.** For many patients, beliefs will generally cluster into one or two of the seven categories described in the Patterns of Problematic Thinking Worksheet. This may suggest a particular cognitive bias or "style" for the patient. If a particular style is apparent, this can help the patient and the clinician to more efficiently identify unhelpful beliefs and to effectively evaluate them. For example, if a patient tends to jump to conclusions (like John), then his or her alternative thoughts will likely need to incorporate situational and contextual factors that the patient may be ignoring. On the other hand, if a patient tends to exaggerate or overgeneralize, alternative thoughts will likely need to address all-or-nothing thinking and/or minimize the use of extreme language (e.g., always, never).

CHAPTER 19

Activity Planning and Coping Cards

Suicidal individuals often experience a greater number of aversive life events than they do pleasurable life events, especially with respect to interpersonal relationships. Suicidal individuals also tend to make decisions and/or engage in behaviors that inadvertently maintain this imbalance, thereby sustaining their emotional distress over time. For example, acutely suicidal individuals may socially withdraw from others or drop out of treatment prematurely, which reduces positive social contact with others. Activity planning is a behaviorally oriented technique designed to target this imbalance. The primary purpose of activity planning is to increase the patient's engagement in those pleasurable and meaningful recreational activities that have been abandoned or reduced during periods of mood disturbance, thereby elevating mood and replacing maladaptive with positive coping responses.

Coping cards are a simple method to support and reinforce the patient's acquisition of skills learned in treatment. Created using 3″ × 5″ index cards, coping cards serve as highly transportable physical reminders of adaptive cognitive and/or behavioral strategies that the patient can keep in his or her pocket, purse, backpack, car, or another convenient location. The coping card is designed to serve as a visual memory aid to remind patients how or when to use a skill, whether the skill is cognitive or behavioral in nature. For example, one coping card might be created to help the patient with the cognitive reappraisal of a particular suicidal or maladaptive belief and another coping card might be created to remind the patient to use a coping skill (e.g., relaxation or mindfulness) in a particular situation (e.g., when craving alcohol or substances). Coping cards therefore serve as a form of "cheat sheet" or quick reference, similar to flash cards created to study for an exam.

RATIONALE

According to behavioral models of depression (e.g., Ferster, 1973; Lewinsohn & Graf, 1973; Lewinsohn & Libet, 1972), the onset of depression is attributable to a decrease in pleasurable events and/or an increase in aversive events. By extension, mood disturbance is maintained over time by the relative imbalance between pleasurable and aversive events in life. From a treatment perspective, this suggests that treatments should target the imbalance between pleasurable and aversive life events, specifically by increasing the frequency and salience of pleasurable life experiences. As the patient experiences a greater number of pleasurable experiences and the ratio of pleasurable to aversive life experiences increases, the patient's mood disturbance will resolve. Increasing the patient's exposure to pleasurable life experience can also serve as a method for reappraising maladaptive core beliefs. For example, experiencing an enjoyable social outing with friends can serve as evidence to counter a suicidal patient's perspective that life is meaningless and that one is a burden on others.

Studying the components of cognitive-behavioral therapy for depression reveals that the activity planning component of treatment may be the primary contributor to recovery from depression. For example, treatments that focus exclusively on increasing engagement in pleasurable activities (referred to as *behavioral activation*) are just as effective at preventing relapse as cognitive therapy (Dimidjian et al., 2006; Gortner, Gollan, Dobson, & Jacobson, 1998). Among patients with more severe depression, increasing pleasurable activities may be especially important for full remission and relapse prevention (Dimidjian et al., 2006). Because most individuals engage in pleasurable activities with others, activity planning may be especially effective with suicidal individuals because it increases social support, a well-established protective factor for suicide (Bryan & Hernandez, 2013; Kaslow et al., 2005). Activities that bring suicidal individuals into contact with peers or supportive others who respect and express concern for the patient are especially important (Bryan & Hernandez, 2013), as such experiences often undermine suicidal core beliefs such as shame, guilt, and perceived burdensomeness. Activities that are personally meaningful (e.g., spending time with family or friends, volunteering, exercising) also have the added benefit of fostering a strong sense of purpose and meaning in life, which has been shown to be associated with decreased suicide risk and positively correlated with social support (Bryan, Elder, et al., 2013).

The primary purpose of coping cards is to serve as a memory aid to facilitate the patient's retention of information and skills outside of treatment. Coping cards therefore support the acquisition of cognitive reappraisal and emotion regulation skills and can be used as an adjunct for most (if not all) of the interventions contained in BCBT.

HOW TO DO IT: ACTIVITY PLANNING

To accomplish activity planning, the clinician asks the patient to identify one or more activities that the patient enjoys. If the patient states that he or she enjoys "nothing" or is unable to identify any pleasurable activities in his or her life, the clinician can ask the patient to identify activities that the patient *used to* enjoy but has since abandoned. For especially distressed or "stuck" patients, an alternative strategy is to ask the patient to identify pleasurable activities that he or she *wishes* to engage in but has not yet done so due to various barriers. Once an activity is identified, the clinician and patient collaboratively develop a specific schedule for the patient to resume or increase engagement in the activity.

The effectiveness of activity planning is largely determined by the clinician's ability to identify and problem-solve solutions to likely barriers to the activity. For example, a commonly scheduled activity in BCBT is exercise, but there are many small, incremental steps that must be taken and considerations to weigh for the patient to successfully meet this goal. For example, the clinician and patient should consider the timing of the exercise (e.g., in the morning prior to work versus the afternoon or evening after work), location of the exercise (e.g., at a gym vs. at home), and preparatory steps needed to exercise (e.g., packing a gym bag). For patients with severe insomnia, waking up early in the morning may be problematic, so planning to exercise in the afternoon or evening might work better. In contrast, for patients with young children at home, planning to exercise at a gym instead of at home may increase their likelihood to exercise without distraction. Another commonly scheduled activity in BCBT is cooking or baking. In order to successfully complete this task, however, the patient may need to purchase all of the necessary ingredients and supplies first. The clinician and patient may therefore need to create a shopping list as a preliminary step to completing the larger activity.

Along these same lines, the clinician and patient should be sure to establish a plan that is specific, measurable, and realistic. Specific plans have detailed and clear parameters for the activity (e.g., timing, frequency, duration, and/or location), measurable plans are quantifiable, and realistic plans are feasible and/or likely to be achieved. For example, "exercising more" is not an ideal activity plan because it is neither specific (i.e., what constitutes "exercise"?) nor measurable (i.e., is a 1-minute walk considered to be "more" exercise?), although it might be realistic. Likewise, "running 10 miles on the weekends" may not be a good goal for a patient who has not exercised in several months because it is not realistic as a first step, although it is specific and measurable. The clinician and the patient may therefore need to "negotiate" the terms of the activity plan to ensure it is meets these three characteristics.

Step 1: Introduce the Concept of Activity Planning

The clinician introduces the concept of activity planning and explains the rationale for the intervention.

> **SAMPLE CLINICIAN SCRIPT**
>
> When we're under a lot of stress it can be easy to let go of meaningful and enjoyable activities because we feel that we don't have enough time for those activities anymore. Another reason for giving up enjoyable activities is that we lose our motivation or interest in them. Although giving up these activities for a short period of time

might make sense when dealing with a short-term stressor, if we continue to experience stress for a long period of time and don't resume those enjoyable activities, our life becomes unbalanced because we end up experiencing lots of stressful events but very few pleasurable events. When this happens, it makes sense that we might see life as pointless and our problems as never-ending. How would you say that this reflects your own life?

Step 2: Identify Pleasurable Activities

The clinician asks the patient to list activities that he or she enjoys. If the patient indicates that he or she is unable to identify pleasurable activities, the clinician asks the patient to identify activities that he or she used to enjoy in the past.

SAMPLE CLINICIAN SCRIPT

An easy way to counter this imbalance is to increase or resume those enjoyable activities in life. The challenge for most people is that when they've been feeling stressed, depressed, or suicidal, they often feel that they can't do these activities, but the good news is that most of us can do these activities and regain balance in our life even if we don't feel like it or don't think that we can. What are some activities that you enjoy but maybe don't do as often as you would like or often as you used to?

[If the patient is unable to identify enjoyable activities:] What are some things that you used to enjoy doing, even if you don't do them anymore?

Step 3: Develop a Plan for Engaging in the Activity

The clinician and the patient collaboratively establish a plan for engaging in the identified activities.

SAMPLE CLINICIAN SCRIPT

[Possible open-ended questions to facilitate the creation of an activity plan:]

Would you be willing to create a schedule for doing this activity?

How often do you currently do this activity?

How often did you used to do this activity?

How often would you like to do this activity?

When do you think you would be able to start this activity?

How often do you think you could do this activity?

How long do you think you could realistically do this activity each time?

Is there anyone who could do this activity with you?

Where could you do this activity?

Is there anything you need to do to prepare for this activity?

Step 4: Elicit Patient Buy-In

Once a schedule has been finalized, the clinician asks the patient to rate the likelihood that he or she will engage in the activities as scheduled on a scale ranging from 0 to 10, with 0 indicating "not at all likely" and 10 indicating "very likely."

SAMPLE CLINICIAN SCRIPT

This seems like a pretty good plan. What do you think? Using a scale from 0 to 10, with 0 indicating "not at all likely" and 10 indicating "very likely," how likely is it that you'll follow this plan?

[If rating is lower than 7 out of 10:] Is there any part of this plan that reduces your likelihood for using it? What could we change about this plan to make it more likely that you would use it?

ILLUSTRATIVE CASE EXAMPLE

Because of Janice's tendency to isolate herself at home and avoid others, her clinician introduced activity planning as a way to increase her engagement in activities and connectedness with others. The clinician first sought to identify some activities that Janice had previously found enjoyable but had subsequently abandoned. Janice indicated that exercise was an activity that she had a strong desire to resume. The clinician therefore helped Janice to develop a specific, measurable, and realistic plan for resuming this activity. During the process of developing this plan, the clinician helped Janice to identify and avoid potential roadblocks and barriers:

CLINICIAN: I think exercise would be a great place to start for increasing your activity level. What would be a good initial goal for exercise?

JANICE: Well, I'd like to eventually get back to working out every day. When I was exercising that often, I felt so much better about myself.

CLINICIAN: How long has it been since you exercised on a daily basis?

JANICE: Oh, I don't know. Years. Many, many years.

CLINICIAN: How often do you exercise now?

JANICE: I haven't worked out in a long time. I don't really exercise at all now.

CLINICIAN: OK, I see. So when you say that you want to work out every day, is that something you're wanting to do right now, or is that more of a long-term goal?

JANICE: Well, I'd like to do that right now but I know that isn't going to happen.

CLINICIAN: Yeah, you may be right. If daily exercise isn't a realistic goal right now, what would you say is a good place to start, then?

JANICE: Well, maybe if I did something like go for a walk a few days a week and maybe do some yoga classes. That would probably be a good start.

CLINICIAN: When you say "a few days a week," is that 2 days, 3 days, 4 days?

JANICE: I'd say 3 days a week. That would be pretty regular but also give me some off days. I'll probably be tired and sore at first.

CLINICIAN: That's a good point. OK, so 3 days a week to start. And is that a mix of walking and yoga?

JANICE: Yeah, but I'll have to sign up for yoga classes somewhere, assuming I can afford them.

CLINICIAN: OK, so starting yoga right away might not be possible, but maybe in the next few weeks?

JANICE: Yeah.

CLINICIAN: So then should we start with walking 3 days a week? Or are you just wanting to walk 2 days a week but then save the third day for yoga?

JANICE: I think I should start with 3 days of walking, then later on I can switch out one of the days for yoga. I think I need to just get in the habit of exercise on a regular basis, so going for a walk would probably help me get in that habit.

CLINICIAN: OK, sounds good. Which 3 days of the week should we plan for?

JANICE: Monday, Wednesday, and Friday for sure, before I go to work. I'll walk around the neighborhood for 15 minutes.

CLINICIAN: Those sound like good days. Since you're going to go for a walk for 15 minutes each morning before work, what time will you need to wake up in the mornings now to make that happen?

JANICE: Oh, I hadn't thought of that. I don't know if I would be able to wake up early. It's hard enough already to get up in time for work.

CLINICIAN: Yeah, I was wondering about that. We've talked about that quite a bit together, and we've made some progress on your sleep already.

JANICE: Yeah, I don't want to mess that up.

CLINICIAN: OK, then. If not in the morning before work, what other times might work?

JANICE: Well, I could do it after work. There's actually a really nice park on the way home from work and lots of people are there walking in the evenings. Every time I drive past there I think about how nice it looks.

CLINICIAN: Oh, that sounds like a great option. I really like that. Do you think you'd be able to stop off at that park on Monday, Wednesday, and Friday on your way home from work to go for a 15-minute walk?

JANICE: Definitely. I think that would be really fun, actually.

CLINICIAN: OK, well, let's write this down then, so we don't forget. Something else we should talk about is what you'll need to take with you for these walks.

JANICE: What do you mean?

CLINICIAN: Well, you'll be coming from work, right?

JANICE: Yes.

CLINICIAN: Are the clothes you wear to work suitable for an afternoon or evening walk?

JANICE: I see what you're saying. I guess they would be OK, but now that you mention it I wouldn't want them to get sweaty or anything, so I should take a change of clothes. I'll also need to take my tennis shoes so I have more comfortable shoes and don't get blisters or anything like that.

CLINICIAN: Yeah, we definitely wouldn't want that.

JANICE: No, definitely not.

CLINICIAN: Since this is a new activity for you, you're probably not yet in the habit of taking these extra items to work with you. What do you think about creating a checklist of things you'll need to pack to take with you so you don't end up at the park without the things you need?

JANICE: That's a good idea.

CLINICIAN: OK, then let's write this down as well. What are the things you'll need to take with you to work on Mondays, Wednesdays, and Fridays in order to take a walk in the afternoons?

JANICE: I'll need a T-shirt, some shorts or workout pants, socks, and shoes.

CLINICIAN: OK, good. And is it your plan to pack that all up the morning of, the night before, or another time?

JANICE: I'll do it the night before so I don't forget. I have a gym bag I can use.

CLINICIAN: Great! And once you're all packed up, where will you put that gym bag so you don't forget it when you leave in the morning?

JANICE: I'll hang it on the doorknob of the door to my garage. That way I won't miss it.

CLINICIAN: Good idea. Can you think of anything else we need to plan for to make this happen?

JANICE: No, I don't think so.

CLINICIAN: Me neither. Last question: when are we going to start this plan?

JANICE: Tomorrow. I'll pack up tonight and will go for the first walk tomorrow.

HOW TO DO IT: COPING CARDS

Coping cards are ideally handwritten by the patient on an index card provided by the clinician. In order to focus the patient's attention on a smaller number of skills and to accelerate mastery, no more than two or three coping cards should be created for the patient at any given time. In BCBT, coping cards are most often used to reinforce change in the patient's belief system and behaviors. In cognitively oriented coping cards, suicidal or maladaptive beliefs are written on one side of the card and an alternative perspective or counterpoint is written on the reverse side. A patient using one of these coping cards might be instructed to review the cards several times per day at regular intervals (e.g., during meals, when using the restroom, in between classes) as well as when he or she experiences the maladaptive thought. When used in this manner, the coping card functions similar to the ABC Worksheets, Challenging Questions Worksheets, and Patterns of Problematic Thinking Worksheets.

Behaviorally oriented coping cards often describe a specific event or situation on one side of the card and on the reverse side lists several concrete steps to be taken by the patient in response to this situation. Note that the coping card breaks down the desired behavioral response into discrete steps that are specific, measurable, and easily achieved. Coping cards can be very useful for increasing the likelihood that a patient will engage in a new response pattern by breaking down the behavior into a sequence of smaller steps that can reduce the perceived complexity or difficulty of the behavior. When used in this manner, the coping card functions similar to a crisis response plan; indeed, the crisis response plan can be conceptualized as a very specific type of coping card.

Once created, the coping cards can be laminated to enhance their durability and to increase their personal meaningfulness. The patient should be directed to review the coping cards multiple times per day, even if he or she is not experiencing the triggering event or cue, as this promotes mental rehearsal and, by extension, faster learning and integration of the card's content.

Step 1: Introduce the Concept of the Coping Card

The clinician introduces the concept of the coping card and explains its rationale a memory aid to facilitate the mastery of a new skill.

SAMPLE CLINICIAN SCRIPT

Let's create a coping card to help you remember this and learn it faster. A coping card is a memory aid, kind of like a flash card that you might create when you're studying for an exam. What we can do with this coping card is write down the most essential parts of the skill you just learned onto an index card. You can keep the index card in your purse, your pocket, your backpack, or somewhere else convenient and easily accessible. That way you can grab it and review it as a quick reminder of what you've been working on.

Step 2: Create the Coping Card

The clinician assists the patient in creating a coping card, making sure to connect the content of the coping card directly to another intervention in BCBT.

SAMPLE CLINICIAN SCRIPT

[For cognitively oriented cards:] This belief seems to be a really important one, and it seems like it'll take a lot of attention and practice. What do you think about making a coping card that focuses on this particular belief, so you have a sort of "cheat sheet" that you can quickly review to remember what we've talked about today?

On this first side of the card, go ahead and write down the belief. Now flip the card over and on this side write down the new response to this belief that we just discussed.

[For behaviorally oriented cards:] It sounds like this particular situation poses a unique challenge for you, and remembering to use a new skill will be challenging. What do you think about making a coping card that can remind you what to do when you're in that situation, sort of like a "cheat sheet"?

On this first side of the card, go ahead and write down the situation. Now flip the card over and on this side let's write down the new behavior that you're going to start using in this situation. Sometimes it's helpful to break things down into smaller steps, kind of like reading an instruction manual when you're putting together a new piece of furniture like a cabinet or something. Do you think it would be helpful to break this new skill down into some smaller steps?

Step 3: Develop a Plan for Reviewing the Coping Card in between Sessions

The clinician and patient collaboratively develop a plan for the patient to review the coping card on a regular basis in between sessions. The clinician explains that the coping card should be reviewed as scheduled even if it is not needed at the scheduled times because this facilitates faster learning. The clinician then gauges buy-in by asking the patient to rate the likelihood that he or she will review the coping card as scheduled on a scale ranging from 1 to 10, with 0 indicating "not at all likely" and 10 indicating "very likely."

SAMPLE CLINICIAN SCRIPT

What I'd like for you to do is take this card out and review it on a regular basis several times per day as well, even if you aren't experiencing the triggering cue. The reason for this is because it's practice. Even though you don't "need" the card at that moment in time, you should take a few seconds to review it anyway because this helps you to remember it faster. It's kind of like studying for an exam: you review the material over and over again to make sure you remember it before you take the exam so you know the material when the time comes for the exam itself. Does that make sense?

So let's pick some times during the day when you can take this card out and review it. The good news is that it'll take you only a few seconds, so it isn't too time-consuming. When learning a new skill like this, it's often helpful to schedule the practice during times that are very easy to remember and that are going to happen anyway. For example, we might schedule you to review this during breakfast, lunch, and dinner because you're going to eat those meals anyway, so it'll be easy to remember. Or we might schedule you to review this whenever you go to the bathroom. You're going to go to the bathroom at least a few times per day, so reading your card then will make it easy to remember. What do you think would work best for you?

[After finishing the plan:] So it sounds like we have a plan in place: you're going to read your card whenever you experience the triggering cue and you're also going to read your card several times per day to practice. Using a scale from 0 to 10, with 0 indicating "not at all likely" and 10 indicating "very likely," how likely is it that you'll be able to follow this plan?

[If rating is lower than 7 out of 10:] Is there any part of this plan that reduces your likelihood for using it? What could we change about this plan to make it more likely that you would use it?

Illustrative Case Example

As Mike approached the end of treatment, his clinician decided to develop some coping cards to further reinforce Mike's progress in reducing suicidal beliefs and several associated risk factors. Several of Mike's coping cards can be found in Figure 19.1. Cards A and B were intended to reinforce Mike's cognitive reappraisal skills by targeting two especially persistent suicidal beliefs: "I'm worthless" and "People would be better off without me." These

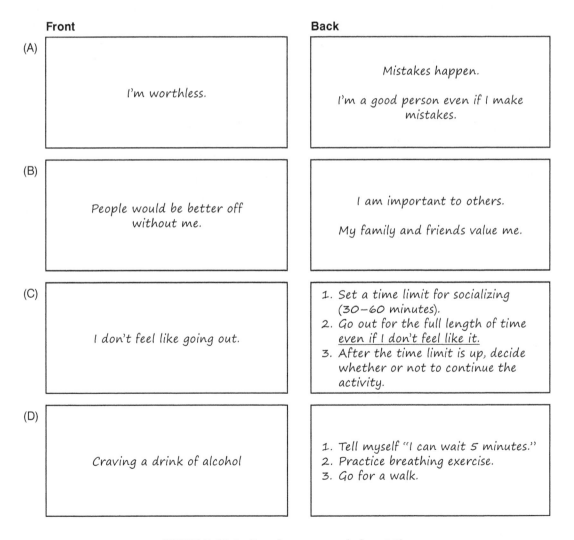

Front **Back**

(A)

I'm worthless.

Mistakes happen.

I'm a good person even if I make mistakes.

(B)

People would be better off without me.

I am important to others.

My family and friends value me.

(C)

I don't feel like going out.

1. Set a time limit for socializing (30–60 minutes).
2. Go out for the full length of time <u>even if I don't feel like it.</u>
3. After the time limit is up, decide whether or not to continue the activity.

(D)

Craving a drink of alcohol

1. Tell myself "I can wait 5 minutes."
2. Practice breathing exercise.
3. Go for a walk.

FIGURE 19.1. Sample coping cards from Mike.

suicidal beliefs were written on the front sides of the index cards, and his alternative beliefs were written on the back sides. These alternative beliefs came from the various worksheets that Mike completed in earlier sessions of BCBT. In addition to these cognitive-oriented cards, Mike and his clinician also developed behavior-oriented cards that aimed at two of Mike's key risk factors: isolating himself when feeling down (Card C), and alcohol use (Card D). On the front sides of these cards, Mike summarized the psychological conditions under which these risk factors tended to emerge: during periods of low motivation and alcohol craving. On the back sides of these cards, Mike listed several steps he could follow to manage these risk factors more effectively.

TIPS AND ADVICE FOR
ACTIVITY PLANNING AND COPING CARDS

1. **Specificity matters.** Specificity in activity planning and coping cards is central to their success. "Exercising more" is too vague to be useful or meaningful as an activity plan. Determining when, where, how often, and with whom a patient will engage in an activity plan will dramatically increase the likelihood that the patient follows through with the plan.

2. **Plan ahead, and don't forget the details.** The most common barriers to carrying out an activity plan involve small details that are easily overlooked during the planning stage. These small details typically entail intermediary steps that are prerequisites for achieving the ultimate goal. For example, if a patient wants to bake a cake as an enjoyable activity, he or she will most likely need to go grocery shopping first. Clinician should help patients to think about these intermediary steps and plan to account for them so the odds of success are raised. This was demonstrated by Janice's clinician, who took into account intermediary steps such as packing a change of clothes and developed a plan with Janice to ensure that she did not overlook them.

PART V

PHASE THREE

Relapse Prevention

CHAPTER 20

The Relapse Prevention Task
and Ending Treatment

The relapse prevention task is the final procedure of BCBT, and is designed to ensure the patient has acquired sufficient competence in the applied use of emotion regulation and cognitive reappraisal skills. The relapse prevention task additionally serves to foster the patient's cognitive flexibility by challenging him or her to successfully adapt to challenges as they are presented. Finally, the relapse prevention task serves as an assessment tool for the clinician to determine if the patient has acquired sufficient skills competence across BCBT, which serves as the basis for determining treatment completion. In the relapse prevention task, the patient imagines him- or herself in a suicidal crisis and then imagines him-or herself successfully utilizing one or more skills learned in BCBT to resolve the crisis. This process is repeated multiple times. With each iteration of the task, the clinician increases its difficulty, thereby requiring the patient to flexibly adapt to new and increasingly challenging situations. In this final step of treatment, the patient is therefore asked to synthesize all the information gained in treatment and to demonstrate his or her mastery of the content, akin to a "final exam."

RATIONALE

The relapse prevention task is a mental imagery exercise designed to facilitate procedural motor memory specific to effective skills used. Despite the absence of sensory input from external stimuli, mental imagery nonetheless entails perceptual processes within the brain (Munzert, Lorey, & Zentgraf, 2009). Because the relapse prevention task is specifically focused on the mental rehearsal of behaviors and actions, it taps into the motor imagery system in addition to the basic sensory systems. Motor imagery based on a first-person perspective is associated with activations in the somatosensory and motor areas of the brain that are similar to activations observed when an individual is actually engaging in the motor task (Jeannerod, 2001; Zentgraf et al., 2005). At a neurological level, mental rehearsal of a behavior is therefore equivalent to actually engaging in the behavior itself. This accounts for findings that behavioral preparation for and rehearsal of a suicide attempt are among the strongest and most robust predictors of suicide attempts (Joiner et al., 1997; Minnix et al., 2007). The relapse prevention task therefore provides the patient with the opportunity to repeatedly practice and apply his or her newly acquired skills to crisis situations within a controlled context. In essence, the patient repeatedly practices *not* making a suicide attempt when he or she is emotionally upset.

Upon completion of the relapse prevention task, the clinician assists the patient in transitioning to a lower level of care, whether that entails a complete termination of treatment or a transition into other forms of mental health treatment that are not focused on the acute reduction of risk for suicide attempts. The final session of BCBT is intended to reinforce the patient's progress in treatment and to clearly articulate the patient's plan going forward. As discussed in Chapter 3, BCBT uses a competency-based approach to determining treatment completion. To this end, BCBT is considered complete when the patient demonstrates the ability to effectively use emotion regulation, problem solving, and cognitive reappraisal skills within the specific context of the relapse prevention task. Competency is demonstrated during the relapse prevention task by several observable criteria:

1. **Selection of a skill that is relevant or appropriate to the situation.** The patient must be able to demonstrate the ability to accurately assess his or her needs within a crisis situation and then choose a skill and response that matches those needs. Choosing a skill or a response that does not directly target the patient's underlying need will be ineffective. For example, if the patient's goal is to "calm down" during a crisis, he or she should select an intervention that reduces physiological arousal, enables him or her to reframe the situation, or induces a positive emotional state. Selection of a skill that does not directly help the patient to "calm down" is neither relevant nor appropriate to the situation and is less likely to be helpful. This criterion therefore demonstrates the patient's capacity for self-awareness.

2. **Selection of a skill that is practical within the constraints of the situation.** The patient must be able to demonstrate the ability to accurately assess the parameters of the situation and then choose a skill and response that fits within these constraints. Choosing a skill or a response that is impractical or impossible to implement during a crisis will be ineffective. For example, a patient's preferred coping strategy might be going for a run, but if the patient experiences a crisis during the middle of the work day, this coping strategy may not be feasible at that particular moment. This criterion therefore demonstrates the patient's ability to accurately assess situational demands.

3. **Adaptation in response to situational demands.** The patient must be able to demonstrate the ability to adapt the use of skills in response to changing circumstances. If the

patient selects an appropriate skill for the situation but the skill is rendered ineffective due to an unanticipated or unforeseen reason, the patient must be able to either adjust how the skill is used to make it work better or choose a new skill that will work better within the given parameters. For example, if the patient chooses to go for a motorcycle ride as a coping strategy but discovers a thunderstorm is moving in, he or she may need to select an alternative coping strategy. Likewise, if the patient uses a coping skill such as relaxation but still feels highly emotionally upset afterwards, he or she may need to choose another coping skill to effectively manage his or her distress. This criterion therefore demonstrates the patient's cognitive flexibility.

4. **Rapid selection and implementation of skills.** The patient must be able to demonstrate the ability to quickly select a coping strategy in response to a crisis. In a crisis, speed is a critical factor for success; if the patient takes too long to assess the situation and choose an appropriate response, he or she may become overwhelmed before a solution can be implemented. Because most coping strategies and skills will have some positive effect on resolving the crisis, even if only a very small impact, speed is probably the most important criterion for assessing competence. In short, it is better for the patient to quickly generate a somewhat helpful solution than to take an extended period of time to generate a "perfect" solution.

When the patient has demonstrated these four criteria, the patient is ready to complete BCBT. In most cases, the clinician and the patient conduct the formal treatment completion after the conclusion of the final relapse prevention task; a separate appointment dedicated entirely to treatment completion is not necessary.

HOW TO DO IT: RELAPSE PREVENTION TASK

The relapse prevention task focuses on at least two crises: the index suicidal crisis and a hypothetical future crisis. When the relapse prevention task is first introduced and rehearsed, the clinician should ask the patient to imagine his or her index suicidal crisis and successfully resolve it. After the patient has demonstrated sufficient skill mastery related to the index suicidal crisis, the clinician and the patient collaboratively develop a hypothetical future crisis given the patient's history. The patient then imagines this crisis and successfully resolves it. Once the patient has demonstrated sufficient skill mastery related to the hypothetical crisis, BCBT is considered complete.

The relapse prevention entails several four primary steps: (1) review of skills and strategies learned in treatment, (2) patient education and informed consent, (3) the imagery task, and (4) integration. In the first step of the relapse prevention task, the clinician asks the patient to take out his or her treatment log to review its contents, and then asks the patient to name the many skills and strategies that he or she learned during the course of BCBT to manage emotional distress and suicidal crises. As the patient names the interventions, the clinician writes them onto a whiteboard or a blank sheet of paper. The clinician asks the patient to describe his or her experience with these skills and strategies, whether positive or negative. The purpose of this first step is to make explicit the considerable progress the patient has made in treatment. The written list of learned skills and strategies can also be used as a memory aid for the patient in the event that he or she struggles or "gets stuck" during the imagery task.

The clinician next describes the procedure in detail and explains its rationale. The relapse prevention task can be an emotionally distressing procedure for the patient; the clinician should therefore take extra time to educate the patient to ensure that he or she is fully aware of what to expect in advance, and allow plenty of opportunity for the patient to ask questions and/or to express concerns. Several points for the clinician to cover during the education and informed consent step are outlined in Figure 20.1.

Once the patient understands the procedure and is ready to begin, the clinician asks the patient to close his or her eyes and to imagine him- or herself located in the environment where the index suicidal crisis occurred. The clinician asks the patient to describe in detail what he or she sees and hears to enhance the vividness of the image, and then asks the

---

- You have learned many new skills and strategies in treatment that have improved your ability to effectively manage stress and crises.

- In this final phase of treatment, we want to make sure that you have gained a very high level of mastery of these skills, especially in the area of managing suicidal crises.

- In order to assess skill mastery, we are going to do a procedure called the relapse prevention task.

- In the relapse prevention task, you will be asked to imagine the circumstances of a suicidal crisis. Specifically, you will be asked to imagine the details of the situation, the thoughts and feelings you had at that time, and the actions you took.

- As we do this together, I may ask you some questions or provide some suggestions to increase the vividness, or realism, of the mental image. I will do this because the more realistic it is, the better this procedure will work.

- Although you'll be reliving a particular moment in your life, your task this time is to change the ending by successfully solving the problem using a new skill or strategy you learned in treatment. You can use any of the skills that we have talked about in treatment to change the outcome—whatever you would prefer.

- Before we start, I want to tell you about a risk associated with this procedure. This procedure can be emotionally upsetting for some patients, because you'll be thinking about an upsetting period of time in your life and remembering all of the negative thoughts and painful feelings that you experienced then. However, this risk is not unique to this particular part of the treatment; you have remembered a lot of stressful and negative thoughts throughout our work together. I will be available to support you, just like I have been throughout the entire treatment.

- After we are done with this task, we will discuss the procedure together.

- This procedure will be repeated several times. Each time we practice it, I will make it a little harder for you to solve the problem, so you'll have to figure out a new way to resolve the situation. This will help us to know for sure that you have truly mastered these skills.

- What questions or concerns do you have about the relapse prevention task?

FIGURE 20.1. Components of informed consent for the relapse prevention task.

patient, "What happens next?" to facilitate the progress of the task. During the procedure, the clinician prompts the patient to describe his or her thoughts and feelings to increase the patient's emotional engagement with the task and to elicit the various domains of the suicidal mode. When the patient successfully imagines him-or herself resolving the crisis by describing the appropriate use of a learned skill, the clinician stops the procedure and praises the patient. The clinician then asks the patient for feedback and elicits his or her experience of the procedure. Following sufficient processing of the task, the clinician tells the patient that the procedure will be repeated and that the patient should solve the problem in a different way (e.g., using a skill at a different point during the crisis, using a skill in a different way, using a different skill).

The relapse prevention task is repeated multiple times, with each iteration becoming increasingly difficult for the patient to solve. The purpose of the repetition is to facilitate the effective application of learned skills through practice. By increasing the difficulty of the relapse prevention task each time, the patient is required to demonstrate cognitive flexibility and problem-solving ability—a critical ability for long-term risk reduction. Because crises can emerge in a variety of contexts and be characterized in many different ways, the patient may not always be able to use his or her preferred coping strategy. If the patient is unable to adapt to such situations, he or she will not be able to effectively manage the crisis. Repetition of the relapse prevention task is therefore critical to ensure the patient possesses the ability to quickly and effectively adapt to different contextual circumstances. If, after several iterations of the relapse prevention task, the patient is unable to effectively resolve his or her imagined crises, the clinician should schedule additional sessions to continue rehearsing skills and practicing the procedure until the patient's competency is established.

Step 1: Review the Patient's Treatment Log and Self-Management Strategies

The clinician and the patient review the patient's treatment log together and discuss the self-management strategies the patient has learned and effectively used during the course of BCBT.

SAMPLE CLINICIAN SCRIPT

Before we move into the final stage of treatment, I want to take a bit of time to review what you've learned so far. Do you have your treatment log on you? Let's take that out and go through all the "lessons learned" during the course of this treatment. Over the course of this entire treatment, what are all of the skills and strategies you've learned for managing stress, solving problems, and handling crises? I'm going to write them down on this whiteboard for us.

Very good. Of all these strategies, which would you say are your "top three" strategies to use? What is it about those strategies that you find to be so useful?

It looks like you've learned a wide range of useful skills that have proven to be very helpful for you. Critically, you've started to use these skills in your everyday life to respond more effectively to problems and stress.

Step 2: Provide Informed Consent for the Relapse Prevention Task

The clinician describes the relapse prevention task in detail and elicits the patient's questions and concerns about the procedure.

SAMPLE CLINICIAN SCRIPT

As we've just discussed, you have learned many new skills and strategies in treatment over the past few months that have improved your ability to effectively manage stress and crises. All of those skills are written here on the whiteboard. In this final phase of treatment we're going to do what's called a "relapse prevention task," which is a procedure designed to make sure that you've not only gained knowledge about these skills, especially with respect to managing suicidal crises, but that you've also gained the ability to use these skills effectively. The relapse prevention task is a mental-imagery-based procedure in which you will put all the skills you've learned to use in order to demonstrate the ability to respond to crises without making a suicide attempt. This is sort of like the "final exam" of treatment because you have to show what you've learned and also show that you know how to apply your new knowledge to specific problems. In many ways, this step is very similar to how athletes imagine themselves making the shot, scoring a point, or otherwise performing at their best. By mentally practicing their actions, they are more likely to perform as imagined. The same is true for you: by mentally practicing your skills, you are more likely to use them in the future.

In the relapse prevention task, I'm going to ask you to imagine the circumstances of a suicidal crisis. I'll ask you to imagine the details of the situation, such as where you are at, what things look like around you, and what you can hear. I'll also ask you to imagine the thoughts and feelings you have during the crisis, and the actions you take. You'll verbally describe all of these things to me out loud so I can follow along with your imagination. As we do this together, I may ask you some questions about what you're seeing or doing, or I might provide some suggestions to you about what you're thinking and feeling. I will do this to increase the realism of the image. The more realistic your mental image is, the better this procedure will work.

We will do this imagination piece several times. The first few times we do it, I'm going to have you focus on the suicidal crisis that brought you in to treatment. Although you'll be reliving a particular suicidal crisis, this time what you'll be doing is changing the end of that story by solving your crisis with a skill or strategy you learned in treatment. In other words, you'll be imagining yourself responding more effectively to that situation, sort of like giving you an opportunity for a "do-over." You can use any of the skills that we have talked about in treatment to change the outcome; whatever you prefer.

Before we start, I want to tell you about a risk associated with this procedure. The relapse prevention task can be emotionally upsetting for some patients because you'll be thinking about a very upsetting period of time in your life and remembering all of the negative thoughts and painful feelings you experienced at that time. However, I should note that this particular risk for experiencing painful memories is not unique to this procedure. As you know, you have remembered a lot of stressful memories and negative thoughts during the course of this treatment. Just like I have done throughout the entire treatment, I will be available to help and support you during this procedure. After we are done with the imagery task, we will discuss the procedure together, just like we have any time you've learned a new skill.

As I mentioned before, we will practice this procedure several times. Each time we practice it, I'll make it a little harder for you to solve the problem so that you have to figure out multiple ways to resolve the situation. This will help us to know for sure that you have truly mastered the skills learned in this treatment. After you have shown the ability to solve your original suicidal crisis in several different ways, we'll have you practice this procedure while imagining one or more hypothetical future crises that we think you will likely experience at some point in your life.

Before we proceed any further, I want to pause and give you an opportunity to ask me any questions you might have about this procedure.

Step 3: Conduct the Relapse Prevention Task Focused on the Index Suicidal Crisis

The clinician guides the patient through an imagery task in which the patient recounts the circumstances and steps leading up to his or her index suicidal crisis. The clinician helps the patient to imagine the effective use of a self-management strategy to avoid a suicide attempt.

SAMPLE CLINICIAN SCRIPT

Go ahead and get yourself comfortable in your seat, and close your eyes. Take a moment to think back to the suicidal crisis that brought you in for treatment, and imagine yourself in that situation, wherever the story starts. Can you describe to me where you are and what you see?

[Sample prompts to increase the vividness of the mental image:]

What is happening around you?

What does that sound like?

Describe what it looks like.

What are the exact words the person uses when he/she says that to you?

What emotion do you feel?

What's going through your mind at this point?

Where in your body do you feel that sensation?

What do you do next?

[For patients who struggle to identify or effectively use a self-management skill:]

What is a skill you could use here?

Is there something you've learned in treatment that could help at this point?

Is there something listed on the whiteboard that might be useful in this situation?

Step 4: Process the Experience

After completing the relapse prevention task, the clinician uses guiding questions to help the patient to recognize the effectiveness and value of the procedure.

> **SAMPLE CLINICIAN SCRIPT**
>
> [Sample prompts to facilitate processing:]
>
> > How was that for you?
> >
> > What did you notice while doing that task?
> >
> > What was easy about that task?
> >
> > What was difficult about that task?
> >
> > Why did you choose to use the specific skill you did?
> >
> > What are some other ways you might have solved that problem?

Step 5: Repeat the Relapse Prevention Task Several Times

The clinician guides the patient through multiple iterations of the imagery task but directs the patient to resolve the crisis in a different way each time. With each iteration, the patient recounts the circumstances and steps leading up to his or her index suicidal crisis and imagines the effective use of a self-management strategy to avoid a suicide attempt, and the clinician introduces new barriers that make successful resolution of the crisis more difficult for the patient. Following each iteration, the clinician and the patient process the experience.

> **SAMPLE CLINICIAN SCRIPT**
>
> Great work! OK, like I mentioned at the start, we'll be doing this several times together because the more we practice, the better you'll get. Let's do this another time, but this time I want you to solve the problem in a different way, whether it's using a different skill or it's using the same skill in a new way. As a reminder, as we do this multiple times, I'll be making it more difficult for you to solve the problem. For example, you might select a skill to use but I'll come up with a reason why the skill won't work as planned, so you'll have to figure out something new at that point in response to that new problem. Does that make sense?
>
> OK, good. Go ahead and close your eyes and we'll do this again.

Step 6: Collaboratively Identify a Hypothetical Future Suicidal Crisis

The clinician and the patient discuss possible crises that have a high likelihood for emerging in the future.

SAMPLE CLINICIAN SCRIPT

You're doing fantastic! You've clearly mastered how to use your knowledge and skills to solve the crisis that started treatment for you. What we want to do next is have you practice these skills while thinking of a future crisis that you're likely to experience in life. This might be an argument or conflict with a loved one, receiving disappointing news of some kind, or feeling criticized or let down by a coworker.

Based on what we've talked about over the past few months, what types of situations seem to trigger you the most? What sort of situation is likely to upset you in the future?

Step 7: Conduct the Relapse Prevention Task Focused on the Hypothetical Suicidal Crisis

The clinician guides the patient through an imagery task in which the patient imagines the circumstances leading up to the hypothetical future suicidal crisis. The clinician helps the patient to imagine the effective use of a self-management strategy to avoid a suicide attempt.

SAMPLE CLINICIAN SCRIPT

Now that we have a hypothetical future crisis, we'll do the exact same thing we were doing before to practice your skills. Go ahead and close your eyes and describe to me where you are and what's going on around you.

[Sample prompts to increase the vividness of the mental image:]

What is happening around you?

What does that sound like?

Describe what it looks like.

What are the exact words the person uses when he/she says that to you?

What emotion do you feel?

What's going through your mind at this point?

Where in your body do you feel that sensation?

What do you do next?

[For patients who struggle to identify or effectively use a self-management skill:]

What is a skill you could use here?

Is there something you've learned in treatment that could help at this point?

Is there something listed on the whiteboard that might be useful in this situation?

Step 8: Process the Experience

After completing the relapse prevention task, the clinician uses guiding questions to help the patient to recognize the effectiveness and value of the procedure.

[Sample prompts to facilitate processing:]

How was that for you?

What did you notice while doing that task?

What was easy about that task?

What was difficult about that task?

Why did you choose to use the specific skill you did?

What are some other ways you might have solved that problem?

Step 9: Repeat the Relapse Prevention Task

The clinician guides the patient through multiple iterations of the imagery task but directs the patient to resolve the crisis in a different way each time. With each iteration, the patient recounts the circumstances and steps leading up to his or her index suicidal crisis and imagines the effective use of a self-management strategy to avoid a suicide attempt, and the clinician introduces new barriers that make successful resolution of the crisis more difficult for the patient. Following each iteration, the clinician and the patient process the experience.

ILLUSTRATIVE CASE EXAMPLE

A partial transcript from the case of Janice is provided to demonstrate how the clinician increased the difficulty of the relapse prevention task after several successful task completions. Note that the clinician introduces new challenges that require Janice to "think on her feet," thereby demonstrating the acquisition of enhanced cognitive flexibility:

CLINICIAN: Good job yet again; I think you're getting the hang of it now.

JANICE: Yeah, I think I've got it.

CLINICIAN: OK, then. Let's start over and do it again. This time around, I want to see how you might respond if things don't work out as planned.

JANICE: OK.

CLINICIAN: Go ahead and start at the beginning.

JANICE: OK. I'm at work and my boss is being a real jerk. He's telling me I'm a screw-up and never do anything right, and when I try to defend myself he just dismisses me and says I'm making excuses. I can feel myself getting angry and wanting to cry, and thinking that I don't want to deal with this anymore, so I decide to go get a cup of coffee because that's the first thing on my crisis response plan. So I walk down to the coffee shop on the first floor of my building.

CLINICIAN: What if you get to the coffee shop and they've closed early for the day?

JANICE: Well, I could just walk over to the cafeteria a few buildings away and get some coffee there.

CLINICIAN: OK, good. Describe yourself doing that.

JANICE: Well, I walk out of my building and down the street, then at the stop sign I turn right.

CLINICIAN: Imagine you get a text message and you look at your phone and it's your supervisor asking where you went.

JANICE: I'll just ignore him and keep going to get coffee.

CLINICIAN: Well, what if he texts again?

JANICE: I'll just keep ignoring him.

CLINICIAN: What if he starts calling when you don't respond?

JANICE: (*Sighs*) I'll just turn off my phone and think about my kids for a while.

CLINICIAN: What about them are you thinking about?

JANICE: Well, I'm thinking about how we can make plans to get together for the weekend, and maybe the dogs can play with each other in the backyard.

CLINICIAN: OK. What happens next?

JANICE: I get my coffee and return to the office through the back stairwell so I don't see my boss.

CLINICIAN: What if he's waiting at your office door for you? What then?

JANICE: Well, I guess I can't avoid him then, and I'll just remind myself that he's not a reliable source of information and that I'm a good person even though he's being a jerk. If I start to criticize myself, that's just emotional reasoning and I'll remind myself that sometimes people are going to be jerks, and that doesn't necessarily reflect on me as a person.

CLINICIAN: Wow, great job! Let's go ahead and stop there.

JANICE: Thanks. That was actually a lot easier than I thought.

HOW TO DO IT: ENDING TREATMENT

Upon completion of the relapse prevention task and demonstration of skills mastery, the clinician raises the issue of ending BCBT, which could entail complete treatment termination or some other form of care transition (e.g., continuation of other therapy or treatment). The clinician reviews relapse prevention concepts and informs the patient about follow-up procedures. Critically, the clinician should communicate to the patient that he or she can resume services again in the future if a new suicidal episode emerges.

Step 1: Discuss Relapse Prevention

The clinician discusses the treatment log as a written plan to help the patient manage crises in the future.

SAMPLE CLINICIAN SCRIPT

Well, you've come a long way in a pretty short period of time. Based on your performance in the relapse prevention task, I would say you now have a very clear grasp of how to handle crises in life. What do you think?

In light of your progress, I think we're at a place now where we can formally wrap up BCBT. As a part of this process, I want to highlight a number of important points. First, this treatment log should serve as your formal plan for managing problems in life going forward. This is why we kept referring back to it and writing down all of the most useful lessons learned in treatment. In essence, you have all of the most important information you need written down in here to continue living a life that's worth living. It's sort of like saving a notebook from class so you can go back and review your notes at a later time to refresh your memory after you're done with that class.

Now that we're done with treatment, where do you think you might keep this treatment log? Do you think you would be able to pull this treatment log out and review it when needed in the future?

Step 2: Discuss Follow-Up Procedures and Make Recommendations for Continuing Care

The clinician provides information about how the patient can seek out additional treatment sessions in the future (i.e., "booster sessions") should the need arise and make recommendations for ongoing care, if appropriate.

SAMPLE CLINICIAN SCRIPT

The second thing I want to discuss is how to resume treatment in the future if you need some additional help. Just because we're done with this treatment doesn't mean you can't ever come back for a few booster sessions if you need some support or coaching. It's pretty common that patients will ask to meet again a few times after a few months have passed and they run into a new crisis in life, for instance, and are having trouble navigating it. In most cases, people only need to meet once or twice to get a refresher or a "tune-up," so to speak, but sometimes they need to meet a few more times than that. So if you find yourself in a situation like this in the future, just give me a call and we'll set up an appointment.

Finally, I want to give you some recommendations about what I think your next step should be in treatment.

The clinician provides additional treatment and follow-up recommendations based on the patient's unique circumstances.

ILLUSTRATIVE CASE EXAMPLES

The Case of John

Because John was not engaged in other forms of treatment with other mental health professionals, BCBT completion marked the conclusion of his mental health treatment. When the clinician followed up with John for a routine 1-year check-in, John indicated that he was doing fine and had experienced no other suicidal crises.

The Case of Mike

Mike attended only one session of the relapse prevention session because he had started a new full-time job. Because Mike successfully completed several iterations of the relapse prevention task during this final session, the clinician determined that Mike had demonstrated skills competency and did not need an additional session. Approximately 6 months later, Mike recontacted his clinician to inquire about a possible psychiatric consult. Mike reported continued agitation and irritability, although he noted that he was "way better than when we first started therapy." He and his wife agreed that the symptoms were interfering enough to warrant a consultation with a psychiatrist about possible medications. The clinician helped to facilitate this referral.

The Case of Janice

At the conclusion of BCBT, the clinician recommended that Janice transition to trauma-focused psychotherapy to address her PTSD. Janice agreed to this recommendation, noting that she "finally feels ready to tackle the abuse I've experienced in my life." Janice completed this treatment several months later, at which point she no longer met diagnostic criteria for PTSD. She noted that she occasionally experienced suicidal thoughts during her PTSD treatment, but "I knew how to handle it this time."

TIPS AND ADVICE FOR
THE RELAPSE PREVENTION TASK AND ENDING TREATMENT

1. **Be alert for avoidance.** Emotional avoidance and suppression reduce the impact of the relapse prevention task and serve as risk factors for continued suicidal behavior. Patients can manifest avoidance during the relapse prevention task in several different ways such as glossing over difficult parts of the story or refusing to provide details. Clinicians should be mindful of such behavior, as it could signal ongoing difficulties with emotion regulation and cognitive reappraisal.

2. **Give voice to the patient's suicidal beliefs.** Related to the first point, an especially potent strategy for increasing the emotional salience of the relapse prevention task is to call attention to the patient's suicidal beliefs. If the patient is unwilling to verbalize his or her suicidal beliefs (a sign of avoidance), the clinician should verbalize the beliefs.

3. **Be alert for cognitive rigidity.** While recounting their index suicidal episode, some patients will become locked into the memory and forget that the purpose of the task is to change the outcome. Because a primary goal of the relapse prevention task is to facilitate the patient's ability to engage in appropriate coping skills other than suicidal behavior, clinicians should redirect the patient if he or she struggles to "break the chain" of their suicidal crisis.

APPENDIX A

Patient Forms and Handouts

The Suicidal Mode

The suicidal mode is a way to organize the many different risk and protective factors associated with a suicidal crisis. These factors can be organized into several domains: cognitive (factors related to how and what we think when stressed), behavioral (factors related to the actions we take and things we do in response to stress), emotional (factors related to the feelings we have when stressed), and physical (factors related to biology and body sensations when stressed). Baseline factors are relatively fixed or unlikely to change, whereas acute factors change in response to activating events that happen in our lives.

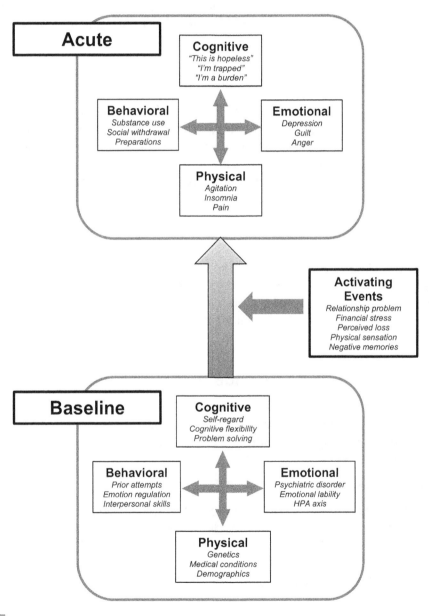

Patient Information Sheet about Brief Cognitive-Behavioral Therapy to Prevent Suicide Attempts

What is the name of the treatment that I am being provided?

Brief cognitive-behavioral therapy (BCBT) to prevent suicide attempts

How and where did my clinician learn to administer BCBT?

[Responses will vary based on the individual clinician but should include information about graduate school, postgraduate experience, and any additional trainings. Clinicians should also describe the amount and nature of the supervision received specific to BCBT.]

How does BCBT compare to other treatments?

In research studies, BCBT has been compared to what is called treatment as usual. Treatment as usual is the typical mental health treatment provided by professionals in the community. In terms of depression, suicidal thinking, and other emotional symptoms, patients in BCBT and treatment as usual improve about the same amount. In terms of suicide attempts and hospitalization, patients in BCBT are about 60% less likely to make a suicide attempt and spend fewer days in a psychiatric hospital.

How does BCBT work?

BCBT is an individual, one-on-one therapy that focuses on teaching you how to solve problems, manage crises, and think about yourself and your life differently. As you learn these new skills, you will find that you are better able to manage crises in your life. To do this, you and your clinician will talk about stressful situations in life and practice new skills to handle these situations differently.

How often will we meet and how long does BCBT last?

BCBT usually lasts for 12 appointments that are scheduled once per week or twice per week, depending on your needs and your clinician's availability. The first appointment is usually 1½ hours long and the remaining 11 appointments are usually 1 hour long.

What are the possible risks associated with BCBT?

The most common risk is feeling upset when talking about stressful or painful situations, thoughts, and feelings. Treatment will involve discussions of emotionally difficult topics that can sometimes increase your distress in the short term. These periods of increased distress tend to be very brief, but they could increase your desire for suicide for short periods of time. Your clinician will work with you to help you get through these periods.

(continued)

Another common risk is suicide attempt. Approximately half of patients who have made a suicide attempt in the past or who start treatment with suicide ideation make a suicide attempt during or soon after treatment. The risk for suicide attempt tends to decline over time, and BCBT has been shown to decrease this risk by more than half.

A much less common but serious risk is death by suicide. Fewer than 2% of patients in outpatient treatment die by suicide. The risk for death by suicide is higher among patients with a history of suicide attempts, especially those who have made multiple suicide attempts. Patients who make a suicide attempt during treatment are at the greatest risk for dying by suicide.

How many patients improve in BCBT? How do you know?

Results of high-quality scientific studies indicate that over 75% of patients who receive BCBT start to see improvements in suicide ideation, depression, hopelessness, and anxiety within the first 3 months of treatment. These improvements tend to last for up to 2 years after treatment. Patients who receive BCBT are also less likely to make a suicide attempt within 3 months of starting treatment. This improvement in risk lasts for up to 2 years after treatment. Patients who receive BCBT also tend to report improvements in other areas of life, such as being less likely to have work problems.

How many patients get worse in BCBT? How do you know?

Results of high-quality scientific studies indicate that few patients will get worse in BCBT, but some patients do not respond as well as others. Anywhere from 15 to 30% of patients will continue to experience significant emotional distress and may make a suicide attempt during or soon after treatment.

How do patients who receive BCBT compare to those who receive no treatment and those who receive other treatments?

The outcomes of patients who receive BCBT have not yet been compared to the outcomes of patients who do not receive any treatment at all.

Over 75% of patients report improvement in emotional distress when receiving BCBT. A similar number of patients report improvement when receiving other forms of therapy and medication. However, only 15–30% of patients who receive BCBT make a suicide attempt during or soon after treatment as compared to 30–60% of patients who receive other forms of therapy and medication. This means that patients in BCBT are half as likely to make a suicide attempt as patients in other treatments.

An alternative treatment that works just as well as BCBT is called dialectical behavior therapy, or DBT. BCBT and DBT have not been directly compared to each other, but like BCBT, DBT reduces emotional distress in most patients and decreases the risk of suicide attempt by approximately the same amount. DBT and BCBT are very similar in terms of teaching skills to solve problems and manage crises. DBT and BCBT are different in terms of length of treatment and treatment modality. DBT includes weekly individual and group therapy sessions that last for 12 months, as well as one 15-minute phone consultation in between weekly sessions, for a total

(continued)

of 52 individual therapy sessions plus 52 group sessions over a year. BCBT includes weekly individual sessions that last for 12 weeks (6 weeks for biweekly sessions).

Another treatment option is psychiatric medication, which might include antidepressants, mood stabilizers, antianxiety medications, or other types of medications. Research suggests that most patients feel their symptoms improve while taking medications, but medications by themselves do not seem to reduce the risk for suicide attempts.

A final treatment option is a combination of therapy and medication. Few studies have compared combined treatment to either therapy or medication by themselves. Most patients who receive BCBT also take medication and recover just as well as patients who receive BCBT but do not take medication.

What do I do if I feel that BCBT is not working?

At the beginning of every appointment, you will be asked to describe how things have been going since the last appointment and will be asked if the new skills and strategies have helped. If a particular strategy is not working, you should say so at that time. Your clinician may be able to help you figure out how to make the strategy work better. In rare cases, you and your clinician may determine the strategy doesn't work and will agree to stop using it to find something else that works better.

Treatment Plan Template

In this treatment, we are going to tailor what we do to your specific needs and interests. It will help us to have a clear plan to follow that is based on those needs and interests. This form is called a treatment plan. The treatment plan summarizes the priorities we will set and gives us a way to keep track of progress. In our work together, we will naturally include "suicide risk" as a problem to be targeted. We will also include "reduce risk for suicidal behaviors" as a goal or objective, but there will likely be other goals that we include, and perhaps add, over the course of treatment.

Problem No.	Problem Description	Goals/Objectives	Intervention	Estimated No. of Sessions	Outcome
1.					
2.					
3.					
4.					

Outcome: 0—Not accomplished; 1—Partially accomplished; 2—Accomplished

Commitment to Treatment Statement

I, _____, agree to make a commitment to the treatment process. I understand that this means I have agreed to be actively involved in all aspects of treatment, including:

1. Attending appointments (or letting my provider know when I can't make it)
2. Setting goals
3. Voicing my opinions, thoughts, and feelings honestly and openly with my provider (whether they are negative or positive, but most importantly my negative feelings)
4. Being actively involved *during* appointments
5. Completing homework assignments
6. Taking my medications as prescribed
7. Experimenting with new behaviors and new ways of doing things
8. Implementing my crisis response plan when needed
9. Any additional terms that my provider and I agree to

I understand and acknowledge that, to a large degree, a successful treatment outcome depends on the amount of energy I devote and the effort I make. If I feel like treatment is not working, I agree to discuss it with my provider and attempt to come to a common understanding as to what the problems are and identify potential solutions.

I also understand and acknowledge that if I do not show up for an appointment without notifying my provider, my provider might contact individuals within my social support network, including my chain of command, in order to confirm my safety.

In short, I agree to make a commitment to treatment, and a commitment to living.

This agreement will apply for the duration of our treatment plan, which will be reviewed and modified on the following date: _____

Patient signature: _____ Date: _____

Provider signature: _____ Date: _____

Means Safety Plan

The means safety plan outlines the steps to be taken to enhance safety and reduce access to potentially lethal means for suicide.

Questions? Contact your provider: _____

Emergencies? Call 911

Patient Name: _____

Support Name: _____

Support's Contact: _____

Safety Plan: _____

_____

_____

_____

_____

_____

_____

_____

_____

_____

_____

Terms for Ending Plan: _____

_____

_____

_____

_____

Patient's Signature: _____

Support's Signature: _____

(to be signed upon implementation of means safety plan)

Crisis Support Plan

Things I can do to assist _____:
(Patient's name)

1. Provide encouragement and support in the following ways:

   -
   -
   -

2. Help _____ follow his/her crisis response plan

3. Ensure a safe environment by doing the following:
   - REMOVE all firearms and ammunition
   - REMOVE or LOCK UP:
     - ✓ All knives, razors, and other sharp objects
     - ✓ All prescription and over-the-counter drugs (including vitamins and aspirin)
     - ✓ All alcohol, illegal drugs, and any related paraphernalia
   - Make sure someone is available to provide personal support and monitor the patient at all times during a crisis and afterward as needed.
   - Pay attention to the patient's stated method of suicide/self-injury/intent to harm others and restrict access to vehicle, ropes, flammables, etc., as appropriate
   - Limit/restrict access to vehicle/car keys as appropriate
   - Identify people who might increase risk for the patient and minimize their contact with the patient
   - Provide access to things the patient identifies as helpful and encourage choices and behaviors that promote health, such as good nutrition, exercise, and rest

If I am unable to continue to provide these supports, or if I believe that the crisis response plan is not helpful or sufficient, I will contact the patient's treatment provider to express my concerns.

If I believe _____ is a danger to self or others, I agree to:

   - Call his/her mental health treatment provider: _____
   - Call the national crisis hotline: 1-800-273-TALK (8255)
   - Help _____ get to a hospital
   - Call 911

I agree to follow this plan until _____

_____   _____
Helper signature   Patient signature

_____
Clinician signature

Improving Your Sleep Handout

1. **Go to bed only when you're sleepy.** There is no reason to go to bed if you are not sleepy. When you go to bed too early, it only gives you more time to become frustrated. Individuals often ponder the events of the day, plan the next day's schedule, or worry about their inability to fall asleep. These behaviors are incompatible with sleep and tend to perpetuate insomnia. You should therefore *delay your bedtime until you are sleepy*. This may mean that you go to bed later than your scheduled bedtime. However, stick to your scheduled rising time *regardless* of the time you go to bed.

2. **Get out of bed when you can't fall asleep or cannot go back to sleep in 15 minutes.** When you recognize that you've become a clock watcher, get out of bed. If you wake up during your sleep and you've tried falling back asleep for 15 minutes and can't, get out of bed. Remember, the goal is to fall asleep quickly. Return to bed *only* when you are sleepy (i.e., yawning, head bobbing, eyes closing, concentration decreasing). The goal is for you to reconnect your bed with sleeping rather than frustration. You will have to repeat this step as often as necessary.

3. **Use your bed for sleep and sex only.** The purpose of this guideline is to associate your bedroom with sleep rather than wakefulness. Just as you may associate the kitchen with hunger, this guideline will help you associate sleep and pleasure with your bedroom. Follow this rule both during the day and at night. *Do not* watch TV, listen to the radio, eat, or read in bed. You may have to temporarily move the TV or radio from your bedroom to help you regain a stable sleep cycle.

SLEEP GUIDELINES

1. **Limit caffeine.** No caffeine 6–8 hours before bedtime. Yes, it's true caffeine disturbs sleep, even for people who do not think they experience a stimulation effect. Individuals with insomnia are often more sensitive to mild stimulants than normal sleepers. Caffeine is found in items such as coffee, tea, soda, chocolate, and many over-the-counter medications (e.g., Excedrin).

2. **Avoid nicotine.** Nicotine is a stimulant. It is a myth that smoking helps you "relax." As nicotine builds in the system it produces an effect similar to caffeine. *Do not* smoke to get yourself back to sleep.

3. **Avoid alcohol.** Alcohol often promotes the onset of sleep, but as alcohol is metabolized sleep becomes disturbed and fragmented. Thus, a large amount of alcohol is a poor sleep aid and should not be used as such. Limit alcohol use to small to moderate quantities.

4. **Limit sleep medications.** Sleep medications are effective only temporarily. Scientists have shown that sleep medications lose their effectiveness in about 2–4 weeks when taken regularly. Over time, sleeping pills actually make sleep problems worse. When sleeping pills have been used for a long period, withdrawal from the medication can lead to an insomnia rebound. Thus, after long-term use, many individuals incorrectly conclude that they "need" sleeping pills in order to sleep normally.

(continued)

5. **Exercise regularly.** Preferably 30 minutes each day. Exercise in the late afternoon or early evening can aid sleep, although the positive effect often takes several weeks to become noticeable. Do not exercise within 2 hours of bedtime because it may elevate your nervous system activity and interfere with falling asleep.

6. **Bedroom environment.** Moderate temperature, quiet, dark, and comfortable. Extremes of heat or cold can disrupt sleep. Noises can be masked with background white noise (such as the noise of a fan) or with earplugs. Bedrooms may be darkened with blackout shades or sleep masks can be worn. Position clocks out of sight since clock watching can increase worry about the effects of lack of sleep. Be sure your mattress is not too soft or too firm and that your pillow is the right height and firmness.

7. **Eating.** Avoid heavy meals soon before bedtime. You should avoid the following foods at bedtime: peanuts, beans, most raw fruits and vegetables (they may cause gas), anything caffeinated (like chocolate), and high-fat foods such as potato chips or corn chips. Be especially careful to avoid heavy meals and spices in the evening. Do not go to bed too hungry or too full. Avoid snacks in the middle of the night because awakening may become associated with hunger. A light bedtime snack, such as a glass of warm milk, cheese, or a bowl of cereal, can promote sleep.

8. **Avoid taking naps during the day.** The sleep you obtain during the day takes away from the sleep you need at night, resulting in lighter, more restless sleep, difficulty falling asleep, or early-morning awakening. If you must nap, keep it brief, and try to schedule it before 3:00 P.M. It is best to set an alarm to ensure you don't sleep more than 15–30 minutes.

9. **Unwind.** Allow yourself at least an hour before bedtime to wind down. The brain is not a light switch that you can instantly turn on and off. Most of us cannot expect to go full speed till 10:00 P.M., then fall peacefully asleep at 10:30. Take a hot bath, read a novel, watch some TV, or have a pleasant talk with your spouse or kids. Find what works for you and make it your routine before bed. Be sure not to struggle with a problem, get into an argument before bed, or do anything else that increases your body's arousal.

10. **Regular sleep schedule.** Maintain a regular schedule, even on weekends and holidays. Spending excessive time in bed has two unfortunate consequences: (1) you begin to associate your bedroom with arousal and frustration and (2) your sleep actually becomes shallow. Surprisingly, it is very important that you cut down your sleep time in order to improve sleep! Set the alarm clock and get out of bed at the same time each morning, weekdays and weekends, regardless of your bedtime or the amount of sleep you obtained on the previous night. You probably will be tempted to stay in bed if you did not sleep well, but try to maintain your new schedule. This guideline is designed to regulate your internal biological clock and reset your sleep–wake rhythm.

ABC Worksheet

The ABC Worksheet is used to identify how thoughts and feelings are connected to each other in response to life events. First, identify a stressful situation and write a summary of this situation in the A box. In the B box, identify the thoughts you had during this situation, and write those thoughts down. In the C box, identify the emotions you felt in that situation and write those emotions down. Next, explain how the thoughts and beliefs you wrote down in the B box are helpful or unhelpful for you. If your thoughts are unhelpful, identify and write down a different way of thinking about the situation that can directly counter what you wrote in the B box.

A Activating Event (What happened?)	B Beliefs (What do I tell myself?)	C Consequences (What emotion do I feel?)

Is the belief above in box "B" helpful?

What is something else I can tell myself in the future when in a similar situation?

Challenging Questions Worksheet

The Challenging Questions Worksheet is used to evaluate your thoughts and beliefs to determine if they are helpful or useful. First, identify a negative belief and write it in the box at the top of the worksheet. Next, review each question as it relates to this belief. Write down your answer to each question in the space provided under the question.

Belief:
1. What is the evidence for and against this idea?
2. Is your belief a habit or based on facts?
3. If someone else had this belief in this same situation, would you consider it accurate?
4. Are you thinking in all-or-none terms?

(continued)

5. Are you using words or phrases that are extreme or exaggerated (i.e., *always, forever, never, need, should, must, can't,* and *every time*)?

6. Are you only focusing on one aspect of the event and ignoring other important facts about the situation that explains things?

7. What is the source of this belief? Is that source reliable?

8. Are you blowing things out of proportion? Or the opposite, minimizing things?

9. Is your belief based on feelings rather than facts?

10. Are you focused on unrelated details of the situation?

Patterns of Problematic Thinking Worksheet

The Patterns of Problematic Thinking Worksheet is used to categorize your thoughts into different "types" or patterns of beliefs. Write your negative thoughts and beliefs under the pattern that best fits them. Note that some thoughts and beliefs fit under multiple patterns.

Jumping to conclusions when the evidence is lacking or even contradictory
Exaggerating or minimizing a situation (blowing things way out of proportion or shrinking their importance inappropriately)
Disregarding important aspects of a situation
Oversimplifying things as good/bad or right/wrong
Overgeneralizing from a single incident (a negative event is seen as a never-ending pattern)
Mind reading (you assume people are thinking negatively of you when there is no definite evidence for this)
Emotional reasoning (you have a feeling and assume there must be a reason)

APPENDIX B

Clinician Tools

APPENDIX B.1

Fidelity Checklists

No	Partial	Yes	Describing BCBT
			Initial symptom/mood check
			Agenda setting
			Reviewed homework and treatment log
			Skills building with practice
			Assigned homework
			Three-phase model of treatment
			Explained role in crisis management, healthy social support, and skill building
			Gauged the patient's understanding about structure for treatment
			Elicited input and feedback about structure for treatment
			Provided an opportunity for the patient to ask questions about the structure of treatment

No	Partial	Yes	Narrative Assessment of Index Suicidal Crisis
			Facilitated narrative description of events leading up to index suicidal episode
			Elicited information about contributory/associated domains, including:
			Predispositions
			Activating Events
			Cognitions
			Emotions
			Behaviors
			Physical
			Identified consistencies across suicidal crises or suicide attempts (where appropriate)

(continued)

No	Partial	Yes	Cognitive-Behavioral Conceptualization
			Explained concept of the suicidal mode using language that is understandable to the patient
			Integrated information from assessment into conceptualization in following domains:
			Predispositions
			Activating Events
			Cognitions
			Emotions
			Behaviors
			Physical
			Gauged the patient's understanding of conceptualization (suicidal mode)
			Elicited agreement from the patient that model is an accurate reflection of his or her experience
			If the patient disagreed, elicited feedback and reconceptualized the model
			Encouraged the patient to record written model of suicidal mode in treatment log

No	Partial	Yes	Treatment Planning
			Explained rationale for treatment plan
			Elicited feedback and input from patient regarding treatment targets
			Core treatment targets emphasized skill development
			Established objective, measurable outcomes for treatment targets
			Identified symptom hierarchy when presented with a mix of prominent symptoms
			Gauged patient's understanding of treatment plan
			Set date for reviewing/revising treatment plan

(continued)

No	Partial	Yes	Commitment to Treatment Statement (CTS)
			Explained rationale for CTS
			Collaboratively reviewed the CTS with patient
			Elicited feedback and input from patient regarding CTS items and expectations
			Invited patient to add or modify CTS
			Gauged patient's understanding of CTS
			Set date for reviewing/revising CTS

No	Partial	Yes	Crisis Response Plan (CRP)
			Written on card (or similar item) that can be easily carried by patient
			Explained rationale for CRP
			Identified and discussed personal warning signs
			Identified and listed self-management skills
			Identified and listed external sources of support
			Identified and listed professional sources of help
			Health care providers
			Suicide crisis hotline
			Emergency department and 911
			Verbally reviewed all steps
			Gauged patient's understanding of CRP

(continued)

No	Partial	Yes	**Means Safety Counseling**
			Explained rationale for means safety
			Discussed impulsivity, cognitive confusion, and poor problem solving when highly distressed
			Identified potential methods for means safety
			Asked about access to firearms
			Collaboratively engaged patient in discussion about means safety
			Elicited feedback and input from patient regarding preferred options for securing means

No	Partial	Yes	**Skills Training**
			Explained rationale for skill
			Explicitly tied skill to suicidal mode/case conceptualization
			Demonstrated/modeled skill
			Practiced skill in session
			Gauged patient understanding and mastery of skill
			Assigned skills practice for between-session practice
			Used treatment journal, including its role as a relapse prevention tool
			Encouraged patient to record lessons learned from the session in treatment journal

No	Partial	Yes	**Relapse Prevention Task (RPT): Informed Consent**
			Explained rationale for intervention
			Elicited feedback and questions about RPT
			Discussed the potential for negative emotional reactions to RPT
			Identified coping strategies and skills for use during RPT
			Obtained the patient's consent to conduct the RPT

(continued)

Fidelity Checklists *(page 5 of 5)*

No	Partial	Yes	Relapse Prevention Task (RPT): Index Crisis
			Encouraged the patient to recount index episode
			Strategically prompted the patient to increase memory vividness
			Focused on beliefs, emotions, behaviors, and circumstances directly related to the crisis
			Facilitated problem solving by introducing new challenges/barriers to skills use
			Encouraged the patient to imagine use of learned skills
			Debriefed the patient

No	Partial	Yes	Relapse Prevention Task (RPT): Future Crisis
			Collaboratively identified likely triggers for future suicidal episodes
			Encouraged the patient to recount future suicidal episodes
			Strategically prompted the patient to increase memory vividness
			Focused on beliefs, emotions, behaviors, and circumstances directly related to the crisis
			Facilitated problem solving by introducing new challenges/barriers to skills use
			Encouraged the patient to imagine use of learned skills
			Debriefed the patient

Suicide Risk Assessment Documentation Template

Y N Suicide Ideation

- Content: _____
- Frequency: Never   Rarely   Sometimes   Frequently   Always
- Intensity: Brief/fleeting   Focused deliberation   Intense rumination   Other
- Duration: Seconds   Minutes   Hours

Y N Recent Intent

- Subjective reports: _____

- Objective signs: _____

Y N Suicide Plan

- How: _____

- When: _____

- Where: _____

Y N Access to Means: _____

Y N Suicide Preparation/Rehearsal: _____

Y N History of Suicide Ideation and Attempts

- Ideation: _____

- Attempts: _____

Y N Impulsivity

- Subjective reports: _____

- Objective signs: _____

Y N Substance Abuse: _____

Y N Significant Loss: _____

Y N Relationship Problems: _____

Y N Health Problems: _____

(continued)

Y   N   Legal Problems: _____

Y   N   Other Problems: _____

Protective Factors

Y   N   Reasons for Living: _____

Y   N   Hope: _____

Y   N   Social Support: _____

Y   N   Meaning in Life: _____

Y   N   Other Protective Factors: _____

Current Assessed Risk Level: **Not Elevated**   **Low**   **Moderate**   **High**

At the current time, outpatient care **can**/**cannot** provide sufficient safety and stability.

Hospitalization **is**/**is not** necessary based on factors above.

Patient agrees to written crisis response plan: Y   N

Plan for securing access to means: _____

_____

_____

_____

_____

_____

_____

_____

_____

_____

_____

_____

_____

_____

_____

_____

_____

Crisis Response Plan Template

The crisis response plan comprises several sections: warning signs, self-management, reasons for living, social support, and crisis and professional services. The crisis response plan can be handwritten on an index card for easy access by patients as a reminder for how to respond effectively to periods of intense stress.

Warning Signs

Pacing
Feeling angry
"I can't take this anymore"

Self-Management

Go for a walk
Listen to some music
Play games on my phone

Reasons for Living

My kids (Tim and Lisa)
My wife (Susan)

Social Support

Call Susan (wife): 555-555-5555
Call John (friend): 555-555-5555

Crisis and Professional Services

Call my doctor and leave a message: 555-555-5555
Call hotline: 1-800-273-TALK
Crisis text line: 838255
Go to hospital
Call 911

Possible Warning Signs

Thoughts	"I'm an idiot." "Here we go again." "This will never end." "It's my fault." "Nobody cares about me." "What's the point?" "I can't take this anymore." "I deserve to be punished." "I'm a failure."
Mental Images	Stressful memories Flashbacks about trauma Reliving uncomfortable situations Seeing myself make a suicide attempt
Emotions or Feelings	Sadness or depression Guilt or remorse Worry Anger
Behaviors or Actions	Pacing Being quiet around others Avoiding others Yelling/screaming Crying Shaking/trembling Aggression Self-injury Practicing/rehearsing the suicide attempt Getting ready for a suicide attempt
Physical Sensations	Headaches or other pain Agitation/feeling on edge Racing heart Muscle tension Nausea Breathing difficulties Insomnia

Common Self-Management Strategies

• Watching a movie	• Relaxation or breathing exercises
• Watching a TV show	• Prayer
• Listening to music	• Puzzles (e.g., crossword, Sudoku, computer games)
• Singing	
• Playing with a pet	• Thinking about a positive upcoming event
• Going for a walk	• Thinking about positive memories
• Exercising	• Looking at pictures of friends
• Taking a warm bath or shower	• Reading letters or e-mails from family members
• Reading a book	• Eating a favorite food (e.g., ice cream, pizza)
• Reading spiritual or religious material	• Cooking or baking
• Meditation	• Playing a sport

Relaxation Script

Note: Ellipses [. . .] indicate places where the clinician should pause for a few seconds.

Let's start by taking a very slow, deep breath in through your nose, so that you fill up your lungs and even feel your belly start to expand . . . And then very slowly let that breath out through your mouth . . . Good . . . Let's repeat that . . . A very slow, deep breath in . . . And then very slowly let it out . . . Very good . . . And you can continue to breathe in this very slow, very deep way . . . In . . . And out . . . In . . . And out . . . Good . . . Just like that.

[Pause for 15 seconds.]

And now with each breath out, what I'd like for you to do is just release the tension and your shoulders and let them slump . . . Sort of like they're getting pulled down by little weights . . . With each slow breath out, just let them slump a little bit more . . . Allowing them to be totally relaxed . . . Good . . . Keep breathing slow and deep . . . Filling up your lungs and your belly . . . And slowly releasing the tension each time you breathe out . . . Over and over . . . again and again . . . Very good.

[Pause for 15 seconds.]

Now that you're in a state of relaxation, I'd like for you to take just one more deep breath in . . . And then slowly let it out . . . And when you're ready you can open up your eyes.

Mindfulness Script

Note: Ellipses [. . .] indicate places where the clinician should pause for a few seconds.

Let's start by slowing down our breathing, nice and slow, so that we're taking slow, steady breaths followed by slow breaths out . . . In . . . And out . . . In . . . And out . . . Very good . . . We'll continue to breathe slowly and deeply, just like this, while we do this attention exercise.

[Pause for 15 seconds.]

Take a moment to really focus your attention on your breathing . . . Notice what the air feels like entering your body . . . Notice what your chest feels like as your lungs fill up with air . . . And then notice what the air feels like as it exits your body . . . Just focus on your breathing . . . In . . . And out . . . If you notice your mind wandering while you do this, that's OK . . . Just notice that and then return your attention back to your breathing.

[Pause for 15 seconds.]

Now shift your attention to the sense of sound . . . Take a moment to notice all of the sounds that you can hear . . . Notice even those in the background that you would normally ignore or filter out . . . If you notice your mind wandering while you do this, that's OK . . . Just notice that and then return your attention back to the sounds . . . Always coming back . . . No matter where your mind wanders to or what it thinks about . . . Just returning your focus to your breathing . . . Again . . . And again . . . And again.

[Pause for 15 seconds.]

Now take a moment to notice the thoughts going through your mind . . . Don't try to change them . . . Don't try to stop them . . . Just look at them move through your mind, sort of like they're on a conveyor belt and just moving past you . . . Sometimes our thoughts are like words or sentences . . . If you have any thoughts that are words or sentences, just put those words on the conveyor belt and watch the words move past you . . . Sometimes our thoughts are like pictures or images . . . If you have any thoughts that are pictures or images, just put those on the conveyor belt as well and watch the images move past you . . . Anytime you notice a thought, just watch it move through your mind without trying to interfere with it . . . Now shift your attention back to the sense of sound . . . Notice how you can shift your focus from your thoughts to something else, whenever you want . . . You'll probably notice that more thoughts keep popping into your head, which is fine . . . Just watch them move past you and then return your focus to your breathing . . . Repeat this process whenever a thought comes into your mind, even if the thought is a stressful thought or a bothersome thought . . . Again . . . And again . . . And again . . . Always returning your attention to your breathing.

(continued)

[Pause for 15 seconds.]

Now take a moment to think about something stressful . . . Perhaps it's a problem you're facing or it's something you've been worrying about . . . Just watch that stressful thought move past you like all the other thoughts, and then return your focus to your breathing . . . Oftentimes our stressful thoughts will keep coming back into our mind, and we'll notice them again . . . That's fine . . . Whenever that happens, just look at the thought and watch it move past, then return to your breathing . . . Do this over and over . . . Again and again . . . Anytime a thought comes into your mind . . . Just noticing and then focusing on your breathing . . . Good.

[Pause for 15 seconds.]

Go ahead and take one more slow, deep breath in . . . And then slowly let it out . . . And when you're ready, you can open up your eyes.

References

Aharonovich, E., Liu, X., Nunes, E., & Hasin, D. S. (2002). Suicide attempts in substance abusers: Effects of major depression in relation to substance use disorders. *American Journal of Psychiatry, 159*(9), 1600–1602.

Akiskal, H. S., & Benazzi, F. (2005). Psychopathologic correlates of suicidal ideation in major depressive outpatients: Is it all due to unrecognized (bipolar) depressive mixed states? *Psychopathology, 38*(5), 273–280.

Allen, J. P., Litten, R. Z., Fertig, J. B., & Babor, T. (1997). A review of research on the Alcohol Use Disorders Identification Test (AUDIT). *Alcoholism: Clinical and Experimental Research, 21,* 613–619.

Bagge, C. L., Conner, K. R., Reed, L., Dawkins, M., & Murray, K. (2015). Alcohol use to facilitate a suicide attempt: An event-based examination. *Journal of Studies on Alcohol and Drugs, 76,* 474–481.

Barraclough, B., & Pallis, D. (1975). Depression followed by suicide: A comparison of depressed suicides with living depressives. *Psychological Medicine, 5,* 55–61.

Bastien, C. H., Vallieres, A., & Morin, C. M. (2000). Validation of the Insomnia Severity Index as an outcome measure for insomnia research. *Sleep Medicine, 2,* 297–307.

Baumeister, R. F. (1990). Suicide as escape from self. *Psychological Review, 97,* 90–113.

Beck, A. T. (1972). *Depression: Causes and treatment.* Philadelphia: University of Pennsylvania Press.

Beck, A. T., Brown, G. K., & Steer, R. A. (1997). Psychometric characteristics of the Scale for Suicide Ideation with psychiatric outpatients. *Behaviour Research and Therapy, 35,* 1039–1046.

Beck, A. T., Kovacs, M., & Weissman, A. (1979). Assessment of suicidal intention: The Scale for Suicide Ideation. *Journal of Consulting and Clinical Psychology, 47,* 343–352.

Beck, A. T., & Steer, R. A. (1991). *Manual for the Beck Scale for Suicide Ideation.* San Antonio, TX: Psychological Corporation.

Beck, A. T., Steer, R. A., & Brown, G. K. (1996). *Beck Depression Inventory–II.* San Antonio, TX: Psychological Corporation.

Bedics, J. D., Atkins, D. C., Comtois, K. A., & Linehan, M. M. (2012). Treatment differences in the therapeutic relationship and introject during a 2-year randomized controlled trial of dialectical behavior therapy versus nonbehavioral psychotherapy experts for borderline personality disorder. *Journal of Consulting and Clinical Psychology, 80*(1), 66–77.

Benazzi, F. (2005). Suicidal ideation and bipolar-II depression symptoms. *Human Psychopharmacology: Clinical and Experimental, 20*(1), 27–32.

Benazzi, F., & Akiskal, H. S. (2006). Psychometric delineation of the most discriminant symptoms of depressive mixed states. *Psychiatry Research, 141*(1), 81–88.

Bennett, B. E., Bricklin, P. M., Harris, E. C., Knapp, S., VandeCreek, L., & Younggren, J. N. (2006). *Assessing and managing risk in psychological practice.* Washington, DC: American Psychiatric Association.

Berman, A. L. (2006). Risk management with suicidal patients. *Journal of Clinical Psychology, 62*(2), 171–184.

Bernert, R. A., Joiner, T. E., Cukrowicz, K. C., Schmidt, N. B., & Krakow, B. (2005). Suicidality and sleep disturbances. *Sleep, 28*(9), 1135.

Bond, G. R., Becker, D. R., & Drake, R. E. (2011). Measurement of fidelity of implementation of evidence-based practices: Case example of the IPS fidelity scale. *Clinical Psychology: Science and Practice, 18*(2), 126–141.

Borges, G., Walters, E. E., & Kessler, R. C. (2000). Associations of substance use, abuse, and dependence with subsequent suicidal behavior. *American Journal of Epidemiology, 151*(8), 781–789.

Bostwick, J. M., & Pankratz, V. S. (2001). "Omission of suicide data": Reply. *American Journal of Psychiatry, 158*(11), 1935.

Boudreaux, E. D., Miller, I., Goldstein, A. B., Sullivan, A. F., Allen, M. H., Manton, A. P., et al. (2013). The Emergency Department Safety Assessment and Follow-up Evaluation (ED-SAFE): Method and design considerations. *Contemporary Clinical Trials, 36,* 14–24.

Britton, P. C., Bryan, C. J., & Valenstein, M. (2016). Motivational interviewing for means restriction counseling with patients at risk for suicide. *Cognitive and Behavioral Practice, 23*(1), 51–61.

Brown, G. K., Beck, A. T., Steer, R. A., & Grisham, J. R. (2000). Risk factors for suicide in psychiatric outpatients: A 20-year prospective study. *Journal of Consulting and Clinical Psychology, 68*(3), 371–377.

Brown, G. K., Henriques, G. R., Sosdjan, D., & Beck, A. T. (2004). Suicide intent and accurate expectations of lethality: Predictors of medical lethality of suicide attempts. *Journal of Consulting and Clinical Psychology, 72*(6), 1170–1174.

Brown, G. K., Steer, R. A., Henriques, G. R., & Beck, A. T. (2005). The internal struggle between the wish to die and the wish to live: A risk factor for suicide. *American Journal of Psychiatry, 162,* 1977–1979.

Brown, G. K., Ten Have, T., Henriques, G. R., Xie, S. X., Hollander, J. E., & Beck, A. T. (2005). Cognitive therapy for the prevention of suicide attempts: A randomized controlled trial. *Journal of the American Medical Association, 294*(5), 563–570.

Bryan, A. O., Theriault, J. L., & Bryan, C. J. (2014). Self-forgiveness, posttraumatic stress, and suicide attempts among military personnel and veterans. *Traumatology, 21,* 40–46.

Bryan, C. J. (2016). Treating PTSD within the context of heightened suicide risk. *Current Psychiatry Reports, 18*(8), 1–7.

Bryan, C. J., Andreski, S. R., McNaughton-Cassill, M., & Osman, A. (2014). Agency is associated with decreased emotional distress and suicidal ideation in military personnel. *Archives of Suicide Research, 18*(3), 241–250.

Bryan, C. J., Bryan, A. O., May, A. M., & Klonsky, E. D. (2015). Trajectories of suicide ideation, nonsuicidal self-injury, and suicide attempts in a nonclinical sample of military personnel and veterans. *Suicide and Life-Threatening Behavior, 45*(3), 315–325.

Bryan, C. J., Bryan, A. O., Ray-Sannerud, B. N., Etienne, N., & Morrow, C. E. (2014). Suicide attempts before joining the military increase risk for suicide attempts and severity of suicidal ideation among military personnel and veterans. *Comprehensive Psychiatry, 55*(3), 534–541.

Bryan, C. J., Clemans, T. A., & Hernandez, A. M. (2012). Perceived burdensomeness, fearlessness of death, and suicidality among deployed military personnel. *Personality and Individual Differences, 52*(3), 374–379.

Bryan, C. J., Clemans, T. A., Leeson, B., & Rudd, M. D. (2015). Acute vs. chronic stressors, multiple suicide attempts, and persistent suicide ideation in US soldiers. *Journal of Nervous and Mental Disease, 203,* 48–53.

Bryan, C. J., Corso, K. A., Corso, M. L., Kanzler, K. E., Ray-Sannerud, B., & Morrow, C. E. (2012). Therapeutic alliance and change in suicidal ideation during treatment in integrated primary care settings. *Archives of Suicide Research, 16,* 316–323.

Bryan, C. J., Corso, K. A., Rudd, M. D., & Cordero, L. (2008). Improving identification of suicidal patients in primary care through routine screening. *Primary Care and Community Psychiatry, 13,* 143–147.

Bryan, C. J., Elder, W. B., McNaughton-Cassill, M., Osman, A., Hernandez, A. M., & Allison, S. (2013). Meaning in life, emotional distress, suicidal ideation, and life functioning in an active duty military sample. *Journal of Positive Psychology, 8,* 444–452.

Bryan, C. J., Garland, E. L., & Rudd, M. D. (2016). From impulse to action among military personnel hospitalized for suicide risk: Alcohol consumption and the reported transition from suicidal thought to behavior. *General Hospital Psychiatry, 41,* 13–19.

Bryan, C. J., Gartner, A. M., Wertenberger, E., Delano, K. A., Wilkinson, E., Breitbach, J., et al. (2012). Defining treatment completion according to patient competency: A case example using brief cognitive behavioral therapy (BCBT) for suicidal patients. *Professional Psychology: Research and Practice, 43*(2), 130–136.

Bryan, C. J., Gonzales, J., Rudd, M. D., Bryan, A. O., Clemans, T. A., Ray-Sannerud, B., et al. (2015). Depression mediates the relation of insomnia severity with suicide risk in three clinical samples of U.S. military personnel. *Depression and Anxiety, 32,* 647–655.

Bryan, C. J., Griffith, J., Pace, B. T., Hinkson, K., Bryan, A. O., Clemans, T., et al. (2015, April). *Combat exposure and risk for suicidal thoughts and behaviors among military personnel and veterans: A systematic review and meta-analysis.* Paper presented at the annual meeting of the American Association of Suicidology, Atlanta, GA.

Bryan, C. J., Grove, J. L., & Kimbrel, N. A. (2017). Theory-driven models of self-directed violence among individuals with PTSD. *Current Opinion in Psychology, 14,* 12–17.

Bryan, C. J., & Hernandez, A. M. (2013). The functions of social support as protective factors for suicidal ideation in a sample of air force personnel. *Suicide and Life-Threatening Behavior, 43*(5), 562–573.

Bryan, C. J., Hitschfeld, M. J., Palmer, B. A., Schak, K. M., Roberge, E. M., & Lineberry, T. W. (2014). Gender differences in the association of agitation and suicide attempts among psychiatric inpatients. *General Hospital Psychiatry, 36,* 726–731.

Bryan, C. J., Kanzler, K. E., Grieser, E., Martinez, A., Allison, S., & McGeary, D. (2017). A shortened version of the Suicide Cognitions Scale for identifying chronic pain patients at risk for suicide. *Pain Practice, 17*(3), 371–381.

Bryan, C. J., Kopta, S. M., & Lowes, B. D. (2012). CelestHealth System: A new horizon for mental health treatment. *Science and Practice, 2,* 7–11.

Bryan, C. J., Mintz, J., Clemans, T. A., Leeson, B., Burch, T. S., Williams, S. R., et al. (2017). Effect of crisis response planning vs. contracts for safety on suicide risk in US Army soldiers: A randomized clinical trial. *Journal of Affective Disorders, 212,* 64–72.

Bryan, C. J., Morrow, C. E., Anestis, M. D., & Joiner, T. E. (2010). A preliminary test of the interpersonal-psychological theory of suicidal behavior in a military sample. *Personality and Individual Differences, 48*(3), 347–350.

Bryan, C. J., Morrow, C. E., Etienne, N., & Ray-Sannerud, B. (2013). Guilt, shame, and suicidal ideation in a military outpatient clinical sample. *Depression and Anxiety, 30*(1), 55–60.

Bryan, C. J., Ray-Sannerud, B., Morrow, C. E., & Etienne, N. (2013a). Guilt is more strongly associated with suicidal ideation among military personnel with direct combat exposure. *Journal of Affective Disorders, 148*(1), 37–41.

Bryan, C. J., Ray-Sannerud, B., Morrow, C., & Etienne, N. (2013b). Optimism reduces suicidal ideation and weakens the effect of hopelessness among military personnel. *Cognitive Therapy and Research, 37*(5), 996–1003.

Bryan, C. J., Ray-Sannerud, B., Morrow, C. E., & Etienne, N. (2013c). Shame, pride, and suicidal ideation in a military clinical sample. *Journal of Affective Disorders, 147*(1–3), 212–216.

Bryan, C. J., Roberge, E. M., Bryan, A. O., Ray-Sannerud, B., Morrow, C. E., & Etienne, N. (2015). Guilt as a mediator of the relationship between depression and posttraumatic stress with suicide ideation in two samples of military personnel and veterans. *International Journal of Cognitive Therapy, 8*, 43–155.

Bryan, C. J., & Rudd, M. D. (2006). Advances in the assessment of suicide risk. *Journal of Clinical Psychology, 62*, 185–200.

Bryan, C. J., & Rudd, M. D. (2012). Life stressors, emotional distress, and trauma-related thoughts occurring in the 24 h preceding active duty U.S. soldiers' suicide attempts. *Journal of Psychiatric Research, 46*, 843–848.

Bryan, C. J., & Rudd, M. D. (2015). Response to Stankiewicz et al. [Letter to the editor]. *American Journal of Psychiatry, 172*, 1022–1023.

Bryan, C. J., & Rudd, M. D. (2017). Nonlinear change processes during psychotherapy characterize patients who have made multiple suicide attempts. *Suicide and Life-Threatening Behavior.* [Epub ahead of print]

Bryan, C. J., Rudd, M. D., Peterson, A. L., Young-McCaughan, S., & Wertenberger, E. G. (2016). The ebb and flow of the wish to live and the wish to die among suicidal military personnel. *Journal of Affective Disorders, 202*, 58–66.

Bryan, C. J., Rudd, M. D., Wertenberger, E., Etienne, N., Ray-Sannerud, B. N., Morrow, C. E., et al. (2014). Improving the detection and prediction of suicidal behavior among military personnel by measuring suicidal beliefs: An evaluation of the Suicide Cognitions Scale. *Journal of Affective Disorders, 159*, 15–22.

Bryan, C. J., Rudd, M. D., Wertenberger, E., Young-McCaughon, S., & Peterson, A. (2014). Nonsuicidal self-injury as a prospective predictor of suicide attempts in a clinical sample of military personnel. *Comprehensive Psychiatry.* [Epub ahead of print]

Bryan, C. J., Sinclair, S., & Heron, E. A. (2016). Do military personnel "acquire" the capability for suicide from combat?: A test of the interpersonal-psychological theory of suicide. *Clinical Psychological Science, 4*, 376–385.

Bryan, C. J., Stone, S. L., & Rudd, M. D. (2011). A practical, evidence-based approach for means-restriction counseling with suicidal patients. *Professional Psychology: Research and Practice, 42*(5), 339.

Bryan, C. J., & Tomchesson, J. (2007, April). *Clinician definitions of common suicide-related terms.* Poster presented at the annual meeting of the American Association of Suicidology, New Orleans, LA.

Bryant, F. (2003). Savoring Beliefs Inventory (SBI): A scale for measuring beliefs about savouring. *Journal of Mental Health, 12*(2), 175–196.

Budman, S. H., & Gurman, A. S. (2002). *Theory and practice of brief therapy.* New York: Guilford Press.

Burns, D. D. (1989). *The feeling good handbook: Using the new mood therapy in everday life.* New York: Morrow.

Busch, K. A., Fawcett, J., & Jacobs, D. G. (2003). Clinical correlates of inpatient suicide. *Journal of Clinical Psychiatry, 64*, 14–19.

Bush, K., Kivlahan, D. R., McDonell, M. B., Fihn, S. D., & Bradley, K. A. (1998). The AUDIT alcohol consumption questions (AUDIT-C): An effective brief screening test for problem drinking. *Archives of Internal Medicine, 158,* 1789–1795.

Bush, N. E., Dobscha, S. K., Crumpton, R., Denneson, L. M., Hoffman, J. E., Crain, A., et al. (2015). A virtual hope box smartphone app as an accessory to therapy: Proof-of-concept in a clinical sample of veterans. *Suicide and Life-Threatening Behavior, 45,* 1–9.

Buysse, D. J., Reynolds, C. F., Monk, T. H., Berman, S. R., & Kupfer, D. J. (1989). The Pittsburgh Sleep Quality Index: A new instrument for psychiatric practice and research. *Psychiatry Research, 28, 1* 93–213.

Centers for Disease Control and Prevention. (2016). Web-based Injury Statistics Query and Reporting System (WISQARS) [Online]. Retrieved from *www.cdc.gov/injury/wisqars/index.html.*

Cha, C. B., Najmi, S., Park, J. M., Finn, C. T., & Nock, M. K. (2010). Attentional bias toward suicide-related stimuli predicts suicidal behavior. *Journal of Abnormal Psychology, 119,* 616–622.

Chang, S., Stuckler, D. S., Yip, P., & Gunnell, D. (2013). Impact of 2008 global economic crisis on suicide: Time trend study in 54 countries. *British Medical Journal, 347,* f5239.

Cipriani, A., Pretty, H., Hawton, K., & Geddes, J. R. (2005). Lithium in the prevention of suicidal behavior and all-cause mortality in patients with mood disorders: A systematic review of randomized trials. *American Journal of Psychiatry, 162*(10), 1805–1819.

Cook, D. A. (2009). Thorough informed consent: A developing clinical intervention with suicidal clients. *Psychotherapy Theory, Research, Practice, Training, 46,* 469–471.

Coombs, D. W., Miller, H. L., Alarcon, R., Herlihy, C., Lee, J. M., & Morrison, D. P. (1992). Presuicide attempt communications between parasuicides and consulted caregivers. *Suicide and Life-Threatening Behavior, 22,* 289–302.

Cordero, L., Rudd, M. D., Bryan, C. J., & Corso, K. A. (2008). Accuracy of primary care medical providers' understanding of the FDA black box warning label for antidepressants. *Primary Care and Community Psychiatry, 13,* 109–114.

Crits-Christoph, P., Ring-Kurtz, S., Hamilton, J., Lambert, M. J., Gallop, R., McClure, B., et al. (2012). Preliminary study of the effects of individual patient-level feedback in outpatient substance abuse treatment programs. *Journal of Substance Abuse Treatment, 42,* 301–309.

Crosby, A., Ortega, L., & Melanson, C. (2011, February). *Self-directed violence surveillance: Uniform definitions and recommended data elements, version 1.0.* Atlanta, GA: Centers for Disease Control and Prevention.

Dawes, R., Faust, D., & Meehl, P. (1989). Clinical versus actuarial judgment. *Science, 243,* 1668–1674.

Dimidjian, S., Hollon, S. D., Dobson, K. S., Schmaling, K. B., Kohlenberg, R. J., Addis, M. E., et al. (2006). Randomized trial of behavioral activation, cognitive therapy, and antidepressant medication in the acute treatment of adults with major depression. *Journal of Consulting and Clinical Psychology, 74,* 658–670.

Dogra, A. K., Basu, S., & Das, S. (2011). Impact of meaning in life and reasons for living to hope and suicidal ideation: A study among college students. *Journal of Projective Psychology and Mental Health, 18,* 89.

Eddleston, M., Buckley, N. A., Gunnell, D., Dawson, A. H., & Konradsen, F. (2006). Identification of strategies to prevent death after pesticide self-poisoning using a Haddon matrix. *Injury Prevention, 12,* 333–337.

Ellis, T. E., & Rufino, K. A. (2015). A psychometric study of the Suicide Cognitions Scale with psychiatric inpatients. *Psychological Assessment, 27,* 82–89.

Erisman, S. M., & Roemer, L. (2010). A preliminary investigation of the effects of experimentally induced mindfulness on emotional responding to film clips. *Emotion, 10,* 72–82.

Esposito-Smythers, C., Spirito, A., Kahler, C. W., Hunt, J., & Monti, P. (2011). Treatment of co-occurring substance abuse and suicidality among adolescents: A randomized trial. *Journal of Consulting and Clinical Psychology, 79,* 728–739.

Fawcett, J. (1999). Profiles of completed suicides. In D. Jacobs (Ed.), *The Harvard Medical School guide to suicide assessment and intervention* (pp. 132–148). San Francisco: Jossey-Bass.

Ferster, C. B. (1973). A functional analysis of depression. *American Psychologist, 28,* 857–870.

Forman, E. M., Berk, M. S., Henriques, G. R., Brown, G. K., & Beck, A. T. (2004). History of multiple suicide attempts as a behavioral marker of severe psychopathology. *American Journal of Psychiatry, 161,* 437–443.

Franklin, J. C., Ribeiro, J. D., Fox, K. R., Bentley, K. H., Kleiman, E. M., Huang, X., et al. (2017). Risk factors for suicidal thoughts and behaviors: A meta-analysis of 50 years of research. *Psychological Bulletin, 143*(2), 187–232.

Frey, L. M., & Cerel, J. (2015). Risk for suicide and the role of family: A narrative review. *Journal of Family Issues, 36,* 716–736.

Gable, S. L., Reis, H. T., Impett, E. A., & Asher, E. R. (2004). What do you do when things go right?: The intrapersonal and interpersonal benefits of sharing positive events. *Journal of Personality and Social Psychology, 87,* 228.

Garland, E. L., Gaylord, S. A., Boettiger, C. A., & Howard, M. O. (2010). Mindfulness training modifies cognitive, affective, and physiological mechanisms implicated in alcohol dependence: Results of a randomized controlled pilot trial. *Journal of Psychoactive Drugs, 42,* 177–192.

Ghahramanlou-Holloway, M., Bhar, S. S., Brown, G. K., Olsen, C., & Beck, A. T. (2012). Changes in problem-solving appraisal after cognitive therapy for the prevention of suicide. *Psychological Medicine, 42,* 1185–1193.

Gortner, E. T., Gollan, J. K., Dobson, K. S., & Jacobson, N. S. (1998). Cognitive–behavioral treatment for depression: Relapse prevention. *Journal of Consulting and Clinical Psychology, 66,* 377–384.

Green, K. L., Brown, G. K., Jager-Hyman, S., Cha, J., Steer, R. A., & Beck, A. T. (2015). The predictive validity of the Beck Depression Inventory suicide item. *Journal of Clinical Psychiatry, 76,* 1683–1686.

Grove, W. M. (2005). Clinical versus statistical prediction: The contribution of Paul E. Meehl. *Journal of Clinical Psychology, 61,* 1233–1243.

Guan, K., Fox, K. R., & Prinstein, M. J. (2012). Nonsuicidal self-injury as a time-invariant predictor of adolescent suicide ideation and attempts in a diverse community sample. *Journal of Consulting and Clinical Psychology, 80,* 842–849.

Gujar, N., Yoo, S., Hu, P., & Walker, M. P. (2011). Sleep deprivation amplifies reactivity of brain reward networks, biasing the appraisal of positive emotional experiences. *Journal of Neuroscience, 31,* 4466–4474.

Gysin-Maillart, A., Schwab, S., Soravia, L., Megert, M., & Michel, K. (2016). A novel brief therapy for patients who attempt suicide: A 24-months follow-up randomized controlled study of the attempted suicide short intervention program (ASSIP). *PLOS Medicine, 13*(3), e1001968.

Hall, M. H. (2010). Behavioral medicine and sleep: Concepts, measures, and methods. In A. Steptoe (Ed.), *Handbook of behavioral medicine: Methods and applications* (pp. 749–765). New York: Springer.

Hall, R. C., Platt, D. E., & Hall, R. C. (1999). Suicide risk assessment: A review of risk factors for suicide in 100 patients who made severe suicide attempts: Evaluation of suicide risk in a time of managed care. *Psychosomatics, 40,* 18–27.

Harmon, S. C., Lambert, M. J., Smart, D. W., Hawkins, E. J., Nielsen, S. L., Slade, K., et al. (2007). Enhancing outcome for potential treatment failures: Therapist/client feedback and clinical support tools. *Psychotherapy Research, 17,* 379–392.

Harris, E. C., & Barraclough, B. (1997). Suicide as an outcome for mental disorders: A meta-analysis. *British Journal of Psychiatry, 170,* 205–228.

Harrison, Y., & Horne, J. A. (2000). The impact of sleep deprivation on decision making: A review. *Journal of Experimental Psychology: Applied, 6,* 236–249.

Harvard University School of Public Health. (n.d.). Lethal means counseling. Retrieved February 8, 2015, from *www.hsph.harvard.edu/means-matter/lethal-means-counseling.*

Hayes, S. C., Wilson, K. G., Gifford, E. V., Follette, V. M., & Strosahl, K. (1996). Experiential avoidance and behavioral disorders: A functional dimensional approach to diagnosis and treatment. *Journal of Consulting and Clinical Psychology, 64,* 1152–1168.

Heisel, M. J., & Flett, G. L. (2008). Psychological resilience to suicide ideation among older adults. *Clinical Gerontologist, 31,* 51–70.

Hendin, H., & Haas, A. P. (1991). Suicide and guilt as manifestations of PTSD in Vietnam combat veterans. *American Journal of Psychiatry, 148,* 586–591.

Hill, R. M., Rey, Y., Marin, C. E., Sharp, C., Green, K. L., & Pettit, J. W. (2015). Evaluating the Interpersonal Needs Questionnaire: Comparison of the reliability, factor structure, and predictive validity across five versions. *Suicide and Life-Threatening Behavior, 45,* 302–314.

Hirsch, J. K., & Conner, K. R. (2006). Dispositional and explanatory style optimism as potential moderators of the relationship between hopelessness and suicidal ideation. *Suicide and Life-Threatening Behavior, 36,* 661–669.

Hirsch, J. K., Conner, K. R., & Duberstein, P. R. (2007). Optimism and suicide ideation among young adult college students. *Archives of Suicide Research, 11,* 177–185.

Hirsch, J. K., Wolford, K., Lalonde, S. M., Brunk, L., & Parker-Morris, A. (2009). Optimistic explanatory style as a moderator of the association between negative life events and suicide ideation. *Crisis, 30,* 48–53.

Horesh, N., Levi, Y., & Apter, A. (2012). Medically serious versus non-serious suicide attempts: Relationships of lethality and intent to clinical and interpersonal characteristics. *Journal of Affective Disorders, 136,* 286–293.

Horvath, A. O., & Greenberg, L. S. (1989). Development and validation of the Working Alliance Inventory. *Journal of Counseling Psychology, 36,* 223–233.

Ilgen, M. A., Harris, A. H. S., Moos, R. H., & Tiet, Q. Q. (2007). Predictors of a suicide attempt one year after entry into substance use disorder treatment. *Alcoholism: Clinical and Experimental Research, 31,* 635–642.

Ingram, R. E., Miranda, J., & Segal, Z. (2006). Cognitive vulnerability to depression. In L. B. Alloy & J. H. Riskind (Eds.), *Cognitive vulnerability to emotional disorders* (pp. 63–91). Mahwah, NJ: Erlbaum.

Inskip, H. M., Harris, E. C., & Barraclough, B. (1998). Lifetime risk of suicide for affective disorder, alcoholism and schizophrenia. *British Journal of Psychiatry, 172,* 35–37.

Jain, S., Shapiro, S. L., Swanick, S., Roesch, S. C., Mills, P. J., Bell, I., et al. (2007). A randomized controlled trial of mindfulness meditation versus relaxation training: Effects on distress, positive states of mind, rumination, and distraction. *Annals of Behavioral Medicine, 33,* 11–21.

Jeannerod, M. (2001). Neural simulation of action: A unifying mechanism for motor cognition. *NeuroImage, 14,* S103–S109.

Joiner, T. E., Jr. (2005). *Why people die by suicide.* Cambridge, MA: Harvard University Press.

Joiner, T. E., Jr., Conwell, Y., Fitzpatrick, K. K., Witte, T. K., Schmidt, N. B., Berlim, M. T., et al. (2005). Four studies on how past and current suicidality relate even when "everything but the kitchen sink" is covaried. *Journal of Abnormal Psychology, 114,* 291–303.

Joiner, T. E., Jr., Pfaff, J. J., & Acres, J. G. (2002). A brief screening tool for suicidal symptoms in adolescents and young adults in general health settings: Reliability and validity data from the Australian National General Practice Youth Suicide Prevention Project. *Behaviour Research and Therapy, 40,* 471–481.

Joiner, T. E., Jr., Rudd, M. D., & Rajab, M. H. (1997). The Modified Scale for Suicidal Ideation: Factors of suicidality and their relation to clinical and diagnostic variables. *Journal of Abnormal Psychology, 106,* 260–265.

Joiner, T. E., Jr., Steer, R. A., Brown, G., Beck, A. T., Pettit, J. W., & Rudd, M. D. (2003). Worst-point suicidal plans: A dimension of suicidality predictive of past suicide attempts and eventual death by suicide. *Behaviour Research and Therapy, 41,* 1469–1480.

Joiner, T. E., Jr., Van Orden, K. A., Witte, T. K., & Rudd, M. D. (2009). *The interpersonal theory of suicide: Guidance for working with suicidal clients.* Washington, DC: American Psychological Association.

Joiner, T. E., Jr., Van Orden, K. A., Witte, T. K., Selby, E. A., Ribeiro, J. D., Lewis, R., et al. (2009). Main predictions of the interpersonal-psychological theory of suicidal behavior: Empirical tests in two samples of young adults. *Journal of Abnormal Psychology, 118,* 634–646.

Joiner, T. E., Jr., Walker, R. L., Rudd, M. D., & Jobes, D. A. (1999). Scientizing and routinizing the assessment of suicidality in outpatient practice. *Professional Psychology: Research and Practice, 30,* 447.

Judd, L. L., Schettler, P. J., Akiskal, H., Coryell, W., Fawcett, J., Fiedorowicz, J. G., et al. (2012). Prevalence and clinical significance of subsyndromal manic symptoms, including irritability and psychomotor agitation, during bipolar major depressive episodes. *Journal of Affective Disorders, 138,* 440–448.

Kabat-Zinn, J., Massion, A. O., Kristeller, J., Peterson, L. G., Fletcher, K. E., Pbert, L., et al. (1992). Effectiveness of a meditation-based stress reduction program in the treatment of anxiety disorders. *American Journal of Psychiatry, 149,* 936–943.

Kanzler, K. E., Bryan, C. J., McGeary, D. D., & Morrow, C. E. (2012). Suicidal ideation and perceived burdensomeness in patients with chronic pain. *Pain Practice, 12,* 602–609.

Kaslow, N. J., Sherry, A., Bethea, K., Wyckoff, S., Compton, M. T., Grall, M. B., et al. (2005). Social risk and protective factors for suicide attempts in low income African American men and women. *Suicide and Life-Threatening Behavior, 35,* 400–412.

Katz, L. Y., Cox, B. J., Gunasekara, S., & Miller, A. L. (2004). Feasibility of dialectical behavior therapy for suicidal adolescent inpatients. *Journal of the American Academy of Child and Adolescent Psychiatry, 43,* 276–282.

Kessler, R. C., Borges, G., & Walters, E. E. (1999). Prevalence of and risk factors for lifetime suicide attempts in the National Comorbidity Survey. *Archives of General Psychiatry, 56,* 617–626.

Klonsky, E. D., & May, A. M. (2015). The three-step theory (3ST): A new theory of suicide rooted in the "ideation-to-action" framework. *International Journal of Cognitive Therapy, 8,* 114–129.

Klonsky, E. D., May, A. M., & Glenn, C. R. (2013). The relationship between nonsuicidal self-injury and attempted suicide: Converging evidence from four samples. *Journal of Abnormal Psychology, 122,* 231–237.

Kopta, S. M., & Lowry, J. L. (2002). Psychometric evaluation of the Behavioral Health Questionnaire-20: A brief instrument for assessing global mental health and the three phases of psychotherapy outcome. *Psychotherapy Research, 12,* 413–426.

Kovacs, M., Beck, A. T., & Weissman, A. (1976). The communication of suicidal intent: A reexamination. *Archives of General Psychiatry, 33,* 198–201.

Kroenke, K., Spitzer, R. L., & Williams, J. B. (2001). The PHQ-9. *Journal of General Internal Medicine, 16,* 606–61.

Lambert, M. J. (2013). Outcome in psychotherapy: The past and important advances. *Psychotherapy, 50,* 42–51.

Lambert, M. J., Morton, J. J., Hatfield, D., Harmon, C., Hamilton, S., Reid, R. C., et al. (2004). *Administration and scoring manual for the OQ-45.* Orem, UT: American Professional Credentialing Services.

Lambert, M. J., Whipple, J. L., Smart, D. W., Vermeersch, D. A., Nielsen, S. L., & Hawkins, E. J. (2001). The effects of providing therapists with feedback on patient progress during psychotherapy: Are outcomes enhanced? *Psychotherapy Research, 11,* 49–68.

Lewinsohn, P. M., & Graf, M. (1973). Pleasant activities and depression. *Journal of Consulting and Clinical Psychology, 41,* 261–268.

Lewinsohn, P. M., & Libet, J. (1972). Pleasant events, activity schedules, and depressions. *Journal of Abnormal Psychology, 79,* 291–295.

Linehan, M. M. (1993). *Cognitive-behavioral treatment of borderline personality disorder.* New York: Guilford Press.

Linehan, M. M., Armstrong, H. E., Suarez, A., Allmon, D., & Heard, H. L. (1991). Cognitive-behavioral treatment of chronically parasuicidal borderline patients. *Archives of General Psychiatry, 48,* 1060–1064.

Linehan, M. M., Comtois, K. A., Brown, M. Z., Heard, H. L., & Wagner, A. (2006). Suicide Attempt Self-Injury Interview (SASII): Development, reliability, and validity of a scale to assess suicide attempts and intentional self-injury. *Psychological Assessment, 18,* 303–312.

Linehan, M. M., Comtois, K. A., Murray, A. M., Brown, M. Z., Gallop, R. J., Heard, H. L., et al. (2006). Two-year randomized controlled trial and follow-up of dialectical behavior therapy vs therapy by experts for suicidal behaviors and borderline personality disorder. *Archives of General Psychiatry, 63,* 757–766.

Luebbert, K., Dahme, B., & Hasenbring, M. (2001). The effectiveness of relaxation training in reducing treatment-related symptoms and improving emotional adjustment in acute non-surgical cancer treatment: A meta-analytical review. *Psycho-Oncology, 10,* 490–502.

Lynch, T. R., Chapman, A. L., Rosenthal, M. Z., Kuo, J. R., & Linehan, M. M. (2006). Mechanisms of change in dialectical behavior therapy: Theoretical and empirical observations. *Journal of Clinical Psychology, 62,* 459–480.

MacLeod, A. K., Rose, G. S., & Williams, J. M. G. (1993). Components of hopelessness about the future in parasuicide. *Cognitive Therapy and Research, 17,* 441–455.

MacLeod, A. K., & Tarbuck, A. F. (1994). Explaining why negative events will happen to oneself: Parasuicides are pessimistic because they can't see any reason not to be. *British Journal of Clinical Psychology, 33,* 317–326.

Mann, J. J., Apter, A., Bertolote, J., Beautrais, A., Currier, D., Haas, A., et al. (2005). Suicide prevention strategies: A systematic review. *Journal of the American Medical Association, 294,* 2064–2074.

Martin, D. J., Garske, J. P., & Davis, M. K. (2000). Relation of the therapeutic alliance with outcome and other variables: A meta-analytic review. *Journal of Consulting and Clinical Psychology, 68,* 438.

May, A. M., & Klonsky, E. D. (2016). What distinguishes suicide attempters from suicide ideators?: A meta-analysis of potential factors. *Clinical Psychology: Science and Practice, 23,* 5–20.

Meltzer, H. Y., Alphs, L., Green, A. I., Altamura, A. C., Anand, R., Bertoldi, A., et al. (2003). Clozapine treatment for suicidality in schizophrenia: International suicide prevention trial (InterSePT). *Archives of General Psychiatry, 60,* 82–91.

Miklowitz, D. J., Alatiq, Y., Goodwin, G. M., Geddes, J. R., Fennell, M. J. V., Dimidjian, S., et al. (2009). A pilot study of mindfulness-based cognitive therapy for bipolar disorder. *International Journal of Cognitive Therapy, 2,* 373–382.

Miller, I. W., Camargo, C. A., Arias, S. A., Sullivan, A. F., Allen, M. H., Goldstein, A. B., et al., for the ED-SAFE Investigators. (2017). Suicide prevention in an emergency department population: The ED-SAFE study. *JAMA Psychiatry, 74*(6), 563–570.

Miller, W. R., & Rollnick, S. (2012). *Motivational interviewing: Helping people change* (3rd ed.). New York: Guilford Press.

Millner, A. J., Lee, M. D., & Nock, M. K. (2017). Describing and measuring the pathway to suicide attempts: A preliminary study. *Suicide and Life-Threatening Behavior, 47*(3), 353–369.

Minnix, J. A., Romero, C., Joiner T. E., Jr., & Weinberg, E. F. (2007). Change in "resolved plans" and "suicidal ideation" factors of suicidality after participation in an intensive outpatient treatment program. *Journal of Affective Disorders, 103,* 63–68.

Munzert, J., Lorey, B., & Zentgraf, K. (2009). Cognitive motor processes: The role of motor imagery in the study of motor representations. *Brain Research Reviews, 60,* 306–326.

Nasir, M., Baucom, B., Bryan, C. J., Narayanan, S., & Georgiou, P. (2017, August). Complexity in speech and its relation to emotional bond in therapist–patient interactions during suicide risk assessment interviews. *Proceedings of the Annual Conference of the International Speech Communication Association, INTERSPEECH*, pp. 3296–3300.

National Action Alliance Clinical Care & Intervention Task Force. (2012). *Suicide care in systems framework*. Washington, DC: National Action Alliance for Suicide Prevention.

National Institute for Health and Clinical Excellence. (2012). *Self-harm: Longer-term management*. Leicester, UK: British Psychological Society.

Nock, M. K., Borges, G., Bromet, E. J., Alonso, J., Angermeyer, M., Beautrais, A., et al. (2008). Cross-national prevalence and risk factors for suicidal ideation, plans, and attempts. *British Journal of Psychiatry, 192*, 98–105.

Nock, M. K., Park, J. M., Finn, C. T., Deliberto, T. L., Dour, H. J., & Banaji, M. R. (2010). Measuring the suicidal mind: Implicit cognition predicts suicidal behavior. *Psychological Science, 21*, 511–517.

Nock, M. K., & Prinstein, M. J. (2005). Contextual features and behavioral functions of self-mutilation among adolescents. *Journal of Abnormal Psychology, 114*, 140.

O'Connor, R. C. (2011). Towards an integrated motivational–volitional model of suicidal behaviour. In R. C. O'Connor, S. Platt, & J. Gorden (Eds.), *International handbook of suicide prevention: Research, policy, and practice* (pp. 181–198). Chichester, UK: Wiley.

O'Connor, R. C., & Noyce, R. (2008). Personality and cognitive processes: Self-criticism and different types of rumination as predictors of suicidal ideation. *Behaviour Research and Therapy, 46*, 392–401.

O'Connor, R. C., & O'Connor, D. B. (2003). Predicting hopelessness and psychological distress: The role of perfectionism and coping. *Journal of Counseling Psychology, 50*, 362–372.

O'Connor, R. C., Rasmussen, S., & Hawton, K. (2010). Predicting depression, anxiety, and self-harm in adolescents: The role of perfectionism and acute life stress. *Behaviour Research and Therapy, 48*, 52–59.

Oquendo, M. A., Galfalvy, H. C., Currier, D., Grunebaum, M. F., Sher, L., Sullivan, G. M., et al. (2011). Treatment of suicide attempters with bipolar disorder: A randomized clinical trial comparing lithium and valproate in the prevention of suicidal behavior. *American Journal of Psychiatry, 168*, 1050–1056.

Owens, D., Horrocks, J., & House, A. (2002). Fatal and non-fatal repetition of self-harm: Systematic review. *British Journal of Psychiatry, 181*, 193–199.

Peterson, L. G., Peterson, M., O'Shanick, G. J., & Swann, A. (1985). Self-inflicted gunshot wounds: Lethality of method versus intent. *American Journal of Psychiatry, 142*, 228–231.

Pigeon, W. R., Britton, P. C., Ilgen, M. A., Chapman, B., & Conner, K. R. (2012). Sleep disturbance preceding suicide among veterans. *American Journal of Public Health, 102*(Suppl. 1), S93–S97.

Pirkola, S., Isometsä, E., & Lönnqvist, J. (2003). Do means matter?: Differences in characteristics of Finnish suicide completers using different methods. *Journal of Nervous and Mental Disease, 191*, 745–750.

Pomerantz, A. M., & Handelsman, M. M. (2004). Informed consent revisited: An updated written question format. *Professional Psychology: Research and Practice, 35*, 201–205.

Poulin, C., Shiner, B., Thompson, P., Vepstas, L., Young-Xu, Y., Goertzel, B., et al. (2014). Predicting the risk of suicide by analyzing the text of clinical notes. *PLOS ONE, 9*, e85733.

Price, R. K., Risk, N. K., Haden, A. H., Lewis, C. E., & Spitznagel, E. L. (2004). Post-traumatic stress disorder, drug dependence, and suicidality among male Vietnam veterans with a history of heavy drug use. *Drug and Alcohol Dependence, 76*(Suppl.), S31–S43.

Pugh, M. J., Hesdorffer, D., Wang, C. P., Amuan, M. E., Tabares, J. V., Finley, E. P., et al. (2013). Temporal trends in new exposure to antiepileptic drug monotherapy and suicide-related behavior. *Neurology, 81*, 1900–1906.

Quoidbach, J., Berry, E. V., Hansenne, M., & Mikolajczak, M. (2010). Positive emotion regulation and well-being: Comparing the impact of eight savoring and dampening strategies. *Personality and Individual Differences, 49,* 368–373.

Resick, P. A., Monson, C. M., & Chard, K. M. (2017). *Cognitive processing therapy for PTSD: A comprehensive manual.* New York: Guilford Press.

Rihmer, Z., & Akiskal, H. (2006). Do antidepressants t(h)reat(en) depressives?: Toward a clinically judicious formulation of the antidepressant–suicidality FDA advisory in light of declining national suicide statistics from many countries. *Journal of Affective Disorders, 94,* 3–13.

Rihmer, Z., & Pestality, P. (1999). Bipolar II disorder and suicidal behavior. *Psychiatric Clinics of North America, 22,* 667–673.

Rudd, M. D. (2006). Fluid vulnerability theory: A cognitive approach to understanding the process of acute and chronic risk. In T. E. Ellis (Ed.), *Cognition and suicide: Theory, research, and therapy* (pp. 355–368). Washington, DC: American Psychological Association.

Rudd, M. D. (2009). Psychological treatments for suicidal behavior: What are the common elements of treatments that work? In D. Wasserman (Ed.), *Oxford textbook of suicidology* (pp. 427–438). Oxford, UK: Oxford University Press.

Rudd, M. D. (2012). Brief cognitive behavioral therapy (BCBT) for suicidality in military populations. *Military Psychology, 24,* 592–603.

Rudd, M. D., Bryan, C. J., Wertenberger, E., Peterson, A. L., Young-McCaughon, S., Mintz, J., et al. (2015). Brief cognitive behavioral therapy effects on post-treatment suicide attempts in a military sample: Results of a 2-year randomized clinical trial. *American Journal of Psychiatry, 172,* 441–449.

Rudd, M. D., Cordero, L., & Bryan, C. J. (2009). What every psychologist should know about the Food and Drug Administration's black box warning label for antidepressants. *Professional Psychology: Research and Practice, 40,* 321–326.

Rudd, M. D., Joiner, T., Brown, G. K., Cukrowicz, K., Jobes, D. A., Silverman, M., et al. (2009). Informed consent with suicidal patients: Rethinking risks in (and out of) treatment. *Psychotherapy, 46,* 459–468.

Rudd, M. D., Joiner, T. E., Jr., & Rajab, M. H. (1995). Help negation after acute suicidal crisis. *Journal of Consulting and Clinical Psychology, 63,* 499–503.

Rudd, M. D., Joiner, T., & Rajab, M. H. (1996). Relationships among suicide ideators, attempters, and multiple attempters in a young-adult sample. *Journal of Abnormal Psychology, 105,* 541–550.

Rudd, M. D., Joiner, T. E., Jr., & Rajab, M. H. (2001). *Treating suicidal behavior: An effective, time-limited approach.* New York: Guilford Press.

Saunders, J. B., Aasland, O. G., Babor, T. F., De la Fuente, J. R., & Grant, M. (1993). Development of the Alcohol Use Disorders Identification Test (AUDIT): WHO collaborative project on early detection of persons with harmful alcohol consumption—II. *Addiction, 88,* 791–804.

Schmitz, W. M., Allen, M. H., Feldman, B. N., Gutin, N. J., Jahn, D. R., Kleespies, P. M., et al. (2012). Preventing suicide through improved training in suicide risk assessment and care: An American Association of Suicidology task force report addressing serious gaps in U.S. mental health training. *Suicide and Life-Threatening Behavior, 42,* 292–304.

Selby, E. A., Anestis, M. D., Bender, T. W., Ribeiro, J. D., Nock, M. K., Rudd, M. D., et al. (2010). Overcoming the fear of lethal injury: Evaluating suicidal behavior in the military through the lens of the interpersonal-psychological theory of suicide. *Clinical Psychology Review, 30,* 298–307.

Shimokawa, K., Lambert, M. J., & Smart, D. W. (2010). Enhancing treatment outcome of patients at risk of treatment failure: Meta-analytic and mega-analytic review of a psychotherapy quality assurance system. *Journal of Consulting and Clinical Psychology, 78,* 298–311.

Silverman, M. M. (2006). The language of suicidology. *Suicide and Life-Threatening Behavior, 36*(5), 519–532.

Simon, G. E., Rutter, C. M., Peterson, D., Oliver, M., Whiteside, U., Operskalski, B., et al. (2013). Does response on the PHQ-9 Depression Questionnaire predict subsequent suicide attempt or suicide death? *Psychiatric Services, 64*, 1195–1202.

Simon, G. E., & Savarino, J. (2007). Suicide attempts among patients starting depression treatment with medications or psychotherapy. *American Journal of Psychiatry, 164*, 1029–1034.

Simon, O. R., Swann, A. C., Powell, K. E., Potter, L. B., Kresnow, M. J., & O'Carroll, P. W. (2001). Characteristics of impulsive suicide attempts and attempters. *Suicide and Life-Threatening Behavior, 32*(Suppl. 1), 49–59.

Simon, W., Lambert, M. J., Busath, G., Vazquez, A., Berkeljon, A., Hyer, K., et al. (2013). Effects of providing patient progress feedback and clinical support tools to psychotherapists in an inpatient eating disorders treatment program: A randomized controlled study. *Psychotherapy Research, 23*, 287–300.

Slade, K., Lambert, M. J., Harmon, S. C., Smart, D. W., & Bailey, R. (2008). Improving psychotherapy outcome: The use of immediate electronic feedback and revised clinical support tools. *Clinical Psychology and Psychotherapy, 15*, 287–303.

Smith, J. C., Mercy, J. A., & Conn, J. M. (1988). Marital status and the risk of suicide. *American Journal of Public Health, 78*, 78–80.

Speca, M., Carlson, L. E., Goodey, E., & Angen, M. (2000). A randomized, wait-list controlled clinical trial: The effect of a mindfulness meditation-based stress reduction program on mood and symptoms of stress in cancer outpatients. *Psychosomatic Medicine, 62*, 613–622.

Stanley, B., & Brown, G. K. (2012). Safety Planning Intervention: A brief intervention to mitigate suicide risk. *Cognitive and Behavioral Practice, 19*, 256–264.

Stetter, F., & Kupper, S. (2002). Autogenic training: A meta-analysis of clinical outcome studies. *Applied Psychophysiology and Biofeedback, 27*, 45–98.

Stewart, A. L., Ware, J. E., Brook, R. H., & Davies, A. R. (1978). *Conceptualization and measurement of health for adults in the Health Insurance Study: Vol. II. Physical health in terms of functioning.* Santa Monica, CA: RAND Corporation.

Strosahl, K., Chiles, J. A., & Linehan, M. (1992). Prediction of suicide intent in hospitalized parasuicides: Reasons for living, hopelessness, and depression. *Comprehensive Psychiatry, 33*, 366–373.

Substance Abuse and Mental Health Services Administration. (2014). *Results from the 2013 National Survey on Drug Use and Health: Mental health findings.* Rockville, MD: Author.

Suicide Prevention Resource Center. (2006). *Core competencies in the assessment and management of suicidality.* Newton, MA: Author.

Swahn, M. H., & Potter, L. B. (2001). Factors associated with the medical severity of suicide attempts in youths and young adults. *Suicide and Life-Threatening Behavior, 32*(Suppl. 1), 21–29.

Tarrier, N., Taylor, K., & Gooding, P. (2008). Cognitive-behavioral interventions to reduce suicide behavior: A systematic review and meta-analysis. *Behavior Modification, 32*, 77–108.

Taylor, D. J., McCrae, C. S., Gehrman, P. R., Dautovich, N., & Lichstein, K. L. (2007). Insomnia. In M. Hersen & J. Rosqvist (Eds.), *Handbook of psychological assessment, case conceptualization, and treatment* (pp. 674–700). New York: Wiley.

Trockel, M., Karlin, B. E., Taylor, C. B., Brown, G. K., & Manber, R. (2015). Effects of cognitive behavioral therapy for insomnia on suicidal ideation in veterans. *Sleep, 38*, 259–265.

VandeCreek, L. (2009). Time for full disclosure with suicidal patients. *Psychotherapy Theory, Research, Practice, Training, 46*, 472–473.

Van Orden, K. A., Cukrowicz, K. C., Witte, T. K., & Joiner, T. E., Jr. (2012). Thwarted belongingness and perceived burdensomeness: Construct validity and psychometric properties of the Interpersonal Needs Questionnaire. *Psychological Assessment, 24*, 197–215.

Van Orden, K. A., Witte, T. K., Gordon, K. H., Bender, T. W., & Joiner, T. E. (2008). Suicidal desire and the capability for suicide: Tests of the interpersonal-psychological theory of suicidal beahvior among adults. *Journal of Consulting and Clinical Psychology, 76*, 72–83.

Wenzel, A., & Beck, A. T. (2008). A cognitive model of suicidal behavior: Theory and treatment. *Applied and Preventive Psychology, 12,* 189–201.

Wenzel, A., Brown, G. K., & Beck, A. T. (2009). *Cognitive therapy for suicidal patients: Scientific and clinical applications.* Washington, DC: American Psychological Association.

Wilcox, H. C., Conner, K. R., & Caine, E. D. (2004). Association of alcohol and drug use disorders and completed suicide: An empirical review of cohort studies. *Drug and Alcohol Dependence, 76,* S11–S19.

Wilkinson, P., Kelvin, R., Roberts, C., Dubicka, B., & Goodyer, I. (2011). Clinical and psychosocial predictors of suicide attempts and nonsuicidal self-injury in the Adolescent Depression Antidepressants and Psychotherapy Trial (ADAPT). *American Journal of Psychiatry, 168,* 495–501.

Williams, J. M. G., Barnhofer, T., Crane, C., & Beck, A. (2005). Problem solving deteriorates following mood challenge in formerly depressed patients with a history of suicidal ideation. *Journal of Abnormal Psychology, 114,* 421.

Woznica, A. A., Carney, C. E., Kuo, J. R., & Moss, T. G. (2015). The insomnia and suicide link: Toward an enhanced understanding of this relationship. *Sleep Medicine Reviews, 22,* 37–46.

Zentgraf, K., Stark, R., Reiser, M., Kunzell, S., Schienle, A., Kirsch, P., et al. (2005). Differential activation of pre-SMA and SMA proper during action observation: Effects of instructions. *NeuroImage, 26,* 662–672.

Index

Note. Page numbers in *italic* indicate a figure or a table.